Improving Newborn Infant Health in Developing Countries

Improving Newborn Infant Health in Developing Countries

Editors

Anthony Costello
University College, London

Dharma Manandhar
Nepal Medical College, Kathmandu

Imperial College Press

Published by

Imperial College Press
57 Shelton Street
Covent Garden
London WC2H 9HE

Distributed by

World Scientific Publishing Co. Pte. Ltd.
P O Box 128, Farrer Road, Singapore 912805
USA office: Suite 1B, 1060 Main Street, River Edge, NJ 07661
UK office: 57 Shelton Street, Covent Garden, London WC2H 9HE

Library of Congress Cataloging-in-Publication Data
Improving newborn infant health in developing countries / editors,
    Anthony Costello, Dharma Manandhar.
        p.   cm.
    Includes bibliographical references (p.   ).
    ISBN 1-86094-097-8
    1. Infants (Newborn) -- Health and hygiene -- Developing countries.
    2. Infants (Newborn) -- Diseases -- Developing countries -- Prevention
    3. Medical care -- Developing countries.   I. Costello, Anthony.
    II. Manandhar, Dharma.
    RJ60.D44I47   1999
    362.1'989201'091724--dc21   99-30272
                                                    CIP

British Library Cataloguing-in-Publication Data
A catalogue record for this book is available from the British Library.

Printed in Singapore by Uto-Print

This book is dedicated to the memory of Dr Shameem Ahmed, an outstanding paediatrician, scientist and mother, who died tragically in an airline accident in Kathmandu, September 1999.

FOREWORD

As we approach the millenium it is useful to take stock of the progress and problems within the health sectors of developing countries. For many, significant progress has been achieved in promoting immunisation and other preventive programmes; in reducing childhood mortality; and in raising life expectancy for adults. But major problems remain. One of the highest health priorities for international agencies, especially those with a primary focus on poverty alleviation, is to help countries achieve further declines in infant mortality, and to improve reproductive health. The British Government Department for International Development which supported the Kathmandu workshop which stimulated the production of this book is committed to helping countries reduce their infant and child mortality rates by two-thirds by the year 2015. They are committed also to help reduce the huge risks to millions of women from a pregnancy-related illness or death. In some countries, women may face a one in 25 lifetime risk of a maternal death — up to 100 times greater than women in industrialised countries.

Safer Motherhood Programmes (of which newborn care is an integral part) are therefore one of the highest investment priorities, but such programmes are often difficult to implement and monitor. It is challenging enough to ensure good emergency obstetric care services at district level linked to an active, effective and mother-friendly primary care referral system. But further problems are faced in reforming health sector management, improving the socio-economic and educational status of women, changing cultural practices which may limit demand for services when they are needed, and in demonstrating the success of Safer Motherhood Programmes in terms of improved health outcomes.

A crucial component is in ensuring that birth does not end in a neonatal death. Such an outcome is still common, represents a tragedy for the family, and exposes the mother to the additional risk of another pregnancy in the near future. Essential newborn care is therefore an integral component of a Safer Motherhood programme, and neonatal outcome one important indicator of success.

Anthony Costello and Dharma Manandhar have collated an extremely important set of papers, mostly from authors working in the south, which provide evidence, experience and ideas for improving newborn care within the framework of Safer Motherhood. The book should be essential reading for professionals working in this area, and I hope many newborn infants will benefit as a result.

Andrew Tomkins
Director
Centre for International Child Health
Institute of Child Health
University College, London

INTRODUCTION

This book arose from a workshop held in Kathmandu in the summer of 1997. We are grateful to the British Government Department for International Development for financial support for the Kathmandu workshop, without which the book could not have been written. Participants were policymakers and professionals, mostly living and working in developing countries, with expertise in maternal and infant care, or in implementing Safer Motherhood (SMP) or essential newborn care programmes. The objectives of the book and the workshop were:

- to review the current status of the newborn infant in the developing world, and especially South Asia where most perinatal deaths occur;
- to consider the evidence-base for interventions included in essential and preventive neonatal care programmes in low income countries;
- to discuss ways of improving perinatal service delivery; and
- to identify priorities for future action and research.

Although the book focuses on the newborn infant, a heavy emphasis, especially in the first two sections, has been placed on maternal health, a major determinant of neonatal survival. The book should be of interest to development workers, public health and tropical medicine specialists, as well as to district health staff, obstetricians and paediatricians. Although most contributors' experience was in Asia, the book should be of interest and relevance to all developing countries, especially in Africa. However the book does *not* address in detail the problems of malaria and human immunodeficiency virus (HIV) in pregnancy, and a number of important studies relevant to newborn care have been published since the Kathmandu workshop. Therefore this introduction summarises these issues below, and points the reader to valuable references.

Until recently, the care of newborn infants in developing countries was low on the list of priorities for policymakers or health professionals. Most mothers in the developing world deliver at home, so newborn infants are 'out of sight, and out of mind.' Further, the images of neonatal care from the industrialised world are of extremely premature infants being rescued by expensive and heroic intensive care, a far cry from the economic realities of health services in the developing world. But times are changing and newborn care has moved up the policymaker's list of priorities. Firstly, the last two decades have seen significant reductions in infant mortality largely because post-neonatal causes of death — diarrhoea, pneumonia, vaccine-preventable infections, malaria — are gradually being tackled. More than 70% of infant deaths now occur in the neonatal period, so further reductions in infant mortality will depend on improvements in neonatal care. Secondly, SMP programmes are receiving welcomed attention and investment, and essential newborn care is an integral part of their success. After all, a pregnancy requires both a healthy mother *and* a healthy infant to be regarded as a success; and newborn infant health outcomes are a valuable proxy measure to monitor SMP progress. Thirdly, the message is slowly sinking in that essential newborn care is potentially a highly cost effective intervention. Simple resuscitation, warmth, early breastfeeding, hygiene, love and the recognition of neonatal illness do not require expensive ventilators, incubators or highly trained staff, but may be incorporated at low cost into existing primary and secondary care programmes. Some of the evidence and experience reviewed by the contributors is difficult to access, drawn as it is from national databases, or 'fugitive documents' from international agencies or non-government organisations. Therefore reference is often made to articles and reports which do not appear in international peer-reviewed journals. The reader must obviously be circumspect in judging the merits of this 'evidence', but we feel it is important to give it the light of day. Readers may also spot discrepancies in reported national statistics e.g. for mortality rates, in different chapters. Sources such as the World Bank, UNDP, UNICEF or national governments, often vary in their reporting of national statistics, as these figures are usually based on estimates derived from different census or national survey data.

Since the Kathmandu workshop in 1997, several important papers on topics relevant to neonatal health in developing countries have been published.

Preterm Birth

Avoiding preterm birth would prevent many neonatal deaths. The role of infection in the aetiology of preterm birth has been of great interest, but remains unclear.[1,2] Abnormal vaginal colonisation could predispose — via induction of cytokines such as TNFa, IL-1b, IL-6, IL-8 — to a prostaglandin driven premature onset of labour, and there is observational evidence for higher risk associated with bacterial vaginosis.[3] This association has not been uniformly supported.[4,5] Trials of screening and treatment have also had variable results[6,7] and meta-analyses have failed to reach firm conclusions.[8] Antibiotic treatment of asymptomatic bacteriuria, on the other hand, appears to be of value in preventing the onset of preterm labour.[9,10] It also prolongs gestation in cases of premature rupture of membranes,[11] although not if membranes are intact:[12] there are issues around the arrest of a process that has already been intitiated, but these will hopefully be addressed in the large ORACLE trial. Wawer and colleagues have conducted a randomised, controlled, community-based trial of intensive sexually transmitted diseases (STD) control, via home-based mass antibiotic treatment, in Rakai district, Uganda. They showed, surprisingly, no effect of the STD intervention on the incidence of HIV-1 infection, contradicting earlier work in Tanzania, but significant effects on the prevalence of bacterial vaginosis and other STDs which might reduce preterm delivery, and a reduction in intrauterine growth retardation.[13]

HIV and Mother to Child Transmission (MTCT)

Whether HIV contributes to neonatal mortality is still unclear. A recent meta-analysis by Brocklehurst[14] concluded that "There appears to be an association, though not strong, between maternal HIV and abnormal perinatal outcome." However many of the studies reviewed had problems with observer bias, losses to follow-up, publication bias, and lack of matching for other confounders. Coovadia and Rollins have recently reviewed the complexities of the HIV epidemic for maternal health and the risks of mother to child transmission (MTCT).[15] Up to one-third of HIV positive mothers will transmit the virus to their infant in the perinatal period. The joint American–French study, ACTG 076, which employed zidovudine (AZT) given from 14 weeks of pregnancy to HIV infected women who subsequently avoided breastfeeding, clearly showed that MTCT was reduced by two-thirds, but the intervention is unaffordable for developing countries.[16] In 1998, results were released of a trial in Thailand, which appeared to be more suited for developing countries. A short course of AZT given orally during the last four weeks of pregnancy, together with oral doses during labour, to non-breastfeeding women, reduced MTCT by 51%, 95% confidence interval 15–71%.[17] The more recent and unfinished PETRA studies in southern Africa suggest a similar reduction can be achieved by treatment starting at delivery and continued during the first postnatal week. Experience with the cheaper and more practical option of vaginal antiseptic douches at delivery to reduce MTCT have not proved efficacious.[18]

Years of successful work to promote breastfeeding and reduce the promotion of breastmilk substitutes are threatened by the risk of transmission of HIV through breastmilk.[19] Yet most babies are infected in utero or during childbirth and not through breastmilk. It seems also from a study in Durban, South Africa that exclusive breastfeeding has a reduced risk of MTCT compared with supplementary feeding with breastmilk substitutes.[20] Nonetheless, policymakers in areas where HIV prevalence is high face difficult decisions in designing appropriate recommendations for infant feeding if mothers know their HIV status.

Malaria Control in Pregnancy and the Perinatal Period

Malaria prophylaxis in pregnancy, and early treatment of congenital infection, is an important and much neglected intervention in many countries with high prevalence.[21] 45 million women live in malarious areas, 23 million in sub-Saharan Africa. Prevalence rates of affected pregnant women may be higher than 75%, especially in primigravidae. The association between malaria infection and intrauterine growth retardation is strong, but effects in the neonatal period depend on the level of malaria transmission.[22] If transmission is high, acquired immunity is also high, so there tends to be placental sequestration and mainly asymptomatic infection. When transmission is low, there is low immunity and hence more acutely ill mothers and congenital malaria cases are reported.

The most important issues for district health staff relate to the promotion of bednet usage by mothers, the use of an effective drug regime for chemoprophylaxis, and how often drug treatment is necessary given the difficulties with compliance. Chemoprophylaxis has been undermined by chloroquine resistance. Drug efficacy studies indicate that pyrimethamine/sulphadoxine (PSD) is now the best first choice, with quinine for complicated malaria, and mefloquine or artemisinin in areas with high resistance to PSD, although there is little data on the use of artemisinin compounds in pregnancy. Despite this evidence, only four countries in Africa (Kenya, Malawi, Botswana and South Africa) have made a change from chloroquine as national policy for chemoprophylaxis. A recent review by a group of the world's leading malaria experts suggests that widespread resistance to chloroquine, and increasing resistance to PSD, means a health calamity looms in the next few years. To avert disaster they recommend that single drug treatment be replaced by combination therapy in the same way as has happened for tuberculosis and AIDS. Artemisinin should be combined with chloroquine and PSD for treatment to reduce the development of resistance.[23] The harsh reality remains that even if health workers recommend antimalarials in pregnancy, few women would take them. As such, one or two opportunistic doses at antenatal visits may be a more realistic practice, with useful effect, than to expect compliance with a weekly regime.[22]

Nutritional Interventions

In the 1960's and 70's, the effect of *food supplementation* on neonatal outcomes was studied, but most groups reported relatively small effects on birth weight and perinatal mortality. The cost effectiveness of food supplementation was questioned because of the expense and leakage of supplements. Cultural taboos about having a big baby may also encourage mothers to "eat down" and deliberately reduce calorie intake.[24] Low birth weight is also determined by many factors prior to conception.[25] For these reasons food supplementation programmes in pregnancy have been largely discredited, and not introduced on a large scale. A recent study from the Gambia has reopened the debate. Ceesay *et al.* gave a large supplement (900 kcals per day) made up of locally prepared high energy biscuits.[26] Using a randomised controlled study design they showed a 136 g increase in birth weight, a small increase (3 mm) in head circumference, a 35% reduction in the low birth weight (LBW) rate, and big effects on stillbirths (55% reduction), perinatal (49% reduction) and neonatal mortality (40%).

Recent studies of different interventions to treat *anaemia* on pregnancy outcomes have demonstrated the beneficial effects of antihelminthic treatment with mebendazole in Sri Lanka,[27] 100 mg per day of supplemental iron on the iron status of both mothers and newborns in Niger,[28] and intermittent sulphadoxine-pyrimethamine to prevent severe anaemia (protective efficacy 39 per cent) in Kenya.[29] Presumably these interventions will have variable but beneficial effects on perinatal and neonatal mortality.

Many studies have evaluated *micronutrient supplementation* on perinatal and neonatal outcomes. An important recent trial is the study by Fawzi and colleagues in Tanzania who screened 14,000 women for HIV, identifying 1806 as HIV positive.[30] All women received iron and folate and weekly chloroquine, and HIV positive women were randomised to receive either multivitamins or vitamin A in a four arm factorial design. They showed no effect with vitamin A supplements on birthweight or neonatal mortality, a finding confirmed by the recent vitamin A supplementation trial in Nepal,[31] but with multivitamin supplements there was nearly a 40% reduction in stillbirths and foetal deaths and also a big reduction in LBW prevalence and IUGR. Nonetheless, the problem with all pregnancy food and micronutrient supplementation research remains: almost no interventions have been translated into national policy or large scale programmes. The effects of various micronutrients are also inter-related. Supplementing iron and folic acid without zinc may not be useful, and zinc administration without copper may lead to hypercholesterolaemia or immunodeficiency. So future interventions should be balanced packages of micronutrients, rather than single nutrients.

Interventions During Delivery

There are many proven, low cost interventions during delivery that are hardly used in developing countries: magnesium sulphate for eclampsia, tocolytic drugs to prevent preterm labour, and antenatal steroids to reduce neonatal hyaline membrane disease. Partography has long been demonstrated to be an efficacious method for the detection of delay in labour, with positive benefits for both mother and baby.[32] An important area for operational research is why the partogram is so rarely used in maternity hospitals, and how organisational change might encourage obstetricians and midwives to make partography a routine practice. It is not enough for researchers to prove the value of interventions; they need active promotion through continuing medical education programmes. A recent study in Zimbabwe has also shown the potential value of amnioinfusion for meconium stained amniotic fluid (MSAF) with a 66% reduction in perinatal deaths.[33] Meta-analysis of available studies on the utility of amnioinfusion in the management of MSAF is less convincing so the procedure is not yet uniformly recommended.

Thermal Protection

Two important issues have arisen in the most recent literature. Firstly, the Kangaroo Care Method (KCM), introduced by Rey and Gomez in Colombia in the 1970s as a means of managing LBW and premature infants, has been shown to improve survival, reduce infection and improve neonatal growth patterns.[34-38] In Asia, KCM lacks widespread cultural acceptance, but many centres are implementing partial KCM, and its widespread adoption is a challenge for the next few years.

Secondly, in industrialised countries, there is current interest in the role of thermal protection (brain cooling methods) for the treatment of infants with neonatal encephalopathy.[39] The results of trials will have implications for developing countries because the methods involved are relatively simple and affordable.

Breastfeeding Promotion

Talukder and Ahmed in their chapters discuss ways to promote exclusive breastfeeding — support and counselling for mothers in hospital and through home visits can be highly effective. Morrow and colleagues have recently reported a randomised controlled trial of home-based support for mothers in Mexico, where exclusivity of breastfeeding is the exception, and report dramatic improvements from 12% exclusive breastfeeding at three months in control mothers to 67% in those visited repeatedly at home.[40] A recent systematic review estimated that in a low income country with a post-neonatal mortality rate of 90 per 1,000 children, the excess number of post-neonatal deaths per million births due to artificial feeding(AF) would range from 11,290 (13%) to 112,900 (59%) depending on a prevalence of AF at six months of age ranging from 10% to 100%.[41] Sadly promotion of breastmilk substitutes by formula milk companies in contravention of the International Code of Marketing of Breastmilk Substitutes in 1981, (which was reaffirmed by all member states at the 1996 World Health Assembly, and endorsed by manufacturers' representatives) continues. Now an Interagency Group on Breastfeeding Monitoring has conducted a large, systematic and random survey of mothers and health professionals to quantify the level of Code violations in four countries: Bangladesh, Poland, Thailand and South Africa.[42,43] The paper provides compelling evidence that Code violations remain widespread.

Neonatal Sepsis and the Study by Bang and Colleagues in Maharashtra

An important study Dr Abhay Bang and colleagues in India will soon be published and readers are strongly advised to study this exciting data in more detail. They have conducted a field trial of home based newborn care management and control of sepsis in an extremely poor district of Maharashtra state where 95% of births occur at home. Bang's data was presented in outline at a conference on global perinatal mortality at Johns Hopkins School of Public Health in May 1999. He found at baseline that 48% of all newborn infants had "high risk morbidities", of which over half was ascribed to sepsis. Village health workers were trained to visit homes, to identify warning signs in newborn infants and to manage cases using gentamicin and penicillin given intramuscularly (using insulin syringes) and cotrimoxazole syrup. Before training there was 17% case fatality, which fell to 2.8% after training. By the third year of the intervention neonatal mortality rate was 26 in intervention and 60 in control areas, a 62% fall. Bang estimated the cost to be $182 per village, or $1.6 per life year saved, better value than almost any other primary care intervention!

Interventions to reduce neonatal mortality are at the cutting edge of child survival programmes. There are many efficacious interventions available but a major problem exists with "getting research into policy and practice". There is always a trade off between impact and sustainability: it is better to have a small effect on a large population than a large effect on a small population. It is therefore essential to evaluate sustainable packages of care, or health promotion interventions, discussed in Bolam's chapter, which might be scaled up quickly even in severely resource deficient countries.[44]

We have many effective interventions for sustainable neonatal care, and low cost approaches can achieve dramatic results. Political commitment and organisational changes are needed if research is to be translated into policy and practice.

Acknowledgements

The authors are grateful to Dr David Osrin and Professor Meharban Singh for their help when preparing this introduction and research update.

References

1. Wawer MJ, Sewankambo NK, Serwadda D, Quinn TC, Paxton LA, Kiwanuka N, Wabwire Mangen F, Li C, Lutalo T; Nalugoda F, Gaydos CA, Moulton LH,

Meehan MO, Ahmed S and Gray RH, "Control of sexually transmitted diseases for AIDS prevention in Uganda: a randomised community trial," Rakai Project Study Group, *Lancet* **353**(9152) (1999): 525–535.

2. Brocklehurst P and French R, "The association between maternal HIV infection and perinatal outcome: a systematic review of the literature and meta-analysis," *British Journal of Obstetrics and Gynaecology* **105** (1998): 836–848.

3. Coovadia HM and Rollins N, "Current controversies in the perinatal transmission of HIV in developing countries," *Seminars in Neonatology* (1999, in press).

4. Connor EM, Sperling RS, Gelber R, Kiselev P, Scott G, O'Sullivan MJ, Van Dyke R, Bey M, Shearer W and Jacobson RL, "Reduction of maternal-infant transmission of human immunodeficiency virus type I with zidovudine treatment," Paediatric AIDS Clinical Trials Group Protocol 076 Study Group, *New England Journal of Medicine* **331** (1994): 1173–1180.

5. Vuthipongse P, Bhadrakom C and Chaisilwattana P, "Administration of zidovudine during late pregnancy and delivery to prevent perinatal HIV transmission — Thailand," *Morbidity and Mortality Weekly Report* **47** (1998): 151–154.

6. Biggar RJ, Miotti PG, Taha TE, Mtimavalye L, Broadhead R, Jutesen A, Yellu F, Liomba G, Miley W, Waters D, Chiphangwi JD and Goedert JJ, "Perinatal intervention trial in Africa: effect of a birth canal cleaning intervention to prevent HIV transmission," *Lancet* **347** (1996): 1647–1650.

7. Latham MC and Greiner T, "Breastfeeding versus formula feeding in HIV infection," *Lancet* **352** (1988): 737.

8. Coutsoudis A, Pillay P, Spooner E, Kuch L and Coovadia HM, "Influence of infant feeding pattermns on early mother to child transmission of HIV-1 in Durban, South Africa," *Lancet* (in press).

9. Foster SO, "Malaria in the pregnant African woman: epidemiology, practice, research and policy," *American Journal of Tropical Medicine and Hygiene* **55**(1) (1996): 1.

10. Steketee RW, Wirima JJ, Slutsker L, Heymann DL and Breman JG, "The problem of malaria and malaria control in pregnancy in sub-Saharan Africa," *American Journal of Tropical Medicine and Hygiene* **55**(1) (1996): 2–7.

11. White NJ, Nosten F, Looareesuwan S, Watkins WM, Marsh K and Snow RW, "Averting a malaria disaster," *Lancet* **353** (1999): 1965–1967.

12. Osrin D and Costello A, "What can be done about intrauterine growth retardation?" *Seminars in Neonatology* (1999, in press).

13. Kramer MS, "Determinants of low birth weight: methodological assessment and meta-analysis," *Bulletin of the World Health Organization* **65**(5) (1987): 663–737.

14. Ceesay SM, Prentice AM, Cole TJ, Foord F, Weaver LT, Poskitt EM and Whitehead RG, "Effects on birth weight and perinatal mortality of maternal dietary supplements in rural Gambia: 5 year randomised controlled trial," published erratum appears in *British Medical Journal* **315**(7116) (1997): 1141.

15. Atukorala TM, de Silva LD, Dechering WH, Dassenaeike TS and Perera RS, "Evaluation of effectiveness of iron-folate supplementation and anthelminthic therapy against anemia in pregnancy, a study in the plantation sector of Sri Lanka," *American Journal of Clinical Nutrition* **60**(2) (1994): 286–292.

16. Preziosi P, Prual A, Galan P, Daouda H, Boureima H and Hercberg S, "Effect of iron supplementation on the iron status of pregnant women: consequences for newborns," *American Journal of Clinical Nutrition* **68**(2) (1998): 404–405; *American Journal of Clinical Nutrition* **66**(5) (1997): 1178–1182.

17. Shulman CE, Dorman EK, Cutts F, Kawuondo K, Bulmer JN, Peshu N and Marsh K, "Intermittent sulphadoxine-pyrimethamine to prevent severe anaemia secondary to malaria in pregnancy: a randomised placebo-controlled trial," *Lancet* **353**(9153) (1999): 632–636.

18. Fawzi W, Msamanga G, Spiegelman D, Urassa E, McGrath N and Mwakagile D, "Randomised trial of effects of vitamin supplements on pregnancy outcomes and T cell counts in HIV-1-infected women in Tanzania," *Lancet* **351** (1998): 1477–1482.

19. West KP, Jr, Katz J, Khatry SK, LeClerq SC, Pradhan EK, Shrestha SR, Connor PB, Dali SM, Christian P, Pokhrel RP and Sommer A, "Double blind, cluster randomised trial of low dose supplementation with vitamin A or carotene on mortality related to pregnancy in Nepal," *British Medical Journal* **318** (1999): 570–575.

20. World Health Organization partograph in management of labour. World Health Organization Maternal Health and Safe Motherhood Programme, *Lancet* **343**(8910) (1994): 1399–1404.

21. Mahomed K, Mulambo T, Woelk G, Hofmeyr GJ and Gulmezoglu AM, "The Collaborative Randomised Amnioinfusion for Meconium Project (CRAMP): 2. Zimbabwe," *British Journal of Obstetrics Gynaecology* **105**(3) (1998): 309–313.

22. Christensson K, Bhat GJ, Eriksson B, Shilalukey Ngoma MP and Sterky G, "The effect of routine hospital care on the health of hypothermic newborn infants in Zambia," *Journal of Tropical Pediatrics* **41**(4) (1995): 210–214.

23. Christensson K, Bhat GJ, Amadi BC, Eriksson B and Hojer B, "Randomised study of skin-to-skin versus incubator care for rewarming low-risk hypothermic neonates," *Lancet* **352**(9134) (1998): 1115.
24. Cattaneo A, Davanzo R, Uxa F and Tamburlini G, "Recommendations for the implementation of Kangaroo Mother Care for low birth weight infants," International Network on Kangaroo Mother Care, *Acta Paediatrica* **87**(4) (1998): 440–445.
25. Kambarami RA, Chidede O and Kowo DT, "Kangaroo care versus incubator care in the management of well preterm infants: a pilot study," *Annals of Tropical Paediatrics* **18**(2) (1998): 81–86.
26. Tessier R, Cristo M, Velez S, Giron M, de Calume ZF, Ruiz Palaez JG, Charpak Y and Charpak N, "Kangaroo mother care and the bonding hypothesis," *Pediatrics* **102**(2) (1998): 17.
27. Edwards AD, Wyatt JS and Thoresen M, "Treatment of hypoxic-ischaemic brain damage by moderate hypothermia," *Archives of Disease in Childhood* **78** (1998): F85–F91.
28. Morrow AL, Lourdes Guerrero M, Shults J, Calva JJ, Lutter C, Bravo J, Ruiz-Palacios G, Morrow RC and Butterfoss FD, "Efficacy of home-based peer counselling to promote exclusive breastfeeding," *Lancet* **353** (1999): 1226–1231.
29. Golding J, Emmett P and Rogers IS, "Breastfeeding and infant mortality," *Early Human Development* **49** Suppl (1997): S143–S155.
30. Taylor A, "Violations of the international code of marketing of breast milk substitutes: prevalence in four countries," *British Medical Journal* **316** (1998): 1117–1122.
31. Costello AM de L and Sachdev HPS, "Protecting breastfeeding from breastmilk substitutes," *British Medical Journal* **316** (1998): 1103–1104.
32. Bolam D, Manandhar S, Shrestha P, Malla K, Ellis M and Costello AM de L, "The effects of postnatal health education for mothers on infant care and family planning practices in Nepal: a randomised, controlled trial," *British Medical Journal* **7134** (1988): 805–810.

CONTENTS

LIST OF CONTRIBUTORS

Ramesh K. Adhikari
Professor of Paediatrics and Child Health
Institute of Medicine, Tribhuvan University
Kathmandu

Shameem Ahmed
Health Scientist, Operations Research Project
International Centre for Diarrhoeal Disease Research Bangladesh (ICDDR,B)
Dhaka, Bangladesh

Santosh K. Bhargava
Former Professor of Paediatrics
University College of Medical Sciences and Safdarjung Hospital
New Delhi, India

O. N. Bhakoo
Professor of Paediatrics
Postgraduate Institute for Medical Education and Research (PGIMER)
Chandigarh, India

Zulfiqar Ahmed Bhutta
Professor of Child Health and Director of Neonatal Services
The Aga Khan University Medical Center
Karachi, Pakistan

Alison Bolam
Research Fellow, Institute of Child Health
London, UK

Anthony Costello
Reader in International Child Health
Institute of Child Health
University of London, UK

Hemang Dixit
Professor of Paediatrics and Director of the Health Learning Materials Centre
Institute of Medicine, Tribhuvan University
Kathmandu, Nepal

Matthew Ellis
Lecturer in Paediatrics
University of Bristol

Dipak K. Guha
Senior Consultant Neonatologist
Sunderlal Jain Hospital
Delhi, India

Therese Hesketh
Research Fellow
Institute of Child Health, London

Simin Irani
Professor of Paediatrics
Bombay, India

Fehmida Jalil
Professor of Social Paediatrics
King Edward Medical School
Lahore, Pakistan

Marta J. Levitt-Dayal
Country Director
Centre for Development and Populations Activities (CEDPA), India

Amali Lokugamage
Honorary Lecturer and Specialist Registrar in Obstetrics and Gynaecology
University College London Medical School
London, UK

Dharma Manandhar
Executive Director, Mother and Infant Research Activities (MIRA)
and Professor of Paediatrics, Nepal
Medical College, Kathmandu

Sophie Mancey-Jones
Research Fellow
Institute of Child Health, London
UK

Sajid Maqbool
Professor of Pediatrics
Shaikh Zayed Medical Complex
Lahore

Susan F. Murray
Lecturer in Maternal Health
Institute of Child Health
London

Nazmun Nahar
Professor of Paediatrics
Dhaka Medical College
Bangladesh

Deb Pal
Research Fellow
Institute of Child Health
University College
London, UK

Catherine Panter-Brick
Reader in Anthropology
Durham University
UK

Carole Presern
Health Adviser
Department for International Development
UK

Siddhartha Ramji
Professor of Neonatal Medicine
Maulana Azad Medical School
Delhi, India

Charles Rodeck
Professor of Obstetrics and Gynaecology
University College London Medical School
London, UK

Harshpal Sachdev
Professor and In-charge, Division of Clinical Epidemiology
Department of Paediatrics
Maulana Azad Medical College
New Delhi, India

Daljit Singh
Professor of Paediatrics
Dayanand Medical College
Ludhiana, India

Meharban Singh
Professor and Head, Department of Paediatrics
WHO Collaborating Centre for Training and Research in Newborn Care
All India Institute of Medical Sciences
New Delhi, India

Hilary Standing
Senior Lecturer in Social Anthropology
University of Sussex
UK

M. Q-K. Talukder
Professor of Paediatrics
Institute of Child and Mother Health
Matuail, Dhaka, Bangladesh

Munu Thapa
Reproductive Health and Gender Coordination
Reproductive Health Project, GTZ

Shyam Thapa
Senior Scientist
Family Health International, North Carolina
At present:
Technical Advisor, Family Health Division, Ministry of Health
and Population Division, Ministry of Population and Environment
Kathmandu, Nepal

Dominique Tillen
Research Fellow
Institute of Child Health
London, UK

Ragnar Tunell
Emeritus Professor of Paediatrics
Stockholm, Sweden

Shashi N. Vani
Professor of Paediatrics
Ahmedabad, Gujarat, India

Ananda Wijekoon
Consultant Neonatologist
University of Peradeniya
Sri Lanka

Shakila Zaman
Consultant in Paediatric Epidemiology
King Edward Medical School
Lahore, Pakistan

Section 1:

Current Status of Newborn Infants and Perinatal Health in South Asia

Chapter 1

CURRENT STATE OF THE HEALTH OF NEWBORN INFANTS IN DEVELOPING COUNTRIES

Anthony Costello
Reader in International Child Health,
Institute of Child Health, University College, London

and

Dharma Manandhar
Consultant Paediatrician, Executive Director,
Mother and Infant Research Activities (MIRA) project,
Kathmandu, Nepal

Only in the past decade has the health of newborn infants in developing countries attracted attention from governments and international agencies. Usually the emphasis is primarily on Safer Motherhood Programmes but, in general, efforts to improve perinatal care will have positive benefits for the health of the newborn infant. Newborn infants, however, deserve their own special focus. Despite a marked downward trend of mortality rates of under-fives in developing countries (and especially South Asia) over the past 20 years, the newborn infant has not had an equal share in this "child survival revolution". This is not a new phenomenon. From 1900 to 1935, perinatal (and maternal) mortality in England and Wales was unchanged and even higher than the average for the developing world today.[1]

3

During the same period, post-neonatal and infant mortality rates fell substantially as a result of improvements in infant nutrition, control of infectious diseases, and better access to infant welfare. But perinatal mortality reduction awaited changes in maternity practices, a better understanding of the physiological needs of the newborn, and the introduction of appropriate newborn care.

Reasons for Neglect of the Newborn

In most developing countries today the health problems of newborn infants remain neglected and interventions to reduce early neonatal mortality are not a high priority for investment. The reasons for this neglect are complex and include cultural adaptation to high neonatal wastage, poor data collection about perinatal deaths, and a widespread misconception that neonatal care is expensive and depends on high technology equipment. It is also partly due to lack of leadership: obstetricians are often responsible for neonatal care but are usually interested solely in the care of mothers, whereas paediatricians have tended to give priority to older infants and children.

Cultural adaptation

Poor awareness among the people, high fertility rates, and fatalistic acceptance of high neonatal mortality have also contributed to the slow development of neonatal care. Societies have culturally adapted to high neonatal casualties by according newborns the status of fully-fledged individuals only after the critical first week of life when a naming ceremony is performed and the birth is "completed". In some communities, there is an erroneous belief that low birth weight is beneficial and protects against an obstructed labour.

Under-reporting

There is also widespread under-reporting of stillbirths and early neonatal deaths which fails to appraise planners of the dimensions of the problem. WHO epidemiologists candidly admit that perhaps 40% or more of early neonatal deaths and stillbirths may go unreported in official data collection. In a study of actual versus officially recorded perinatal mortality in a district in Thailand the measured a rate of 22 perinatal deaths per 1,000 compared with no perinatal deaths reported through official statistics.[2] Even in research studies,[3] analysis of infant mortality may fail to give perinatal causes their due prominence and often being subsumed under the category of "other causes".

A misconception that essential newborn care is expensive

A final crucial reason for neonatal neglect is the widely held misconception that perinatal care depends upon interventions which are too costly or technological for high coverage in poor communities. This attitude has been aggravated by the exposure of professionals to neonatal intensive care units. Yet over 50% of all infant deaths occur in the first month,[4,5] two-thirds in the first few days, and many could be prevented just as easily as later childhood deaths due to diarrhoeal or respiratory diseases. Mothers, health professionals and policymakers all seem to lack education about the simple, low-cost principles of newborn care laid down by the French obstetrician Pierre Budin in his classic work "The Nursling",[6] as shown in Table 1.

Table 1 Principles of essential newborn care.

Air	Resuscitate and maintain an airway.
Warmth	Keep the newborn warm and avoid unnecessary hypothermia or cold stress.
Food	Encourage early breastfeeding, and feed high-risk newborns more frequently.
Hygiene	Maintain hygiene during delivery and cord-cutting; treat infections promptly.
Love	Ensure the newborn infant stays close to its mother, and mothers have open access to their newborn infant if he or she requires special care.

Size and distribution of global perinatal mortality

Table 2 shows the most recent estimates for perinatal, neonatal and maternal mortality rates for different regions of the world. The perinatal mortality rate is the number of stillbirths and deaths in the first seven days of life (of infants more than 28 weeks gestation or > 1,000 g birthweight) per 1,000 births. Stillbirths were slightly more common than first-week deaths in studies from India (50–56%),[7] Nepal (57%),[8] and Ghana (67%).[9] The neonatal mortality rate is the number of deaths ocurring in the first 28 days per 1,000 livebirths, and the maternal mortality rate is the number of maternal deaths occurring in the perinatal period per 100,000 livebirths. All figures from developing countries are based on census or survey estimates so their reliability is open to

Table 2 Perinatal, neonatal and maternal mortality rates worldwide.

	World	More developed countries	Less developed countries	Asia	Africa	Latin America
Perinatal deaths (thousands)	7,636	155	7,480	4,583	2,404	483
Perinatal mortality rate	53	11	57	53	75	19
Neonatal deaths (thousands)	5,080	96	4,984	3,386	1,291	301
Neonatal mortality rate	36	7	39	41	42	25
Maternal deaths (thousands)	585	4	582	323	235	23
Maternal mortality rate	430	27	480	390	870	190

Source: World Health Organization (1995)

question. South Asia is one of the most highly-populated regions of the world with nearly one quarter of the world's population. Although Africa has the highest overall perinatal, neonatal and maternal mortality rates, the greatest number of deaths occur in Asia, especially the South Asia region.

The leading causes of neonatal deaths are usually birth asphyxia, low birth weight (both premature and intrauterine growth-retarded infants), tetanus and other bacterial infections, and jaundice, but the allocation of cause to death during this period can be as difficult as the assignment of mortality by verbal post-mortem in older age groups. The most useful pathophysiological classification described by Wigglesworth[10] has been used in audits of perinatal mortality and is discussed more fully in Chapter 22.

The Importance of Low Birth Weight

Over 70% of neonatal mortality occurs in the low birth weight group (< 2,500 g).[7] The risk factors for intrauterine growth retardation have been well described. In developing countries a low pre-pregnancy maternal weight and height, low caloric intakes, and infections, especially malaria, outweigh the effects of developed country risk factors such as cigarette smoking and primiparity. Preterm infants are at greater risk than growth-retarded infants. In a large longitudinal study in Brazil[11] preterm babies had a perinatal mortality rate 13 times higher than that of babies of appropriate birth weight and gestational age, and two times higher than that of intrauterine growth-retarded babies. But what to do about low birth weight? In India, substantial achievements in reducing severe forms of protein energy malnutrition have not been matched by a decline in low birth weight incidence (see Chapter 4). The national incidence is 30% rising to levels above 50% in urban slum mothers. Supplementation programmes can produce small increases in birth weight but they are expensive to implement. In fact, some authors have questioned whether they confer any significant benefit.[12] There are antenatal interventions which can affect foetal growth but their impact in a developing country setting needs further evaluation (see Chapter 8).

Low birth weight is not only a major risk factor for neonatal death, but also has long-term consequences for health and development in childhood and adult life. Recent epidemiological studies, reviewed in Chapter 17, have identified strong associations between low birth weight and a later risk of cardiovascular and other degenerative diseases such as diabetes. This emphasises the potential cost-effectiveness of perinatal interventions, which may have long-term as well as short-term health benefits.

Birth Asphyxia

Birth asphyxia leading to either stillbirth or hypoxic-ischaemic encephalopathy in the newborn is a major cause of neonatal death and neurodevelopmental sequelae. It is also an important area for future research. We need to know more about the epidemiology, causes and sequelae of asphyxia as well as the most cost-effective interventions for prevention. How can labour be managed better in order to reduce the number of asphyxiated babies? To what extent do postnatal insults like hypothermia and hypoglycaemia contribute to and exacerbate asphyxial mortality and morbidity? Does the higher incidence of perinatal asphyxia in developing countries lead to a higher incidence of minor neurodevelopmental sequelae in survivors, such as motor and learning deficits, or is asphyxia an "all-or-nothing" phenomenon — the asphyxiated infant either dies or makes a full recovery? Is it cost-effective to train community based midwives and birth attendants in neonatal resuscitation? Should they be given a simple bag and mask or be trained in mucous extraction? Or should training for birth attendants be confined to recognition of the mildly asphyxiated infant and postnatal support through avoidance of hypothermia and the establishment of early and frequent breastfeeding? Many of these questions are addressed in Chapters 11 and 12.

Hypothermia

Newborn infants are vulnerable to hypothermia and cold stress, especially those born with a low birth weight. Recent evidence indicates that hypothermia is a common and preventable cause of neonatal morbidity and mortality even in countries with a predominantly warm climate. In many maternity hospitals, preservation of the "warm chain", to ensure a newborn infant is dried, wrapped, breastfed early and nursed in an appropriate ambient temperature, is not maintained. Monitoring methods for thermal control are rudimentary or absent (see Chapters 9 and 10). Skin-to-skin contact and the Kangaroo Care Method are low-cost and effective methods to prevent hypothermia, but still not widely practised.

Infection

Clean surface, clean hands, clean cord-cutting — these are basic principles for the maintenance of hygiene in the perinatal period, but unfortunately they still not practised on a large scale. Newborn infants are especially vulnerable to infection and the signs and symptoms may be non-specific. Prompt recognition of possible infection in a newborn infant, and rapid treatment with appropriate anti-microbial drugs is a key part of essential newborn care. Perinatal transmission of infection from mother to infant is a major area for future preventive action. Syphilis, hepatitis B, and now HIV infection, are of major importance. In sub-Saharan Africa congenital syphilis remains common yet entirely preventable with appropriate antenatal screening. Hepatitis B vaccination has been available since 1982 and is now recommended as part of the Global Programme for Vaccination in many developing countries. So far, virtually no country in sub-Saharan Africa or South Asia has introduced mass vaccination as recommended, even though the cost of the vaccine has fallen substantially. HIV infection is at epidemic proportions in many African countries and is rapidly increasing in South Asia. Therapeutic measures to reduce perinatal transmission have been successful in the West but remain unaffordable elsewhere (see Chapter 13).

Early Breastfeeding

Every year brings new discoveries about benefits that can be derived from breastfeeding (see Chapter 14). Early breastfeeding, starting from the first hour after birth, guarantees that infants receive the anti-infective and immunising effects of colostrum, protection against hypothermia and hypoglycaemia, and a secure bond with their mothers. It is an astonishing fact that over half of all newborn infants in South Asia are not put to the breast at all in the first 24 hours and colostrum is widely discarded. Many innovative strategies to promote breastfeeding have been tried, more recently as part of the Baby Friendly hospital initiative. This has enjoyed considerable success but faces competition from the inappropriate promotion of breastmilk substitutes by formula milk companies, in contravention of the WHO Code on the marketing of breastmilk substitutes ratified by most governments in the 1980s. Many health workers are poorly informed about breastfeeding and lack the skills necessary to tackle problems with lactation.

Perinatal Care: A World Bank Priority for Investment

In the 1993 World Development Report "Investing in Health", published by the World Bank, investment in perinatal care was identified as one of their highest priorities. It was seen as potentially the most important strategy, along with the targeting of acute repiratory infections in infancy, for reducing mortality of under-fives (see Appendix B6 in the report). As the World Bank is the largest health sector donor it is hoped that governments use this investment capital in ways that will strengthen perinatal and neonatal care.

Getting Research into Policy and Practice

How can apparently simple interventions be implemented more effectively to reduce the 7.6 million perinatal deaths each year? Inadequately trained health workers, particularly maldistribution of trained personnel, inadequate resources for medical equipment and supplies, and difficult geographical terrain are major problems in providing good health care for all the people.

Levels of Perinatal Care and Referral Systems

The two main determinants of successful perinatal health care seem to be first, a motivated community based worker with basic training in the management of safe delivery and newborn care, and second, a tiered system of referral.[13] Traditional birth attendant training has many advantages in societies where most births take place at home, but there have been few rigorous evaluations of such training programmes (see Chapters 23 and 24). The coverage of many TBAs may be less than 30 deliveries per year so the need for follow-up refresher training of large numbers of women in remote areas imposes severe logistic difficulties for health planners. A successful referral system must also be physically and economically accessible so that mothers identified as high risk can be transferred to a higher level facility. In remote areas far from district hospitals it may be useful to develop maternity staging posts[14] with trained staff available at all times. But in many countries rapid urbanisation is leading to a sharply increasing demand for institutional delivery so attention is focussing again on the quality of hospital maternity care. Even where referrals take place the conditions of care for infants during transport are grossly inadequate, and audit studies suggest many infants might have have had a better outcome without referral (see Chapter 25).

Special care for high risk infants in hospital need not be expensive (see Chapters 20 and 21). Most life threatening conditions can be treated at low cost for more mature infants. Infants less than 32 weeks gestation may need more expensive care, and in many settings it will be considered inappropriate and not cost-effective to attempt intensive care such as ventilation.

User-friendly Services

The supply of accessible primary care perinatal services is not the only limitation. In India, a lack of demand appears to be a major problem with up to 90% of mothers choosing not to use existing and accessible services.[15] Much of this lack of demand may be accounted for by the services not being "user-friendly". The involvement of mothers in the design and monitoring of these services might improve the situation. Midwives, obstetricians and paediatricians need also to practice evidence-based treatment. There has been extensive analysis of the value of different perinatal interventions, yet too often mothers are subjected to procedures and routines for which there is no proven benefit (see Chapter 26).

More worrying in some countries is the impact of user charges (now widely encouraged by international agencies) on the utilisation of antenatal and perinatal services. In Nigeria, a study of attendance patterns at a district general hospital revealed a sharp and sustained decline in antenatal attendances and hospital deliveries since user charges were introduced in 1984, together with a rising trend in hospital perinatal mortality and morbidity such as neonatal hypothermia and tetanus.[16] In Zimbabwe, maternal mortality rates rose after the introduction of charges for perinatal care. In South Asia, there are often many hidden costs involved in supposedly free maternity services which act as an economic deterrent to users.[17]

Dissemination of Information and Continuing Medical Education

Since 1990 the Baby Friendly Hospital initiative of UNICEF has been an important advance not only to stop the dangerous distribution of free infant formula supplements in maternity hospitals but also to promote good perinatal care to hospital staff in the developing world. More can be done using the principles of medical audit to improve care: agreement on guidelines of good practice, monitoring of actual practice, and implementation of training and management initiatives to bring about changes in care (see Chapter 22).

Modern communication methods make information more accessible and more easily disseminated to remote areas. These methods need to be harnessed so that the population as a whole, rather than an urban elite, can benefit.

Conclusion

Much ill-health in developing countries is often attributed to socio-economic factors beyond the control of health professionals, but for perinatal health there is a real opportunity in the next decade to make progress, led by doctors, midwives and nurses. It is hoped that this book will stimulate readers to improve perinatal care, wherever they are working, by getting research findings into policy and practice.

References

1. "Child Health and Development: Health of the Newborn," In: World Health Organization, EB89/26 (1991).
2. Lumbiganon P, Panamonta M, Laopaiboon M, Pothinam S and Patithat N, "Why are Thai official perinatal and infant mortality rates so low?" *International Journal of Epidemiology* **19** (1990): 997–1000.
3. Chen L, "Primary health care in developing countries: Overcoming operational, technical and social barriers," *Lancet* **ii** (1986): 1260–1265.
4. Ashworth A and Waterlow JC, "Infant mortality in developing countries," *Archives of Disease in Childhood* **57** (1982): 882–884.
5. Costello AM de L, "GOBI and infant mortality," *Lancet* **i** (1988): p. 186.
6. Budin P, *The Nursling*, The feeding and hygiene of premature and full-term infants. Translated by Maloney WJ. The Caxton Publishing Company (1907) London.
7. Bhave SA, "Trends in perinatal and neonatal mortality and morbidity in India," *Indian Pediatrics* **26** (1989): 1094–1099.
8. Malla DS and Johanson RB, "A review of 1,000 cases of stillbirth and neonatal death at the maternity hospital, Kathmandu," *Journal of the Nepal Medical Association* **27A** (1989): 24–34.
9. Fiander A, "Perinatal mortality in a district general hospital, Upper East Region, Ghana, *Tropical Doctor* **22** (1992): p. 82.
10. Wigglesworth JS, "Monitoring perinatal mortality. A pathophysiological approach," *Lancet* **ii** (1980): 684–686.
11. Barros FC, Huttly S, Victora CG, Kirkwood B and Vaughan JP, "Comparison of the causes and consequences of prematurity and intrauterine growth retardation: A longitudinal study in Southern Brazil," *Pediatrics* **90**(2) (1992): 238–244.
12. Garner P, Kramer MS and Chalmers I, "Might efforts to increase birthweight in undernourished women do more harm than good?" *Lancet* **340**(8826) (1992): 1021–1022.
13. Bhargava SK, "Perinatal and neonatal care: The need for reappraisal and action," *Indian Pediatrics* **26** (1989): 1073–1075.
14. Larsen JV, "Reducing the perinatal mortality rate in developing countries," *Tropical Doctor* **22** (1992): 49–51.
15. Bhargava SK, Singh KK and Saxena BN (eds), "A national collaborative study of identification of high risk families, mothers and outcome of their offsprings

with particular reference to the problem of maternal nutrition, low birth weight, perinatal and infant morbidity and mortality in rural and urban slum communities," Indian Council of Medical Research, New Delhi (1990).

16. Owa JA, Osinake AI and Costello AM de L, "Charging for health services in developing countries," *Lancet* **340** (1992): p. 732.

17. Nahar S and Costello AM de L, "The hidden costs of free maternity care in Dhaka, Bangladesh," *Health Policy and Planning* **13**(4) (1998): 417–422.

Chapter 2

RECENT TRENDS IN PERINATAL HEALTH IN SOUTH ASIA

Nazmun Nahar
Professor of Paediatrics, Dhaka Medical College, Bangladesh

Santosh K. Bhargava
Former Professor of Paediatrics, University College of Medical Sciences and Safdarjung Hospital, New Delhi, India

Dharma Manandhar
Senior Consultant Paediatrician, Maternity Hospital, Kathmandu, Visiting Professor, Institute of Medicine, Kathmandu, Nepal

Shakila Zaman
Consultant in Paediatric Epidemiology, King Edward Medical School, Lahore, Pakistan

and

Ananda Wijekoon
Consultant Neonatologist, Univeristy of Peradeniya, Sri Lanka

Introduction

South Asia comprises nearly one quarter of the world's population. Although Africa has the highest overall perinatal, neonatal and maternal mortality rates, most deaths occur in Asia, especially in the southern region. Table 1

15

Table 1 Demographic, health and income indicators of South Asian countries compared with Finland (which has the lowest under-five mortality rate).

Country	Total population 1995 (millions)	Population growth rate 1995 (percent)	GNP per capita 1995 (US$)	Maternal mortality rate 1990–1995 (per 100,000 livebirths)	Life expectancy 1995 (yrs)	Under-five mortality rate 1995	Infant mortality rate 1995
Bhutan	0.7	–	420	–	–	175	–
Pakistan	129.9	2.5	460	340	63	127	91
Nepal	21.5	2.9	200	515	56	131	92
Bangladesh	119.8	1.6	240	887	58	115	80
India	929.4	1.7	340	437	62	95	69
Sri Lanka	18.1	1.2	700	30	73	19	16
Finland	5.1	0.5	20,580	11	76	5	5

From: Sector Strategy Paper. Health, Nutrition and Population (The World Bank, 1997).

shows development indicators for countries in South Asia, including mother and child mortality rates.

Data on perinatal health in developing countries is scanty or difficult to access. In this chapter, perinatal experts from each country report relevant data obtained from research studies, government statistics and national surveys. All data must be treated with caution especially where it is drawn from unpublished studies. The authors have collected interesting up-to-date information on perinatal health indicators and the current status of health services, especially for newborn infants from their own country and its demography.

2.1 BANGLADESH

Nazmun Nahar

Background and Demography

Bangladesh has six administrative divisions, 64 districts, 490 thanas, 4451 rural unions, 119 municipalities (excluding city corporations), and four city corporations. There are nearly 20 million households. More than half of the population (53.5%) is under 16 years of age,[1] 48% of the rural population are below the poverty line, and an additional 25% barely manage to meet basic needs.

Perinatal Health Indicators

Maternal mortality and morbidity

The current level of maternal mortality is uncertain but probably above 500 per 100,000 live births — 80 times higher than the level in developed countries. Population-based studies on maternal mortality over the past 20 years have shown a mortality ratio of 4.4 to 7.7 per 1,000 live births (Table 2).

Koening and colleagues,[2] showed that the percentage of deaths in the reproductive age attributed to maternal cause was 37% in one study area. In survey (1993–94) by BIRPERHT, a Bangladeshi research organisation on reproductive health, interviewed 6,493 mothers to estimate the prevalence of maternal morbidity and mortality in eight rural unions.[3] The major causes of maternal death was eclampsia (40%), haemorrhage (15%), ruptured uterus (11%), obstructed labour (8%), sepsis (4%), and other obstetric causes (22%). They also described maternal morbidities showing that 75% of mothers had morbidity in the antenatal period, 28% in the intrapartum period, 66% in the

Table 2 Maternal mortality ratio reported from various population-based studies in Bangladesh.

Study by	Period	Population size	Maternal mortality ratio
ICDDR,B	1967–68	180,000	7.7
ICDDR,B	1968–70	180,000	5.7
BAMANEH	1982–83	267,000	6.2
Alauddin M.	1982–83	341,000	5.7
BAMANEH Project	1982–83	137,000	4.8
ICDDR,B	1976–85	187,000	5.5
BAMANEH	1985	63,000	4.7
BBS	1987	221,000	6.1
BBS	1988	220,000	5.9
ICDDR,B	1982–90	105,000	4.4

postpartum period and 40% reported chronic conditions. 98% of mothers in this survey had delivered at home. The majority of deliveries (49%) were by an untrained traditional birth attendant (TBA) or by relatives (39%).

An analysis of 19,031 maternity admissions to institutions such as medical colleges, district hospitals and thana health complexes reported 491 deaths (2.6%).[4] The causes of death were similar to the BIRPERHT study.

Eclampsia and perinatal outcome

Eclampsia remains a major cause of death and morbidity in Bangladesh. Shahabuddin and colleagues[5] studied 274 clinically confirmed eclampsia cases at Rangpur Medical College Hospital.[5] 84% of mothers presented antepartum and only 19% of cases were graded as severe. Nonetheless, eclampsia carried a high risk for the mother and foetus: 16% of mothers and 33% of infants died (Table 3).[5]

Table 3 Perinatal and maternal outcome by types of eclampsia.

Outcome	Type of Eclampsia		
	Antepartum (n = 230)	Postpartum (n = 44)	Total (n = 274)
Maternal death	35 (15%)	8 (18%)	43 (16%)
Still birth	66 (29%)	1 (2%)	67 (25%)
Early neonatal death	22 (10%)	1 (2%)	23 (8%)
Total	88 (38%)	2 (5%)	90 (33%)

Neonatal mortality

About 60–70% of infant deaths occur during the neonatal period in rural Bangladesh. Births are usually attended by elderly female members of the family who are not well trained. Less than 10% of rural and only 45% of urban births are attended by a trained person. A national estimate for neonatal mortality rate is 48 per 1,000 live births assuming that 60% of newborn deaths occur in the neonatal period.[6] In the first hour after delivery 12 of every 1,000 live births will die.[7] The common causes of neonatal death are birth asphyxia or injuries, prematurity, low birth weight (LBW), tetanus, pneumonia, and diarrhoea.

Low birth weight (LBW)

Bangladesh has the highest birth prevalence of LBW infants in the world. One-third to half of all newborns have a birth weight of less than 2.5 kg, a reflection on the maternal nutritional status of the country. Other contributing factors are the small stature of the mother, infections during pregnancy, anaemia, and closely spaced pregnancies.[8] LBW infants are two to three times as likely to die in infancy as those of normal weight.

A recent prospective study of 660 live births, recorded within 24 hours of delivery, measured the incidence and associated factors of low birth weight infants in three different communities: urban, urban slum, and rural areas of Bangladesh[8] (Table 4). LBW rates were highest in urban slum areas. The mean birth weight of the total population was 2,789 g (sd 501). There was an increased risk of an LBW infant in mothers living in the urban slum, in those with reduced weight (mothers less than 40 kg particularly), poor educational status, and without any antenatal care. Mothers aged below 20 years and above 35 years were at higher risk of giving birth to LBW infants.

Table 4 Risk factors for LBW infants in Bangladesh.

Variable	NBW > 2,500 g n (%)	LBW < 2,500 g n (%)	Total
Location			
Urban	171 (85)	30 (15)	201 (100)
Rural	174 (79)	46 (21)	220 (100)
Urban slum	151 (63)	88 (37)	239 (100)
Maternal weight (kg)			
30–39	18 (45)	22 (55)	40 (6)
40–49	250 (73)	91 (27)	341 (52)
50–59	164 (79)	44 (21)	208 (32)
< 60	64 (90)	7 (10)	71 (11)
Maternal education			
Never at school	140 (64)	79 (36)	219 (33)
Class I–V	105 (72)	41 (28)	146 (22)
Class VI–X	100 (83)	21 (17)	121 (18)
Class XI and above	151 (87)	23 (13)	174 (26)
Antenatal visits			
None	134 (63)	78 (37)	212 (32)
1–3	113 (74)	39 (26)	152 (23)
4–6	249 (84)	47 (16)	296 (45)
Maternal age			
15–19	28 (57)	21 (43)	49 (7)
20–35	427 (77)	128 (23)	565 (86)
< 35	32 (68)	15 (32)	47 (7)

From Nahar N and Hossain M (1994).

What proportion of LBW infants are preterm? A study of 397 newborns from Dhaka hospitals found that 10% of the infants were preterm and 90% were term.[9] The incidence of LBW infants was 47%, of which 87% were term and only 13% were preterm. Most LBW infants are therefore the result of intrauterine growth retardation (IUGR).

Neonatal morbidity

Perinatal asphyxia

In developing countries, the World Health Organization estimates that 3% of all newborn infants (3.6 million) develop moderate or severe asphyxia, of which 840,000 die and approximately the same number develop severe sequelae such as epilepsy and mental retardation. However, these figures may be inaccurate because of the lack of agreement over the definition of birth asphyxia (see Chapter 11).

There are no good epidemiological studies of birth asphyxia in Bangladesh. A prospective study of 122 infants born with asphyxia in the neonatal care unit of the Institute of Postgraduate Medicine and Research suggested that oxytocin may be a risk factor for asphyxia as 61% of asphyxiated infants had received it.[10] However, the study was uncontrolled.

Neonatal sepsis and tetanus

Septicaemia is an important global cause of neonatal morbidity and mortality. The incidence of neonatal septicaemia is from one to ten cases per 1,000 live births, with a mortality rate of 40–65%.[11] *E. coli* is the most commonly reported organism, followed by *S.aureus, Pseudomonas* spp. and *Klebsiella*.[12]

A study of 39 cases of neonatal septicaemia at the Institute of Postgraduate Medicine and Research showed that 23 out of 32 term infants were LBW.[13] Case fatality rates were much higher for preterm (71%) than full-term infants (12%); the case fatality rate for LBW infants was 30%. Prematurity therefore carries the highest risk of a poor outcome in neonatal septicaemia.

It is estimated there are as many as 550,000 deaths from neonatal tetanus world wide of which approximately 220,000 occur in South Asia. Tetanus is often associated with sepsis and newborn deaths due to sepsis are caused by unclean delivery and cord care practice.

A study of 343 cases of neonatal tetanus admitted to the Infectious Disease Hospital of Dhaka between 1990 to 1991 showed that 98% were from poor families (usually from villages or urban slums), 85% were born to mothers never immunised against tetanus and all but one case arose from umbilical infection.[14]

A study of 73 neonatal tetanus cases in Mymensingh Medical College Hospital during 1992 to 1993[15] showed all cases were delivered at home by family members or by TBAs. The umbilical cord was usually cut using an ordinary razor blade (69%) or bamboo (28%), and 66% of infants had received an application of cowdung, ash or hot poultice to the umbilical stump. 87% of mothers were not immunised and 11% had received only one dose of tetanus toxoid.

A survey of 350 neonatal deaths in Rajshahi Division showed that 112 were due to tetanus.[16] Risk was reduced by training birth attendants to wash their hands and to use a cleaned cord-cutting tool. Risk was not reduced, surprisingly, by a maternal history of two doses of tetanus toxoid, although the estimated efficacy of two doses was 45%.[16] Table 5 summarises the circumstances of delivery for neonatal tetanus deaths compared with controls, i.e. deaths which arose from other causes.

Neonatal jaundice

Two prospective studies of jaundice in neonates admitted to the special care unit at the Institute of Postgraduate Medicine and Research, Dhaka, in 1982 and 1992 determined the prevalance of clinical jaundice, predisposing risk factors and outcome.[17] The incidence of neonatal jaundice over a period of six months was 34% in 1982 and 51% in 1992. In both studies, ABO and Rhesus incompatibility were the commonest causes for neonatal hyperbilirubinaemia. Exchange transfusion was needed in 22% of cases in both studies. The rate of fall of serum bilirubin per 12 hours after exchange

Table 5 Circumstances of delivery for neonatal tetanus cases (n = 112) and matched controls (n = 336).

	Cases No. (%)	Controls No. (%)
Place of delivery		
In hospital or clinic	0 (0)	6 (2)
At home	112 (100)	330 (98)
Birth attendant		
Relative	63 (56)	182 (54)
Unrelated traditional birth attendant	23 (21)	84 (25)
Health care worker	0 (0)	8 (2)
Self (delivered without assistance)	26 (23)	62 (18)
Delivery practices[a]		
Attendant washed hands	45 (40)	182 (54)
Perineum washed	41 (37)	146 (44)
Mustard oil applied to vagina	22 (20)	69 (21)
Coconut oil applied to vagina	9 (8)	12 (4)
Safe delivery kit used	2 (2)	7 (2)
Cord-cutting tool cleaned before use	55 (49)	231 (69)
Multiple cord ties used	41 (37)	89 (27)
Mother's vaccination status at delivery		
History of TT2[b]	33 (30)	122 (36)
No history of TT2	79 (71)	214 (64)

[a]Figures exceed total (100%) because categories are not exclusive.
[b]Two doses of tetanus toxoid at least four weeks apart, with the second dose at least 30 days before delivery.

transfusion was 4 mg in 1982 and 10 mg in 1992. The mortality rate after exchange transfusion was 36% in 1982 and only 5% in 1992. In the 1982 study, 84% of the neonates made a full recovery, 14% died and 2% had neurological sequelae on discharge from hospital. In the 1992 study, 97% had immediate good prognosis and mortality rate was 2.8%. These results show that the outcome of treatment and the results after exchange transfusion had improved markedly over the decade.[1]

Newborn Care Services

The average Bangladeshi household spends less than 1% of their income on health and education. There are 919 hospitals of which 396 are thana health complexes.[1] The total number of hospital beds is 35,795 and the ratio of person per bed is 3,288. The total number of medical colleges is 20, 13 of which are government and the rest are in the private sector. The number of registered physicians is about 25,000, with a person per physician ratio of 4,725. The total number of nurses is under 10,000 and of midwives is nearly 8,000. There are 96 maternity and child welfare centres. The governments total expenditure in health including the family planning sector is about US$300 million per year.

Is prevention enough?

Despite all the preventive approaches taken up by mothers like antenatal, postnatal care, referral of high risk pregnancies, MCH based family planning services, and an extensive TBA programme countrywide, maternal and neonatal mortality rates remain high in Bangladesh. The study by Fauveau and colleagues (Table 6) showed that even in a rural area (Matlab) where intensive antenatal interventions have been introduced, neonatal mortality was reduced by onlynine per 1,000 in comparison with a control population.[18] Neonatal tetanus reduction through better immunisation coverage was the main cause of this decline.

The need for emergency obstetric care services

Policymakers in Bangladesh now realise that without proper facilities for case management of major obstetric complications, the lives of mothers cannot be saved.[4] Maternal mortality cannot be substantially reduced unless women have access to emergency obstetric care (EOC), where they will get prompt and adequate medical treatment. UNICEF and OGSB have launched an EOC project in Bangladesh since 1994.[19] Table 7 summarises the potential role of interventions to improve maternal health status in Bangladesh.

Table 6 Causes of death among neonates (less than 31 days) in study and comparison areas of Matlab 1986–87 (rates per 1,000 live births).

Cause of death	Study area (6,663 live births)			Comparison area (7,677 live births)			Difference between rates
	No.	Rate	%	No.	Rate	%	
Complications of small size at birth	132	19.8	44.1	144	18.8	34.8	1.0
Birth trauma	43	6.5	14.4	44	5.7	10.6	0.8
Neonatal tetanus	20	3.0	6.7	85	11.1	20.5	−8.1***
Neonatal pneumonia	30	4.5	10.0	42	5.5	10.1	−1.0
Acute watery diarrhoea	1	0.2	0.3	3	0.4	0.7	−0.2
Acute non-watery diarrhoea	0	0.0	0.0	3	0.4	0.7	−0.4
Persistent diarrhoea	1	0.2	0.3	0	0.0	0.0	0.2
Other neonatal infections	32	4.8	10.7	36	4.7	8.7	0.1
Other neonatal disorders	7	1.1	2.3	9	1.2	2.2	−0.1
Impossible to specify	33	5.0	11.0	48	6.3	11.6	−1.3
All causes	299	44.9	100	414	53.9	100	−90*

*p < 0.05; ***p < 0.001. Some totals do not add up because of rounding.

Table 7 Influence of interventions to improve maternal health status in Bangladesh.

Cause of Death	Relative influence of interventions			
	Family planning	Antenatal care	Trained TBA	Case management
Haemorrhage		+	+	+++
Induced abortion	++		+	+++
Eclampsia		++	+	+++
Puerperal sepsis		+	++	+++
Obstructed labour		+	+	+++

+ = advocative, ++ = preventive, +++ = life saving

EOC services can be classified into three levels:

(a) Obstetric first aid only: giving a parenteral oxytocic drug (ergometrine), parenteral antibiotics, sedatives/anticonvulsants.
(b) Basic EOC: all functions of obstetric first aid, plus manual removal of placenta and assisted vaginal delivery (vacuum extraction, forceps).
(c) Comprehensive EOC: basic EOC plus surgery (e.g. caesarean section, curettage, etc.) and blood transfusion.

Facilities

In Bangladesh, provision for neonatal care in institutions remains poor and there is very limited access to good quality obstetric services. There is no structured training in neonatal care at any level of health care provider. In the eight old medical colleges and postgraduate research institute there are small neonatal units but most lack essential equipment.

Conclusion

Despite many preventive measures delivered through the MCH-based family planning services and an extensive TBA training programme, maternal and neonatal mortality remain high in Bangladesh. Policymakers realise the need for better case management for high risk mothers and newborns, and various initiatives have been started like the Emergency Obstetric Care Programme, the Mother and Baby Package, the Baby Friendly Hospital initiative, and various nutritional projects targeted towards vulnerable mothers.

However, 80% of the population are rural so midwife training and undergraduate teaching for doctors must be modified to be needs-based and community-oriented. A combined service delivery programme has been launched recently: it is expected that health and nutrition care for 70% of the population of Bangladesh will be covered, and hopefully mortality of newborn infants and mothers will continue to fall in the next decade.

References

1. *Statistical Pocket Book of Bangladesh*. Bangladesh Bureau of Statistics, Ministry of Planning, Government of Bangladesh.
2. Koening MA *et al.*, "Maternal mortality in Matlab, Bangladesh, 1976–1985," *Studies in Family Planning* **19**(2) (1988): 69–80.
3. Ahmed YH and Rahman MH, "A report on a baseline survey for assessment of emergency obstetric care services in Bangladesh," BIRPHERT (1995).
4. Akhter HH, "Situation analysis of maternal health in Bangladesh," paper presented at National Conference on Safe Motherhood, December 1994.
5. Shahabuddin AKM, Hasnat M *et al.*, "Perinatal outcome of eclampsia in a Medical College Hospital," *Bangladesh Journal of Child Health* **20**(1) (1996).
6. Progothir P. *Achieving the Mid-Decade Goals for Children in Bangladesh*. Bangladesh Bureau of Statistics with assistance from UNICEF (1996).
7. Talukder MQK and Kabir L, "Situation analysis of child health in Bangladesh," paper presented in National Conference on Safe Motherhood, December 1994.
8. Nahar N, Hossain M *et al*, "Incidence of low birth weight and associated factors, comparison between different communities," Bangladesh Medical Research Council Project (1994).
9. Rahman S and Akhtar M, "Incidence of low birth weight, term and preterm infants in institutional deliveries of Dhaka city," *Bangladesh Journal of Child Health* **16**(3/4) (1992): 79–83.
10. Khatoon SA and Kawser CA *et al*, "Risk factors, clinical profile and hospital outcome of birth asphyxiated infants," *Bangladesh Journal of Child Health* **13**(1) (1989): 7–15.
11. Siegel JDM and McCracken GH, "Sepsis neonatorum," *New England Journal of Medicine* **304** (1981): 642–647.
12. Chandna A and Rao MN *et al*, "Rapid diagnostic test in neonatal septicaemia," *Indian Journal of Pediatrics* **55** (1988): 947–953.
13. Khatoon S and Khatoon M, "Clinical and bacteriological profile of neonatal septicaemia and their outcome," *Bangladesh Journal of Child Health* **17**(2) (1993): 48–53.
14. Mohiuddin M and Hossain AM, "A study on neonatal tetanus in the infectious disease Hospital, Dhaka," *Journal of Preventive and Social Medicine* **12**(2) (1993): 44–47.
15. Haque M and Begum W *et al.*, "Neonatal tetanus — A declining trend," *Mymensingh Medical Journal* **3**(1) (1994): 9–13.

16. Hlady WG and Bennett JV *et al.*, "Neonatal tetanus in rural Bangladesh. Risk factors and toxoid efficacy," *American Journal of Public Health* **82** (1992): 1365–1369.

17. Ahmed S and Parvin M *et al.*, "Jaundice in the newborn in Bangladesh. A comparison of data 10 years apart," *Bangladesh Journal of Child Health* **18**(2) (1994): 46–50.

18. Fauveau V *et al.*, "The effect of maternal and child health and family planning services on mortality: Is prevention enough?" *British Medical Journal* **301** (1990): 103–107.

19. OGSB, UNICEF, "Emergency obstetric care. Intervention for the reduction of maternal mortality," URC Bangladesh (1995).

2.2 INDIA

Santosh K. Bhargava

Background and Demography

In the 1991 census India's population was 846.3 million; by the turn of the century it will cross the unenviable mark of a billion. India has 451 districts with 74% of the population living in rural areas. It has a predominantly Hindu population (84%). The female-to-male ratio is 927 per 1,000 males, the annual population growth rate below 2%, life expectancy is 61 years, and the crude birth rate 29 per 1,000. The overall literacy rate is 53% for males and 39% for females but there is marked geographical variation.[1,2]

Historic perspective on newborn care and traditional practices

Current trends in neonatal health and care must be viewed in the light of traditional practices and development progress in contemporary India. There are numerous traditional cultural practices, rituals and celebrations with the birth and survival of a newborn (see Chapter 7). Women and children were of deep concern in Ayurveda, the most ancient Indian system of medicine, which developed into three branches: the Atreya School (medicine), Susruta School (surgery), and Kashyap School (obstetrics and pediatrics). In the more recent past, however, women's health became, and remains in many communities, a subject of neglect. A parturient mother and her newborn may be considered unhygienic and untouchable by the family. The delivery may take place in the darkest, dingy corner of the house, on dirty and discarded clothes, and the birth attended by an untrained, socially outcast woman. The pregnancy, method of delivery, maternal care after birth, and care of the newborn in the first few weeks of life is often accompanied by harmful traditional practices.

Unfortunately, the neglect of pregnant women and particularly the neonate has continued even in contemporary post-independence India. The newborn is considered a mere appendage of her mother and not even accorded the status of a hospital bed. Maternal and neonatal deaths were considered as "God's wish".[4] It is only in the last few years that the special needs of the newborn have been accepted and "Essential Newborn Care" included as part of a national programme.

Newborn care in contemporary India

At the time of independence in 1947, India had virtually no basic health services. The country opted to develop a network of primary health centres and sub-centres for its vast rural population. These were provided with basic amenities, and medical and paramedical professionals were allocated according to population size. Today, these centres are the nucleus for providing primary health and family welfare services in rural areas, and are linked to community health centres and district hospitals. In urban areas, health care is provided through family welfare, maternal and child welfare centres, and hospitals.

A national health policy was only enunciated by the Government of India in 1983, which set goals for the year 2000, including those for essential newborn care.[5] India is rapidly shifting from vertical to integrated health care programmes, e.g. the Universal Immunization programme was integrated into the Child Survival and Safe Motherhood Programme in 1992,[6] and Essential Newborn Care was added in 1993.[7]

Perinatal Health Indicators

Table 8 shows perinatal health indicators in India and selected states which reflect poor, average and good development progress. The birth and total fertility rates are gradually declining but population stabilisation remains a major problem. 30% of the population is below a national poverty line. The age of marriage for females is still low. The low birth weight prevalence is about 30% (see Chapter 4). 80% of pregnant mothers receive some form of antenatal care and 86% are immunised against tetanus. 74% of births occur at home of which 9.1% are conducted by qualified health professionals, 35.1% by traditional birth attendants and the remaining 30% by relatives.[8]

Table 8 Perinatal health indicators in India and selected states reflecting poor, average and good development status.

Indicator	India	Orissa (poor)	Tamil Nadu (average)	Kerala (good)	National goal by year 2000
Female literacy, 1991 (%)	38	34	52	87	–
Age at marriage (mean, years)	18.3	19	20.2	21.8	–
Total fertility rate, 1991	3.4	1.8	2.5	2.5	2.2
Perinatal mortality rate, 1993	44	66	48	17	–
Neonatal mortality rate, 1993	47	78	46	10	–
Infant mortality rate, 1993	74	126	57	17	below 60
Maternal mortality rate, 1993 (per 100,000)	400	–	–	–	below 200
Home deliveries (%)	74	86	36	12	–
Trained attendant at birth (%)	49	19	57	74	100

Sources: Ramji S[12] (1989); Health Information of India (1994), Ministry of Health and Family Welfare; Registrar General of India (1991). Note that the data for trained birth attendants is from 1993 for the national figure and from 1985 for the state figures.

Maternal mortality

The current national maternal mortality rate is 437 per 100,000 births but varies from state to state. The prevalence of different causes varies in different age groups but abortions, puerperal sepsis, and malposition remain the leading causes.[8]

Perinatal mortality

The current national perinatal mortality rate (PNMR) is 44 per 1,000 births. It varies in different samples but is generally higher in hospitals compared to the community. The National Neonatology Forum (NNF) neonatal and perinatal data base reported a PNMR of 71.6 with a stillbirth rate of 39.1 and early neonatal mortality of 32.5.[9] The ICMR national collaborative study recorded it as 57.5 in rural and 52.0 in urban slum areas. The PNMR is influenced by family socio-economic status, maternal education, biological factors, nutritional status, parity, bad obstetric history, previous preterm birth, place of birth, and person conducting the delivery. Amongst fetal and neonatal factors birth weight, gestational age, cry at birth, and congenital malformation showed a relationship with PNMR.[10-12] Antepartum haemorrhage, toxemia and maternal disease are common clinicopathological causes of perinatal death, with asphyxia, pulmonary conditions and birth trauma as necropsy causes of perinatal deaths (Table 9).

Neonatal mortality

The 1993 national neonatal mortality rate is 47.2 which shows a slow decline from 66.7 in 1982. The NMR varies from state to state, between urban and rural areas, and from community to hospital births. It is lowest in the state of Kerala (at 10) and highest in Orissa state (at 78) (Table 8). The urban NMR is 28.9 and rural 52.3. The NNF neonatal perinatal hospital data base[11] recorded it as 37.7 and the district newborn care project as 18.9 in the districts studied.[13]

Table 9 Causes of neonatal deaths in India from different data sources: hospital necropsy study; National Neonatology Forum survey of hospital deaths; national survey of reported rural deaths.

Cause	Necropsy data, Delhi n = 547 (%)	NNF clinical survey, 1995 n = 1400	India	Orissa	Kerala
	Ghosh and Bhargava, 1983	NNF neonatal database	Annual survey of causes of death, 1994, "causes peculiar to infancy."		
Birth asphyxia	13	24	–	–	–
Pulmonary	30	20	16	17	29
Septicaemia or infection	10	19	12	3	21
Prematurity	–	11 (extreme)	50	70	21
Congenital malformation	10	10	3	1	7
Birth trauma	17	1	3	1	0
Intraventricular bleed	–	6	–	–	–
Other	19	8	15	8	22

Sources: Ghosh and Bhargava (1983); NNF database (1995); Survey of causes of death (rural), Annual Report (1994), Registrar General, India.

Causes of neonatal mortality

The causes of neonatal death show striking differences depending upon the location of the study and the method used to ascertain cause. There has been no acceptance of a uniform classification for causes of death. In general, prematurity/low birth weight, asphyxia and infections (including tetanus) have been reported as the main causes of neonatal deaths in community based studies (Table 9).[14] While intrapartum anoxia, birth trauma, pneumonia and aspiration syndrome, infections, and congenital malformations continue to remain as leading causes,[11] hyaline membrane disease and intraventricular haemorrhage appear to be emerging problems in hospital births, reflecting the increasing survival of premature and very low birth weight infants.

Factors contributing to neonatal mortality

These include socio-economic status (income, housing, literacy, age at marriage), maternal biological factors (age, parity and nutritional status — pregravid weight and height), pregnancy care and complications, intranatal factors (place and person conducting the birth), and neonatal factors (birth weight, gestational age and facilities for newborn care at birth).[10,12,15] Many of these factors contribute to the occurrence of low birth weight or preterm birth, which together account for more than 70% of neonatal mortality.

NMR is also influenced by the knowledge, attitude and practices of expectant women and the person or professionals involved in her care. Habits such as tobacco chewing, smoking, and consumption of alcohol are significantly prevalent in both urban and rural populations.[10] Similarly, unhygenic measures such as not washing hands before conducting deliveries, use of non-sterilized cutting instrument, immediate bath after birth, and

Table 10 Perinatal care practices by poor mothers in India.

	Urban slum (%)	Rural (%)
Mother working	40	38
Betel nut chewing	13	5
Tobacco chewing	12	5
Smoking	2	3
Alcohol consumption	2	3
No visit of health functionary	79	78
No utilisation of health services	83	94
No washing of hands before delivery	46	44
Harmful practices for umbilical cord care at birth	7	54
Bathing after birth within eight hours	87	31
Use of a prelacteal feed	73	98
Time of first feed during first eight hours	41	53

Source: National Collaborative Study; Indian Council of Medical Research (1990).

offering prelacteal feeds and first feed after eight hours of birth were some examples of practices affecting neonatal mortality (see Table 10).[3,10] Poor utilisation of existing available facilities and the absence of even primary newborn care facilities, such as warming, suction and resuscitation equipment, have been other major determinants of high neonatal mortality across the country.[10,15]

Low Birth Weight (LBW)

Low birth weight remains the single most important problem for neonatal health in India because of its high prevalence, its contribution to neonatal mortality and sequelae in surviving infants, and because of the lack of good special care facilities.

The prevalence of low birth weight in different parts of the country and in different studies varies from 10–56% (see Chapter 4).[16–19] LBW rates have not significantly declined in national reports, although a recent report recorded a significant fall from 27–16% in the same population.[20] LBW infants comprise two groups: the preterm (short gestation) and the intrauterine growth-retarded (IUGR), which can occur at any gestational age. The preterm comprise from 7–22%, and IUGR at all gestation ages from 30–85% of newborn infants.[21–23]

Distribution by birth weight and gestation

There have been many studies of the distribution of births by birth weight.[9,10,21–23] This varies with the nature of the study and population. Amongst LBW infants 70–90% are born in birth weight group 2,000–2,499 g, 5.8–15% below 2,000 g, 1.4% below 1,500 g and 0.5–1% below 1,000 g.

7–22% of births in India are preterm (< 37 weeks), 72–97% term (37–41 weeks), and 6–14% postterm (42 weeks or more).[9,11,19] A comparison of births at different weeks of gestation with similar studies from developed countries shows interesting variation.[24,27] In India, more births occur at each week of gestation up to 36 weeks compared with Western countries, with maximum births occurring at 38 and 39 weeks. These findings suggest that labour amongst Indian women occurs earlier than in their more affluent counter parts. This phenomenon is universal to all groups of the population and has significant epidemiological implications: if the gestation curve is only shifted by one week to the right it will result in a significant fall in preterm and LBW prevalence.

A two-way distribution by birth weight and gestation has shown that in the birth weight group of 1,500–2,000 g, 30–35% of the infants are preterm and in the birth weight group 2,001–2,500 g only 13–15% are preterm.[21,22]

Distribution by fetal growth

Several fetal growth curves studies have classified infants as appropriate for gestation, small for gestation and large for gestation.[27,29] Bhargava *et al.* have proposed a classification by standard deviation score to identify a separate group of IUGR infants with birth weight between −1SD and −2SD. These constitute 85% of births in the birth weight group 2,001–2,500 g which contribute maximally to low birth weight prevalence.[19−28]

Surrogates to birth weight

Measuring birth weight in the community, where two-thirds of births occur, is a problem. In India, villages and houses are scattered widely and often a sub-centre or primary health centre is located at a distance. The absence of suitable portable weighing scales, and beliefs that weighing/or undressing will harm the baby, are common constraints to recording birth weight. To overcome this problem Bhargava *et al.*[30] in a community based study demonstrated a strong relationship between mid-arm circumference (MAC) obtained at birth with birth weight, and outcome. Almost 98% of infants with birth weight 2,000 g or less and 79% of LBWs had an MAC 9.0 cm or less. Neonatal mortality showed an inverse relationship with MAC. Other studies have evaluated measurements such as chest circumference, thigh circumference and foot length.[31] Kumar *et al.* used a bangle with an internal diameter of 8.5 cm and 7.5 cm for identifying LBW infants with birth weight less than 2,500 g and 2,000 g respectively.[32]

Aetiology of low birth weight

Several studies have demonstrated the association of socio-environmental factors such as income, housing, type of family, number of living rooms, education of mother, smoking, tobacco chewing, and consumption of alcohol, with low birth weight.[10]

Pregravid maternal nutritional status and nutrition during pregnancy are known to affect fetal growth. Pregravid weight of 45 kg or less, height 145 cm or less, a low Body Mass Index, weight gain of less than 9 kg during pregnancy, poor dietary intake, hypoalbuminemia, and maternal anemia are associated with LBW.[32] Interesting studies by Ramachandran *et al.*[34] and Bhargava *et al.*[35] on low maternal haemoglobin and ferritin levels have demonstrated their relationship with LBW. Khan *et al.*[36] recorded the adverse influence of performing physical labour, without rest at home, with causation of low birth weight perhaps due to excess energy expenditure.

Personal habits in teenage pregnancy, successive births with an interval of less than two years, previous preterm or low birth weight sibling, parity, and pregnancy complications such as toxemia, antepartum haemorrhage have been recorded as significant causes of LBW.[10,18,37-43] While urinary tract infection has been reported as a significant cause, Indian literature is scanty on the effects on LBW of infections like malaria and amoebiasis.[10] In a recent study coitus during pregnancy has also been reported to contribute to this problem[43] (for further details see Chapters 4 and 17).

Mortality and outcome of low birth weight infants

The mortality of LBW infants is still high but is showing a significant change specially at the institution and hospital level.[10,11,18,21-23,45-47] It is inversely related to birth weight and gestation (see Tables 11 and 12).

Longitudinal studies from birth to 18 years have recorded significant mortality and morbidity in LBW children (see Chapter 17). Cognitive development seems to be affected in very low birth weight infants. An increasing developmental lag in language development was observed between preterm and IUGR, and controls, in follow-up studies from birth to ten years.[48-51]

Table 11 Early neonatal mortality in relation to birth weight.

Source	NNF Perinatal database, 1995	Ghosh, 1979	Bhargava, 1977
Place	Multicentre hospital study, national	Delhi, community	Delhi hospital, urban
Sample size	37,082	5,598	25,878
Mortality by weight group (%)			
< 1,000 g	78	100	97
1,001–1,500 g	40	38	85
1,501–2,000 g	12	9	25
2,001–2,500 g	3	1	1
> 2,500 g	3	1	1

Table 12 Trends in neonatal survival (%) at selected regional referral institutions.

	PGI, Chandigarh		AIIMS, Delhi		KEM, Pune		MAMC, Delhi		SL Jain, Delhi	
	1975	1989	1982	1986	1983	1993	1981	1992	1988	1996
Birth weight										
< 1,000 g	12	60	–	16	3	22	0	0	0	40
1,001–1,500 g	35	39	36	56	47	57	24	60	57	75
1,501–2,000 g	72	87	85	89	68	86	62	87	87	92

Sources: Postgraduate Institute, Chandigarh; All India Institute of Medical Sciences, New Delhi; King Edward Medical College, Pune; Maulana Azad Medical College, Delhi; Sunder Lal Jain Hospital.

Neonatal morbidity

In a recent district newborn care project co-ordinated by the NNF and the government of India covering births in 24 districts from different parts of the country, asphyxia, hypothermia and infections were the main causes of morbidity.[13] The prevalence varied slightly between districts and between first referral unit and primary health centre. In comparison, the ICMR national collaborative study in urban slum and rural populations[10] recorded respiratory problems as the commonest morbidity and a much higher prevalence of infections and asphyxia. The NNF neonatal perinatal database studies[9] showed infections, respiratory distress and CNS problems but the nature of these varied.

Asphyxia

Asphyxia contributes significantly to neonatal morbidity and mortality. The prevalence is reported to vary from 6–24%.[9–13,51,52] Epidemiological studies on causes and prevention are few and mostly hospital-based. The national rural sample survey does not list asphyxia as a cause of morbidity or mortality.[8] In a prospective study of 35,959 births, Kumari et al.[52] recorded a prevalence of low Apgar score (< 6 at one minute) as 7.6%. Its prevalence increased from 5.8% in 1982 to 8.9% in 1986 and declined to 7.2% in 1988. The initial increase was ascribed to better recording and the fall to early intervention. However, while Mishra et al.[53] noted inadequate antenatal care, prematurity and IUGR as important factors, the same was not reported by Kumari et al. Both the studies recorded a high caesarian section rate, abnormal presentation and hypertensive disease of pregnancy as common causes. These studies suggest the need for common protocols for studies in rural and urban slum communities where most births occur at home and are attended by trained or untrained birth attendents (see Chapter 11).

Infections

10–12% of maternal deaths are caused by puerperal sepsis and 10–25% of neonatal deaths are caused by pneumonia, septicemia, diarrhoea and meningitis.[9,10] Nosocomial infections may be as high as 25%.[54–56] *E. coli, Klebsiella* and *Staphylococcus* are the common offending organisms.[9] *Salmonella* has been reported as endemic and a common organism in nursery epidemics, *Chlamydia* has been reported in conjunctival infections, but Groups B and D *Streptococci* have not been found to be prevalent. There are hardly any studies on causation by *Listeria monocytogenes* and *Haemophilus influenza* (see Chapter 13).[57]

The high prevalence of superficial and systemic infection in India have been reported to be associated with multiple factors including living conditions, socio-cultural patterns, and traditional practices. Low income, single-room dwelling, an unprotected water supply, poor maternal nutritional status, inadequate antenatal care, delivery by untrained birth attendants, poor hand washing practices, unhygienic care of the mouth and umbilical cord, and overcrowding in nurseries have been associated with high infection rates.[9,11,57]

Neonatal jaundice

Neonatal jaundice occurs commonly — from 53% in term infants to over 80% in preterms and IUGR. The prevalence of hyperbilirubinaemia (serum bilirubin > 12 mg/dl in term and > 15 mg/dl in preterm infants) is 5–7%. ABO haemolytic disease and infections have been the commonest causes in most studies, but G-6PD deficiency and Rhesus (RH) haemolytic disease have shown considerable variation in studies from different parts of the country and even in the same city.[58–60] G6-PD was reported by Bhargava *et al.*[58] in 42% against 0.6% and 0.9% in other series. Rh haemolytic disease was recorded in 33% by Ahmad *et al.*[59] but was not observed by Bhargava *et al.* and seen in only 4.8% by Chaturvedi *et al.*[60]

Hypothermia and thermal regulation

Hypothermia as a cause of neonatal morbidity is hardly reported in India. The NNF perinatal database[9] reported its occurrence in 1% of hospital births and the NNF district care project as 2.5%.[13] It usually goes unrecognised as it is a common practice to keep infants covered and low-reading thermometers (< 95° F) are not used in newborn care. Hypothermia is usually caused by the use of harmful traditional practices such as an early bath, inadequate clothing, and not keeping the room warm. However, further community based studies will be needed to establish its prevalence (see Chapters 9 and 10).

Primary cold injury in newborn was described for the first time from tropical countries by Bhargava *et al.* in 1971 during the winter months at a temperature of 31–49° F.[61] Since then it is being increasingly recognised in different parts of the country — especially in north India and the coastal areas. Hypothermia, coldness to touch, and bradycardia are key features of the disease which affects multiple systems and has been seen in infants from eight hours of age to 21 days. Mortality occurs due to massive pulmonary haemorrhage.

Heat injury in the newborn was first described by Bhargava *et al.* in 1977[62] after a prolonged heat wave in Delhi. The disease resulted from non air-conditioned or air-cooled post-natal wards. The diagnosis was established by exclusion of other causes of fever and the presence of high fever ($> 39.4°C$) with or without other symptoms. The critical environmental temperature which caused the heat injury was 42.5°C or above. It caused widespread multiple-system involvement with electrolyte disturbance. Mortality was high and excessive weight loss, hypertonia and bleeding signified a poor prognosis.

Congenital malformations

The prevalence of congenital malformation has been reported to vary from 1.6–2.8% of births.[9,10,63] The prevalence rates varied because of the classification, place of birth, and person conducting the neonatal examination. In a prospective community based study on urban births Ghosh and Bhargava[63] recorded a prevalence of all types of congenital malformations as 26.2/1,000.[18] NNF neonatal perinatal data from different hospitals in the country reported it as 2.2%.[9] Musculoskeletal, central nervous system and genitourinary are the most frequent major malformations reported. Skin and its appendages are the most common minor malformations. In an interesting follow-up study of the cohorts from birth to five years of age the incidence of congenital malformation increased from 22.6/1,000 to 40.3/1,000 births.[63]

Newborn Care Services

In India, even in the 1990s, three quarters of births occur at home. Most newborns are therefore cared for by the family and/or birth attendants. Those born in institutions receive care by health professionals, some of whom may not have received training in newborn care.

Domiciliary care

The family, grandmother, or sometimes another elderly lady in the house will determine the care for the mother and her newborn. They decide on the place where they are to be nursed, the method of warming the room or otherwise, the type of food for the mother, and the time and type of the first feed for the newborn. Similarly, bathing, massage, type of clothes, and application of *kajal* to the eyes for the newborn will be decided. These practices are almost universally practiced in one form or another in different parts of the country.[3] An NNF survey showed that most newborn resuscitation measures were unsatisfactory and immediate bath after birth was customary in all urban births. *Kajal* application to eyes occurred in over 80% and massage in 67–96% of infants. Rural and urban newborns were fed within the first six hours in 75% of mothers studied, and first feeding was done in six to 12 hours in 55% of tribal births. The nature of the first feed varied, but breast milk was offered as the first feed by less than 10–12% of mothers![3,10]

The health professionals who provide advice to families must be aware of these practices and the sensitivity of families to them. For example, most families give a bath and massage, apply *kajal*, and offer honey as a first feed to the newborn. Under the circumstances the most readily acceptable advice might be not to give any honey, apply *kajal* after the ceremony, delay the bath, and massage in a warm ambient temperature. To condemn or berate these practices totally may antagonise the family.

Newborn care at primary level

Until recently, government primary care services in rural areas have had no special provision or facility for newborns such as warming, oro-pharyngeal suction, weighing, or temperature measurement. There was no training for primary care workers for the care of a normal or sick newborn. In 1993, the Government of India, under the technical advice of the National Neonatology

Forum, developed a package for "Essential Newborn Care" as part of the national programme of "Child Survival and Safe Motherhood". This defined the components of care at birth, in the immediate neonatal period, the provision of training to health professionals, and the establishment of neonatal units at primary health centres and at first referral units such as community health centres and district hospitals. In a pilot project the National Neonatology Forum established newborn care units in 24 districts of the country and monitored newborn care and the utilization of training and equipment provided.[13] The results of the project were widely acclaimed and essential newborn care is now being extended to all districts of the country based on this model.

Newborn care at institutional level

The past decade has seen rapid development in the care of the newborn at institutional level. The concept that newborn infants requires primary care and that at-risk or sick newborn infants need special care has been accepted. This has resulted in neonatal special care units being set up in both govenment and private hospitals across the country. The National Neonatology Forum and Government of India, Ministry of Health, and the Family Welfare task force on Minimum Perinatal Care suggested a tiered system of care.[64] It defined the care as:

- primary or level 1,
- secondary or level 2, and
- tertiary or level 3

based on an infant's birth weight, gestational age, condition at birth, sickness, etc. It further elaborated on equipment and personnel norms for the different levels of care.[64,65]

The impact of sustained advocacy for the needs of the newborn in past decade, the provision of essential newborn care, and creation of special baby care unit or level 1 nurseries is already resulting in improved quality newborn care and better survival. Table 12 compares the trends of survival status in tertiary institutions and shows a significant change in survival for all birth weight groups.[45-47]

It is difficult to quantify the number of personnel who have been trained in newborn care or the number of institutions which provide neonatal care. NNF has a system of accreditation of newborn units and a recent report suggest there are 29 accredited level 2 units.[67] This is likely to be a gross underestimate because many units do not apply for accreditation.

Referral services have not yet developed even though at district level a linkage is supposed to exist between the district hospital and primary care services (see Chapter 25). The feasibility of a referral system between an apex hospital and rural primary centre was adequately demonstrated by Bhargava *et al.* in 1983.[66]

What of the future in newborn care in India?

Recent developments such as the recognition of pediatrics as a separate subject for undergraduate teaching, television and audio net working at district level, and increasing utilization of the information highway, offer an opportunity to expand provision of perinatal and neonatal care at different levels. India has a unique opportunity to explode the myths regarding neonatal care in the community, to allow participation and monitoring of newborn care by the community, and to develop appropriate curricula for training and education for health professionals, and to promote good newborn care in the home. What is needed is strong advocacy and commitment from those whose concern is the care of the newborn.[68]

References

1. Health Information of India (1994).
2. *The State of the World's Children.* Unicef, Oxford University Press (1997).
3. National Neonatology Forum, Proceedings of a national workshop on traditional practices of neonatal care in India (1991).
4. Bhargava SK, "Neonatal care: A newborns' right and not a luxury," *Indian Pediatrics* **18** (1981): p. 687.
5. National Health Policy, Government of India, Ministry of Health and Family Welfare (1985).
6. National Child Survival and Safe Motherhood programme, Government of India, Ministry of Health and Family Welfare (1992).

7. National Child Survival and Safe Motherhood Programme. Integrated clinical skills course for Physicians, MCH division, Ministry of Health and Family Welfare (1993).

8. Sample Registration System, Registrar General of India (1991).

9. National Neonatology Forum: Neonatal-Perinatal database (1995).

10. "A national collaborative study of identification of high risk families, mothers and outcome of their offsprings with particular reference to the problem of maternal nutrition, low birth weight, perinatal and infant morbidity and mortality in rural and urban slum communities," Indian Council of Medical Research (1990).

11. Ghosh S, Bhargava SK, Saxena HMK *et al.*, "A study of perinatal mortality with reference to maternal, fetal and neonatal factors from a clinical, biochemical, bacteriological and pathological point of view," Indian Council of Medical Research report (1977).

12. Ramji S, "Socio-economic and environmental determinants of perinatal and neonatal mortality in India," *Indian Pediatrics* **26** (1989): 100–105.

13. National Neonatology Forum and Government of India, Ministry of Health and Family Welfare, District Newborn Care Project (1996) *personal communication*.

14. "Survey of causes of death (rural)," Annual Report (1994) Registrar General, India.

15. "Evaluation of quality of family welfare services at primary health centre level," Indian Council of Medical Research report (1991).

16. Madhavan S and Taskar AD, "Birth weight of Indian babies born in hospitals," *Indian Journal of Pediatrics* **36** (1969): 193– 204.

17. Bhargava SK, Sachdev HPS, Ramji S *et al.*, "Low birth weight: Aetiology and prevention in India," *Annals of Tropical Paediatrics* **3** (1983): 115–119.

18. Ghosh S, Bhargava SK and Moriyarna IM, "Longitudinal study of the survival and outcome of a birth cohort. Phase 1," NCHS, USA (1979).

19. Bhargava SK, Sachdev HPS, Iyer PU and Ramji S, "Current status of infant growth measurement in the perinatal period in India," *Acta Paediatr. Scand. Suppl.* **319** (1985): 103–110.

20. Antosainy B, Rao PSS and Sivaram M, "Changing scenario of birth weight in South India," *Indian Pediatrics* **34** (1994): 931–937.

21. Bhargava S, Ghosh S and Lall UB, "A study of low birth weight infants in an urban community," *Health and Population Perspective and Issues* **2** (1979): 5–10.

22. Bhargava SK, Sachdeva HPS and Ghosh S, "Distribution of live births and early neonatal mortality in relation to gestation and intrauterine growth," *Indian Journal of Medical Research* **82** (1985): 95–99.

23. Bhargava SK, Iyer PU, Nafde S, Datta V, Ramji S and Sachdev HPS, "Perspective in low birth weight survival and outcome," In: *Proceedings of National Neonatology Forum* (1985): 44–52.

24. Babson SG, Behrman E and Lessel R, "Liveborn birthweight for gestational age of white middle class infants," *Pediatr.* **45** (1970): 937–942.

25. Bjerkedahl T, Bakketeig L and Lehmann E, "Percentiles of birth weights of single live births at different gestation periods," *Acta Pediatr. Scand.* **62** (1973): 1449–1454.

26. Sheth P and Merchant SM, "Fetal growth in two socioeconomic groups," *Indian Pediatrics* **9** (1972): 650–657.

27. Ghosh S, Bhargava SK, Madhava S, Taskar AD, Bhargava V and Nigain SK, "Intrauterine growth of north Indian babies," *Indian Pediatrics* **47** (1971): p. 826.

28. Bhargava SK and Ghosh S, "Nomenclature of the newborn," *Indian Pediatrics* **11** (1974): p. 443.

29. Singh MB, Gili SK and Ramachandran K, "Intrauterine growth curves of liveborn single babies," *Indian Pediatrics* **1**(1) (1974): 475–479.

30. Bhargava SK, Ramji S, Kumar A, Manmohan, Marwah J and Sachdev HPS, "Mid arm chest circumference measurements at birth as predictors of low birth weight and neonatal mortality in the community," *British Medical Journal* **291** (1985): 1617–1619.

31. Ramji S, Marwah J, Satyanaryana I, Kapani V, Man M and Bhargava SK, "Neonatal thigh circumference: An alternative indicator of low birth weight," *Indian Journal of Medical Research* **83** (1986): 652–653.

32. Kumar A., Manmohan, Ramji S *et al.*, "The bangle as a screening technique for identification of low birth weight neonates," *Indian Journal of Medical Research* **86** (1987): 621–623.

33. Bhargava SK and Dadhich JP, "Maternal nutrition and fetal outcome," In: *Nutrition in Children*, eds Sachdev HPS and Choudhary P, New Delhi (1994): 34–35.

34. Rarnachandran P, "Nutrition in pregnancy," In: *Women and Nutrition in India*, eds Gopalan C and Kaur S, New Delhi, Nutrition Foundation of India (1989): 153–193.

35. Bhargava M, Kumar R, Iyer PU, Kapani V, Bhargava SK, "Effect of maternal anemia and iron depletion on fetal iron stores, birth weight and gestation," *Acta Pediatr. Scand.* **78** (1989): 321–322.

36. Khan E, Infant mortality in Uttar Pradesh — A micro level study," In: *Infant Mortality in India. Differential and Determinants*, eds Jain AK and Visaria P, New Delhi, Sage Publications (1988): 227–246.

37. Pachuri S, Shah SM and Rao NSN, "A multifactorial approach of the study of factors influencing birth weight in an urban community of New Delhi," *Indian Journal of Medical Research* **59** (1971): 1318–1383.

38. Rainan L, "Fetal effects of maternal disorders," *Indian Journal of Pediatrics* **47** (1980): 9–17.

39. Srikantia SG and Iyengar L, "Effects of nutrient supplements in pregnancy on birthweight of the newborn," *Proc. Nat. Soc. India* **11** (1972): 27–37.

40. Kewal K, "Tobacco chewing in pregnancy," *British Journal of Obstetrics and Gynaecology* **85** (1978): 726–728.

41. Verrna RC, Chansoriya M and Kaul KK, "A study of the effect of tobacco chewing on fetal outcome," *Indian Pediatrics* **20** (1983): 105–111.

42. Sharina U, Indrani N and Saxena S, "Effects of maternal medical diseases on the newborn," *Indian Journal of Pediatrics* **45** (1978): 154–167.

43. Sudershan K *et al. Personal communication* (1996).

44. Mittal SK, Singh PA and Gupta RC, "Intrauterine growth and low birth weight criteria in Punjabi infants," *Indian Pediatrics* **13** (1976): 678–682.

45. Bhargava SK, "Trends in neonatal survival at a private regional neonatal referral unit," *Indian Pediatrics* (in press).

46. Singh M, "Hospital based data on perinatal and neonatal mortality in India," *Indian Pediatrics* **23** (1986): 579–584.

47. Bhakoo ON, Kajuria R, Desai A and Narang A, "Lessons from improved neonatal survival at Chandigarh," *Indian Pediatrics* **26** (1989): 234–241.

48. Bhargava SK, Sudershan K and Choudhary P, "Outcome of low birth weight infant," *Acta Pediatr. Scand.* **73** (1984): 403–407.

49. Bhargava SK, Kumari S, Pandit, Prabhhakar AK, Lama IMS, Ghosh S and Nanda S, "Outcome of low birth weight children: A longitudinal study of growth and development from birth to six years," *Annals IAMS* **11** (1975): p. 77.

50. Bhargava SK, Banedee SK, Chaudhary P and Kumari S, "A longitudinal study of morbidity and mortality pattern from birth to six years of age in infants of varying birth weight," *Indian Pediatrics* **16** (1979): 967–971.

51. Bhargava SK, Kumari S and Datta I, "Outcome of low birth weight children. A longitudinal study of survival, sequelae, growth and intellectual performance from 0–10 years," Indian Council of Medical Research. Final Report (1982).

52. Kumari S, Sharrna M, Yadav M *et al.*, "Trends in neonatal outcome with low Apgar score," *Indian Journal of Pediatrics* **60** (1993): 415–422.

53. Mishra PK, Kapoor RK, Sharma B *et al.*, "Perinatal asphyxia: Clinico-epidemiological factors — An analysis," in: *Abstracts of 8th Asian Congress of Pediatrics*, eds Chaudhary P, Sachdev HPS, Puri RK *et al.*, Jaypee Brothers, Medical Publishers (P) Ltd. (1994).

54. Kumari S, Bhargava SK, Sibal A *et al.*, "Neonatal sepsis with special reference to maternal factors," in: *Abstracts of 8th Asian Congress of Pediatrics*, eds Chaudhary P, Sachdev HPS, Puri RK *et al.*, Jaypee Brothers, Medical Publishers (P) Ltd. (1994): p. 26.

55. Malakar B, "The spectrum of infections in Level II nurseries with special reference to nosocomial infections," in: *Abstracts of 8th Asian Congress of Pediatrics*, Jaypee Brothers, Medical Publishers (P) Ltd. (1994): p. 23.

56. Parmanantham P, Andadan S and Raju BB, "Environmental factors and bacterial isolates in the hospitalised," In: *Abstracts of 8th Asian Congress of Pediatrics*, Jaypee Brothers Medical Publishers (P) Ltd. (1994): p. 23.

57. Bhargava SK, "Epidemiology of feto-maternal bacterial infections in India," in: *Abstracts Books*; *XIX International Congress of Pediatrics* (1989): p. 38.

58. Bhargava SK, Dinesh J, Suri N and Sood SK, "Neonatal hyperbilirubinemia and G-6PD deficiency in North India," *Current Topics in Pediatrics*, Interprint, New Delhi (1977): p. 335.

59. Ahmed SH, Sethi AS, Buch NA *et al.*, "Neonatal hyperbilirubineniia," in: *Abstracts of 8th Asian Congress of Pediatrics*, Jaypee Brothers, Medical Publishers (P) Ltd. (1994): p. 31.

60. Chaturvedi P, Panwar A and Banerjee K, "Neonatal hyperbilirubinemia," in: *Abstracts of 8th Asian Congress of Pediatrics*, Jaypee Brothers, Medical Publishers (P) Ltd. (1994): p. 16.

61. Bhargava SK, Kumari S, Ghosh S and Sanyal SK, "Primary cold injury in the newborn," *Indian Pediatrics* **8** (1971): p. 762.

62. Bhargava SK, Mittal SK, Kumari S and Ghosh S, "Heat injury in the newborn," *Indian Medical Association* **69** (1977): p. 1.

63. Ghosh S, Bhargava SK and Bhutani R, "Congenital malformations in a longitudinally studied birth cohort in an urban community," *Indian Journal of Medical Research* **82** (1985): p. 427.

64. Government of India, Report of the task force on minimum perinatal care (1982).

65. National Child Survival and Safe Motherhood Programme.

66. Bhargava SK, Rahrnan F and Aryal HV, "Triage system of neonatal care: Experience at Safdarjung Hospital, New Delhi. Recommendations of education and training in neonatology," Published by the National Neonatology Forum, New Delhi (1982).

67. "NNF — Accredited neonatal units," In: *Bulletin National Neonatology Forum*, eds Deorari AK **10** (1996): p. 1.

68. Bhargava SK, "NNF Award Oration," *XVI Annual Convention of the National Neonatology Forum*, Chandigarh, Nov. 1997.

2.3 NEPAL

Dharma Manandhar

Background and Demography

Nepal lies between two large countries, China to the north and India to the south. The country is physically divided into the terai plains in the south, valleys and hills in the central region, and the great Himalayan mountains in the north. Poverty is widespread with nearly 60% of the population under the poverty line. The GNP per capita was estimated to be only US$200 per annum in 1995. The population numbered 18.5 million in the 1991 census with a population growth rate of above 2.0%.[1] Nearly 45% of the population is under 16 years of age. Road communications are poorly developed. The overall literacy rate is still low at 26%, with female literacy at only 13%.

The crude birth rate has been estimated to be 39.6/1,000, so over 800,000 infants are born every year. The fertility rate has been estimated to be 5.6. Important demographic, health and socio-economic indicators are shown in Table 1.

Perinatal Health Indicators

Maternal mortality

Nepal has one of the highest maternal mortality rates in the world. A study of maternal deaths in different hospitals within Nepal carried out in 1989–90 revealed a maternal mortality rate (MMR) ranging from 72 per 100,000 live births in the maternity hospital in Kathmandu to 1,810 per 100,000 in Bheri zonal hospital, Nepalgunj. The mean MMR in the hospitals studied was 291/100,000 live births.[2] MMR recorded at the maternity hospital in

Kathmandu between 1994 and 1995 was 95 per 100,000.[3] A sample survey of maternal deaths in the remote Jumla district of Nepal recorded an MMR of 2,000 per 100,000 live births.[4] The very high maternal death in the far west is explained by the fact that the provision of health services, particularly obstetric care, in that region is very limited.

Infant deaths

The infant mortality rate (IMR) of Nepal has fallen from 102/1,000 live births in 1991[5] to 92 per 1,000 live births in 1995.[6,7] Again there is a great geographical variation in IMR; the highest rate at 201 was reported from Mugu district in the far west compared with 34 from Kathmandu district. On the whole, districts in the west and far west of the country have an IMR above 100 while districts in the central and eastern regions have rates less than 100. The results of correlation coefficients generally show an inverse association between socio-economic development and infant mortality in the districts. Female literacy is the most important factor in accounting for variations in infant mortality; other factors of importance are availability and use of health services.

Perinatal mortality

An official national perinatal mortality rate (PMR) is not available although the 1996 Nepal Family Health Survey of 8,429 women reported a PMR of 63 per 1,000 stillbirths and livebirths in the period 10–14 years before the survey, compared with 52 in the period 0–4 years before the survey — a decline of 17%. PMR rates were higher in rural than urban areas, and especially in mothers whose inter-pregnancy interval was short (see Chapter 6).[16]

A multi-centre study of perinatal mortality in Nepal in 1989–1990 found PMR levels of 48.0 and 23.7 per 1,000 births respectively at the maternity hospital and Patan hospital (a mission-funded general hospital in Kathmandu), and a PMR of 96.2 and 42.5 in the rural settings of Jumla and Patan respectively.[6,8,10] Women who attend Patan hospital are generally from a

Table 13 Perinatal mortality by weight at Patan Hospital in Kathmandu, in the year 1994–95.[8]

Weight (kg)	No. of birth	Stillbirths	Neonatal deaths	PNMR
< 1	1	1	0	1,000
1–1.2	22	5	5	454.5
> 1.2–1.5	37	9	8	459.5
> 1.5–2	109	7	13	183.5
> 2–2.5	627	12	15	43.1
> 2.5	3,507	25	11	10.3
Total	4,303	59	52	25.8

better socio-economic class. 93% of women who delivered in this hospital had antenatal check-ups compared with less than 50% of women who delivered at the maternity hospital in Kathmandu. As expected, PMR was highest in the very low birth weight group and least in the group whose birth weight was over 2.5 kg. Table 13 gives the PMR according to different birth weight groups in Patan hospital.[10]

Perinatal mortality at the Tribhuvan University Teaching Hospital (TUTH) in 1995–96 was found to be 29.8/1,000 births.[11] Very low birth weight, severe birth asphyxia, respiratory distress, septicaemia, intraventricular haemorrhage, and severe congenital anomalies and maternal conditions like antepartum haemorrhage and pre-eclampsia were the main causes of perinatal deaths. A PMR of 139/1,000 was reported from Bheri zonal hospital, Nepalgunj, in the far west of Nepal, but this very high rate may reflect the proportion of complicated cases which arrive from remote areas.[12]

Neonatal morbidity

There is little published data on neonatal morbidity in Nepal. An analysis of 1,063 consecutive admissions to the Special Care Baby Unit (SCBU)

Table 14 Causes of admission of 1,063 newborns to the Special Care Baby Unit of the maternity hospital in Kathmandu (April–September 1996).

Cause	Number (%)
Low birth weight	372 (35)
Birth asphyxia	309 (29)
Respiratory distress	86 (8)
Neonatal jaundice	60 (6)
Fever	38 (4)
Congenital anomalies	27 (3)
Meconium aspiration	25 (2)
Poor sucking	19 (2)
Diarrhoea/vomiting	17 (2)
Miscellaneous	110 (10)
Total	1,063 (100)

of the maternity hospital in Kathmandu in 1996 revealed that low and very low birth weight, birth asphyxia, neonatal jaundice, feeding problems, congenital anomalies, and hypothermia were the main causes for admission (see Table 14).

After admission for some other reason, 58 infants developed significant jaundice (i.e. total serum bilirubin > 15 mg/dl), 29 infants were diagnosed to have septicaemia including one with meningitis, two infants had congenital heart disease, two others had oesophageal atresia, and one partial intestinal obstruction. However, neonatal tetanus, which is a significant problem causing neonatal morbidity and mortality in the southern terai region, is virtually never seen in Kathmandu.

Table 15 gives data on 1,063 newborns admitted over a six-month period in 1996 to the SCBU of the maternity hospital in Kathmandu. 50% were LBW infants (birth weight of < 2,500 g) and 6% below 1,500 g. Most low birth weight infants were therefore in the weight group of 1,500 to 2,500 g. Most were also term infants, with less than 10% below 32 weeks of gestation.

Table 15 Distribution by weight and gestational age of 1,063 newborns, and causes of 141 early neonatal deaths admitted to the SCBU at the maternity hospital in Kathmandu (April–September 1997).

Weight (g)	*Number* (%)
< 1,000	12 (1)
1,000–1,499	53 (5)
1,500–1,999	222 (21)
2,000–2499	244 (23)
2,500 and above	532 (50)
Total	**1,063 (100)**
Gestational age (*weeks*)	
< 28	12 (1)
28–32	88 (8)
33–36	241 (23)
37–41	633 (60)
> 41	89 (8)
Total	**1,063 (100)**
Cause of death	
Severe birth asphyxia	44 (31)
RDS[a]	40 (28)
Septicaemia	18 (13)
Extreme prematurity	14 (10)
Haemorrhages[b]	9 (6)
Congenital anomalies	7 (5)
Aspiration	3 (2)
Hypothermia	2 (1)
Miscellaneous[c]	4 (3)
Total	**141 (100)**

[a]RDS — respiratory distress syndrome. Includes respiratory distress due to severe meconium aspiration.
[b]includes three each of intracranial, pulmonary and g.i. haemorrhage.
[c]includes one each of Hydrops fetalis, severe diarrhoea, congestive cardiac failure, and cot death.

Most infants (52%) were term and appropriate for gestational age in size, 30% were term and small-for-dates, 16% were preterm, 2% were preterm as well as small-for-dates, and 0.3% were large-for-dates.

Low birth weight newborns (LBW)

There is a high prevalence of low birth weight infants in Nepal. Hospital based studies tend to underestimate the size of the problem because they select from a relatively privileged population. For example, in 1988–89 a study at the maternity hospital in Kathmandu reported that 21% of infants were LBW;[13] in 1989, at the University Teaching Hospital,[14] 21% were also LBW; and Patan hospital reported a significant decline in LBW infants from 29% in 1993–94 to 18% in 1994–95.[10] However, a large and systematic study of term newborns in 1993 at the maternity hospital in Kathmandu showed that 32% of them were LBW infants.[15] The inclusion of preterm infants would have increased this figure by at least 5–8%. This gives one of the highest prevalence rates of LBW infants in the world. The high incidence of LBW infants in the latter study conducted at the maternity hospital could reflect the influx of poor migrant workers who came to Kathmandu for work, and who chose to deliver at the maternity hospital because user charges are low. The earlier study of the maternity hospital was on mothers who were the residents of two better-off urban localities close to the hospital.

Neonatal deaths

Deaths within four weeks of birth (neonatal deaths) account for over 60% of infant mortality. The latest report from the Ministry of Health gives a neonatal mortality rate (NMR) of 50 per 1,000, which constitutes 64% of IMR.[16] Table 15 gives the causes of early neonatal deaths seen at the maternity hospital in Kathmandu. Over 75% of early neonatal deaths occurred in LBW infants; among those weighing above 2,500 g at birth, severe birth asphyxia was the commonest cause of death. Neonatal tetanus is an important cause of death particularly in the terai region, but this condition is rarely observed in hospital deliveries in Kathmandu.

Newborn Care Services

Most infants are born at home so the mother is the prime care provider during the newborn period. Other family members, particularly her own mother and sisters and mother-in-law, provide great help. With increasing urbanisation, a significant proportion of infants in urban areas are now born in hospital. In the Kathmandu valley, it has been estimated that nearly 65% of births occur in the hospitals.[17]

That special care services should be provided to sick newborns has been appreciated only recently. Healthy newborns are generally looked after by the delivering obstetricians or midwives, and they manage minor problems as well. It is only when a newborn infant becomes sick that paediatricians are requested to manage the infants. Even among paediatricians, only a few have experience and proper training in the management of sick newborns.

Facilities for the care of sick newborns are very limited in Nepal. There are only about 60 cots available in the country for the special care of sick newborns, and almost all of these are in Kathmandu. Most sick newborns that reach secondary care are managed in general paediatric wards of regional, zonal and district hospitals. There is virtually no functioning referral system. There is still a very high risk for hospitalised infants not only because they are brought in late but also because of the lack of facilities for the in-patient care and a lack of experience among physicians, nurses and other health personnel. With an increasing trend towards smaller families, particularly among the middle class, and an increased awareness of better health care among the population, a parent's expectation for newborn infant survival has increased. Until recently there was no countrywide programme for the care of newborns. The government's decision in 1993 to undertake a Safe Motherhood Programme (SMP) in ten districts of the country has given a boost to neonatal care, as the SMP package includes the care of newborns. District hospitals will be upgraded not only to provide emergency obstetric services for mothers but also "Essential Neonatal Care" for the newborns.

References

1. *Statistical Year Book of Nepal 1993*. HMG, National Planning Commission Secretariat, Central Bureau of Statistics.

2. Malla DS, "Study report on prevention of maternal mortality," (in selected hospitals of Nepal) (1991).
3. Malla K and Padhye S, "Maternal mortality at the maternity hospital, Kathmandu," paper presented at the Ninth Workshop of the Federation of Asia and Oceania Perinatal Societies at Lahore (1995).
4. World Health Organization (WHO), "Maternal mortality rate — A tabulation of available information," Geneva (1986).
5. HMG Ministry of Health. Health Information Bulletin (1992).
6. Thapa S, "Infant mortality and its correlates and determinants in Nepal: A district-level analysis," *Journal of the Nepal Medical Association* **34**(118) and (119) (1996): 94–109.
7. *UNICEF The State of the World's Children*, Oxford University Press (1995).
8. Geetha T, Chenoy R, Stevens D and Johanson RB, "A multicentre study of perinatal mortality in Nepal," *Paediatric and Perinatal Epidemiology* **9** (1995): 74–89.
9. Manandhar DS *et al.*, "A study of perinatal mortality at the Maternity Hospital, Kathmandu," in: *Proceedings of International Workshop on Women and Health*, Kathmandu (1991).
10. Adhikari N and Sharma P, "Care of the newborn at Patan hospital," paper presented at XVI Annual Convention of National Neonatology Forum, Chandigarh, India (1996).
11. Shrestha PS. *Personal communication.*
12. Pradhan DP and Shah U, "Perinatal mortality in Bheri Zonal Hospital," *Journal of the Nepal Medical Association* **35**: 146–149.
13. Malla DS. The final report on the study of low birth weight and infant morbidity and mortality, Maternity hospital, Kathmandu (1992).
14. Dali SM, Shrestha PN, Rijal B, Shrestha P and Koirala S, "Low birth weight — A study of 1,000 live birth at Tribhuvan University Teaching Hospital," Institute of Medicine, Kathmandu (1989).
15. Manandhar DS, Rajbhandari S, Pal D and Costello AM de L, "Anthropometry of term newborn and postnatal mother in Nepal," *Journal of the Nepal Medical Association* **35** (1997): 150–157.
16. Nepal Family Health Survey. Preliminary report; Family Health Division, Ministry of Health, His Majesty's Government Nepal., (eds) Pradhan A *et al.*, New Era, Kathmandu, Macro International Inc. Maryland, March 1997.
17. Manandhar DS, Bolam A., Shrestha P, Manandhar B, Malla K, Shrestha LN, Ellis M and Costello AM de L, "Maternity care utilisation in the Kathmandu valley: A community based study," *Journal of the Nepal Medical Association* **35** (1997): 122–129.

2.4 PAKISTAN

Shakila Zaman

Background and Demography

Pakistan has a diverse geographical profile, ranging from mountainous areas to plains and the sea coast. The estimated population for 1996, based on the Census of 1981 with the prevalent growth rate, is 134 million. In the absence of the 1991 Census, the estimates of the population vary between 133–140 million with varying growth rates of 2.8% to 3.4%.[1] Pakistan is likely to double its population within 25 years if it keeps on growing at the same rate. The rural population is 68% of the total, but the size of the urban population is increasing rapidly and will reach over 50% by the year 2020 if the annual growth rate remains 3.9 to 4.2%.[1,2]

Important demographic and mortality data for Pakistan has been shown in Table 1. Life expectancy is now 61 years, the total fertility rate is estimated to be between 5.2 and 6.2, and the crude birth rate remains high at 39 per 1,000 (estimated for 1990–95). Fertility rates have not shown a considerable change since 1974–75. An estimated female population of 46.7% in 1990 will increase to 49.4 in 2010.[2] Population growth remains the highest in the region at 3.1%. Female literacy is still low, with only 35% of women above 15 years able to read or write. 31% of the population are below the poverty line and the GNP per capita is US$420.

Perinatal Health Indicators

Mortality

The infant mortality rate has decreased from 106 per 1,000 live births in 1984–85 to 91 per 1,000 live births in 1995 (Table 1). The Pakistan

Table 16 Neonatal, infant and child mortality rates in Pakistan expressed per 1,000 livebirths for three six-year periods prior to the survey, by area and maternal education.

Years preceding survey	Neonatal	Postnatal	Infant	Child*	Under-five
0–5	51	39	91	30	117
6–11	57	40	97	30	124
12–17	63	44	107	41	144
	Mortality rates for the ten-year period preceding the survey				
By area of residence					
Total urban:	41	34	75	21	94
Major city	40	34	74	20	92
Other urban	42	34	76	22	96
Rural	59	44	102	33	132
By maternal education					
No education	56	43	99	33	128
Primary	50	41	90	18	107
Middle	44	37	80	8	87
Secondary	27	19	46	4	50

*Child mortality = deaths between 1–5 years of age.

Demographic and Health survey was conducted in 1990–91[6] based on a 2% household sample. Infant mortality was studied in three six-year time periods prior to the survey. The trends in mortality are sufficiently acceptable given the sampling and non-sampling errors caused by under-reporting early deaths or misreporting the age at death. Keeping in mind these problems and the constraints of socio-cultural influences, the trends in infant and child mortality are shown in Table 16.

Table 17 Neonatal and under-five mortality rates per thousand livebirths showing the relationship with the maternal care received during the antenatal and delivery period.

Medical maternity care	Neonatal	Postnatal	Infant	Child	Under-five
No antenatal care or natal care	57	47	104	32	133
Either antenatal or delivery care	33	32	65	41	103
Both antenatal and delivery care	47	23	70	11	79

Table 16 shows that the period immediately prior to the survey had a much lower under-five mortality, declining by 18% compared to the 12–17 years period. There is a slower rate of decline in more recent periods. Mortality rates are higher in the rural setting and where mothers were illiterate compared to those who were literate, especially above the secondary level of education.

The use of basic health care services available for the mothers during antenatal or natal period can affect the outcome of delivery, or even later (Table 17). Neonatal mortality rises in the group receiving both antenatal and delivery care, which may indicate that the mothers who receive antenatal care do not also seek delivery care unless there is a problem related to the pregnancy. The post-neonatal and child mortality is lower in this group compared to the other two groups. This may reflect on the availability and quality of delivery care available in the country.[7]

Table 18 shows that males are more likely than females to die during the neonatal period, although later deaths become more equal. This may indicate a male-preference bias in the social and cultural outlook of the communities. Maternal age at the time of birth indicates a U-shaped relationship between deaths at all ages shown. The pace of childbearing affects the infant mortality in a way that we can easily understand. The death rates increase if the interbirth interval is less than two years as compared to four years or more (see Chapter 6). Birth size was measured by the mothers' perception of the baby at birth: this shows deaths as higher among the very small infants at birth.

Infant mortality has been studied in various country based surveys and in community based studies.[8–10] There is indication of a high infant mortality,

Table 18 Neonatal and under-five mortality rates for the ten-year period preceding the survey, by selected demographic characteristics.

Biological or demographic characteristics	Neonatal	Postnatal	Infant	Child	Under-five
By sex of the child					
Males	60	42	102	22	122
Females	46	39	86	37	119
By mother's age at birth					
< 20	70	51	121	27	145
20–29	51	40	91	29	117
30–39	49	35	84	32	125
40–49	56	50	107	27	136
Previous birth interval					
< 2 years	74	19	133	43	170
2–3 years	39	26	65	26	89
4 years or more	14	16	30	15	44
*Birth size**					
Very small	91	41	131	31	158
Small	42	58	100	23	121
Average or larger	40	32	72	28	97

*Rates are for the five-year period before the survey. Birth size indicates the perception of mothers.

from 88 to114/1,000 livebirths. Early neonatal mortality constitutes more than 50% of infant deaths; 86–96% of infant deaths occur before nine months of age.

Causes of neonatal and infant deaths

The major reported causes of death vary depending on the source of information, i.e. either doctor or other health professionals, hospital records or from the impressions of the mothers. In the Demographic and Health survey,[6] the cause of deaths reported for the neonatal period show a disparity between the mothers impressions and the doctors' determination of the cause of death. Although, fever is reported as a cause of nearly 16% of newborn deaths, the underlying cause may be septicaemia or other infections, while deaths reported due to convulsions may well have been due to tetanus neonatorum.

Causes of death among infants were assessed by the Government of Pakistan through a population growth survey in 1971,[11] which described the major cause of death as infective and parasitic diseases (60%) followed by congenital anomalies and birth anoxia (20%). In a longitudinal study[9] in Lahore of households from urban, periurban and rural areas, 1,476 newborns were followed for 24 months by monthly home visits. Information on mortality and morbidity was collected during these visits. The cause of death identified in the early neonatal period (less than seven days) was asphyxia neonatorum (23/47), septicaemia (8/47), respiratory infections (4/47), tetanus neonatorum (4/47), and other causes. From seven to 28 days, diarrhoea was also an important cause of death. Both acute and chronic diarrhoeal illness was then responsible for most deaths (56/159) after this age and up to 24 months of age. An important observation was that although the number of deaths in the upper middle class group was only four out of 159, these deaths were due to asphyxia neonatorum.[9] This indicated that despite the best of available health facilities at private level, newborns are still prone to this risk.

Another study done at the Aga Khan University[10] in Karachi showed that for those dying by 28 days of life the main causes were low birth weight and prematurity (26%) while 14% died of asphyxia or birth trauma followed by pneumonia or diarrhoea (14%) and unknown causes (29%).

Lady Wallingdon Hospital in Lahore is one of the largest maternity hospitals in Pakistan with nearly 13,000 deliveries each year. The hospital has a neonatal nursery which is attached to the Paediatrics department at King Edward Medical College in Lahore. Two to three trained paediatricians who are trained in neonatology are on 24-hours duty supervised by a senior paediatrician. The report from 1994 indicates an admission of 941 newborns to the unit with 577 (61%) full-term newborns, 344 (36%) as preterms and 20 (2.4%) post-term newborns. Of those admitted, 65% were discharged while 282/941 (30%) died and the rest were referred to the larger unit. The two major reasons for their admission were asphyxia neonatorum and prematurity. The number of deaths contributed by asphyxia neonatorum was 95/282 (34%) and by prematurity was 154/282 (55%). From the 13 infants who had sepsis eight died (62%), indicating a high fatality (*personal communications*). The low birth weight rate was reported as 21% in this population.

Breastfeeding practices

Breastfeeding is a common practice in Pakistan. Over 94% of infants have been found to be breastfed. However, initiation of breastfeeding is often delayed to three days with use of prelacteals as a common practice.[5–7,12] The Pakistan Demographic and Health Survey[6] reported 98% infants as ever being breastfed, but only 9% was initiated within the first hour, and 26% were only put to the breast on the first day. Prelacteals were introduced early and a variety of foods and fluids were given depending on the social customs and economic situation. Exclusive breastfeeding was rare, with only 25% of infants fed in this way for at least four months. The median duration of breastfeeding was 22 months to 28 months.[6,12,13]

However, practices can change with the right promotion and policy. Since 1994, breastfeeding steering committees in all four Provinces of Pakistan have introduced and implemented breastfeeding policies for health facilities. In a follow-up cohort study in Lahore[14] where breastfeeding promotion and support was actively introduced in communities, and was later taken up as a universal programme for promoting optimal breastfeeding practices, 94% of the mothers were found to have initiated breastfeeding within six hours after the birth of the child without any prelacteals and bottle feeding. These mothers exclusively breastfed and 84% were still doing so at four months of age. The duration of breastfeeding also increased from 18 to 22 months in the village and from 14 to 18 months in urban populations.[14] There are more than ten hospitals in Pakistan which have been declared as Baby-Friendly hospitals, i.e. where optimal breastfeeding practices are actively carried out.

Nutritional status of newborn infants

Birth weight less than 2,500 g has been reported through hospital based data and a national LBW figure of 25% is quoted. However, in the Lahore study — where 964 newborns were examined within 72 hours after birth and their body measurements were taken — low birth weight babies, i.e. all those lying below −2SDS, ranged from 12.4% (wealthier area) to 31.5% (poorer area).[8]

Maternal Care Indicators

Antenatal care

In national surveys done in 1990 and 1992, showed that nearly 83% of pregnant mothers in villages did not receive antenatal care compared to 40% in urban mothers.[6,7] 85% of the mothers delivered at home while 13.4% delivered at a health facility. The trend in the rural areas was to deliver at home (94%) compared with urban mothers (85%). Among rural mothers, attendants at birth were usually (88%) either a trained birth attendant or a traditional birth attendant or other family members. Only 8.2% were assisted at birth by a trained personnel. 56% of urban mothers sought assistance at birth from traditional or trained birth attendants while 42% went to a doctor or a Lady Health Visitor (see Table 19).

Table 19 Mothers receiving antenatal care, place of delivery, and birth attended by type of attendants, as reported by various studies.

	Received antenatal care (%)	Place of* delivery (%)	Birth attended by trained health personnel (%)
PCPS (1984–85)			
Pakistan	26	8	23
Major urban	49	34	30
Other urban	35	8	29
Rural	20	3	21
PDHS (1990–91)			
Major urban	70	46	70
Other urban	43	14	43
Rural	16	5	24

PCPS = Pakistan Contraceptive Prevalence Survey, 1984–85.
PDHS = Pakistan Demographic and Health Survey, 1990–1991.
*Health facility as the place of delivery.

Contraceptive knowledge and use

The Pakistan Contraceptive Prevalence survey (1984–1985)[17] interviewed currently married women regarding contraceptive knowledge and use. Knowledge about at least one contraceptive method was found for 61.5%, and 88% among the more educated women. Current use of contraceptives was low, although it increased from 2% rural and 8% urban women in 1979 to 5% rural and 18% urban women by 1984–85. This can be explained to some extent by the availability of Family Planning services and supplies in the country. Although many mothers want to space their births, non-availability of the services may still hinder this desire.

Utilisation of perinatal health care services

An evaluation study of the utilisation of basic health services was published by the Pakistan Medical Research Council in 1993, when a 2% household sample was taken by stratified probability sampling. 89 institutions were chosen from all over Pakistan; three were locked at the time of survey so a sample size of 86 institutions was investigated.[19] The absence rate of the medical officers was 36%; 70% of posts for male medical officers were filled, but only 48% of the female posts. 61% of the doctors did not know their job description. No trained gynaecologist or paediatrician were posted at this level of health care facility and no training in neonatology was provided to the doctors or lady health visitors. The bed occupancy rate was only 16%. No birth or death records were maintained at these centres. Facilities for immunisation and growth monitoring were provided by 40% and 9% of the primary care institutions. Antenatal care was provided at 7–62% of the health facilities and generlly the attendance rate was very low. High risk pregnancies were not recorded at most facilities. The deliveries were conducted mainly by the private *dais*, while a lady health visitor or a doctor conducted between four to six deliveries per health provider per month. The family planning services were minimal due to either lack of drugs or communication. Only 7% of the women were practicing family planning. Postnatal care was minimal (see Table 20).

Table 20 Antenatal and delivery care by type of facility in Pakistan.

	Rural health centres n (%)	Basic health units n (%)	MCH centres n (%)
Persons conducting deliveries			
Births reported	49	129	22
Private *dais*	35 (71)	86 (67)	12 (55)
Government *dais*	3 (6)	11 (9)	2 (9)
Lady health visitors	2 (4)	4 (3)	2 (9)
Lady doctor	7 (14)	7 (5)	2 (9)
Others	2 (4)	21 (16)	4 (18)
Facilities providing postnatal care			
Facility utilisation of postnatal care in past month	23	58	8
0–9 mothers	10	18	5
10–19	2	2	1
> 20	0	1	0

Source: Utilization of Rural Basic Health Services in Pakistan (1993).

Health Services

The Government of Pakistan has endeavoured to provide a comprehensive health care system through a network of Rural Health Centres (RHCs) and Basic Health Units (BHUs). Since 1982, a medical officer has been posted at each BHU while two male medical officers and a female medical officer were posted at the RHCs.[4]

The national network for health services, as reported in 1995, consisted of 823 hospitals, 4,205 dispensaries, 4,925 Basic Health Units (BHUs), 856 Maternity and Child Health Centres (MCHs), 498 Rural Health Centres (RHCs) and 260 Tuberculosis Centres. There were 85,552 beds available in hospitals, BHUs and RHCs. In 1994, there were 69,694 doctors, 2,753 dentists and 22,531 nurses registered with the Ministry of Health. The private sector also contributes to health care by providing over 11,000 practitioners.[5]

Conclusion

Birth rates and the population growth rate remain high in Pakistan. Five to six million illiterate, unskilled, malnourished and impoverished people will be added to the country every year.[20] Pakistan is already the seventh most populous country in the world and will rank number three by 2050.[21] The Ministry for Population and Welfare aim to bring down the growth rate from 2.9% to 2.6% and to increase services for family planning and safe motherhood.[22]

Neonatal and perinatal mortality in Pakistan is also high. The causes of perinatal and early neonatal mortality are dependent on the health of the mother. Neonatal mortality is related to the health of the mother before and during pregnancy, and the utilisation of antenatal care, care at the time of delivery and postnatal care to prevent subsequent complications and infections. The percentage of LBW infants reflects the nutritional status of mothers and short interpregnancy intervals.

Caring for the high risk mothers (5–15% of the total mothers) requires that appropriate measures be taken to provide good antenatal care, identifying highrisk mothers and providing them proper care. Prevention of complications during the antenatal period and during labour will reduce maternal, perinatal and early neonatal deaths. Timely referrals of highrisk pregnancies and sick newborns to appropriately equipped hospitals will prevent many unnecessary deaths of mothers and their newborn infants.

Providing safe delivery by trained birth attendants at homes in the rural areas should improve health. Female education is perhaps the most important determinant of ill-health and mortality.[20] Illiteracy is the hallmark of under-developing countries and poor perinatal health. Countries like Sri Lanka, Singapore, South Korea, Malaysia and Thailand have invested heavily in education and health care for national development. Investment in literacy and health, including reproductive health, also helped to produce the conditions for later sustained economic growth.[21]

Despite recent political instability, a realistic realisation of the problem of maternal and perinatal care could bring changes in the health care delivery system in order to meet the actual needs of mothers and newborn infants.

References

1. Population Census Organization. *Handbook of population Census Data*, Government of Pakistan.
2. Ministry of Population Welfare. Population projections of Pakistan, Provinces, FATA and Islamabad. National Institute of Population Studies, Islamabad (1994).
3. *A World Bank Book. Social Indicators of Development*. Johns Hopkins University Press, Baltimore and London (1994).
4. Finance Division, Economic Advisors Wing. *Economic Survey 1995–1996*. Government of Pakistan.
5. Planning Commission, Government of Pakistan. *Seventh five year Plan 1998–1993 and Perspective Plan 1988–2003*. Report of the Working Group on Health and Nutrition. July 1987.
6. National Institute of Population Studies. *Pakistan Demographic and Health Survey*, 1990–1991. IRD/Macro International Inc. Columbia, Maryland.
7. UNICEF and Government of Pakistan. "Situation analysis of children and women in Pakistan, 1992," (1992).
8. Jalil F, Lindblad BS, Hanson LÅ, Yaqoob M and Karlberg J. "Early child health in Lahore, Pakistan. IX. Perinatal events," *Acta Paediatrica* Suppl **390** (1993): 95–107.
9. Khan SR, Jalil F, Zaman S, Lindblad BS and Karlberg J, "Early child health in Lahore, Pakistan. X. Mortality," *Acta Paediatrica* Suppl **390** (1993): 109–117.
10. "Maternal and Infant Mortality. Policy and Interventions," Report of an International Workshop at The Aga Khan University. Feb. 7–9 (1994).
11. *Population Growth Survey, 1971*, Government of Pakistan.
12. Ashraf RN, Jalil F, Khan SR, Zaman S, Karlberg J, Lindblad BS and Hanson LÅ, "Early child health in Lahore, Pakistan. V. Feeding patterns," *Acta Paediatrica* Suppl **390** (1993): 47–61.
13. UNICEF, "The State of the World's Children 1996," Oxford University Press (1996).
14. Ashraf RN *et al.* "Impact of breastfeeding motivation programme in a village and urban slum," (in press).

15. Nutrition Cell of Planning and Development Division, Government of Pakistan, *Micronutrient Survey of Pakistan, 1976–1977.*
16. Nutrition Cell of Planning and Development Division, Government of Pakistan, *Micronutrient Survey of Pakistan, 1988.*
17. Ministry of Population *Welfare. Pakistan Contraceptive Prevalence Survey, 1994–95. Basic Findings*, The Population Council, Islamabad.
18. Population Welfare Division. Ministry of Planning and Development. *Pakistan Contraceptive Prevalence Survey, 1984–85.*
19. Pakistan Medical Research Council, *Utilization of Rural Basic Health Services in Pakistan*, Report of Evaluation Study (1993).
20. Nafis S, "Population imperatives," In: *Business Recorder*, Feb. 28, 1996.
21. Hassan M, Population Welfare programme. In: *Muslim* Oct. 8, 1995.
22. Ministry of Population Welfare. *Population Welfare Programme, 1993–1998.* Government of Pakistan.

2.5 SRI LANKA

Ananda Wijekoon

Background and Demography

Sri Lanka has a total population of 18.1 million with 367,000 births per year. As shown in Table 1 development and health indicators are generally good. Total fertility is low (2.4%), contraceptive prevalence high (62%) and female literacy almost universal (above 85%).[1,2] With a strong political commitment and a health infrastructure that permeates into the remotest areas of the country it has made great strides in health parameters such as neonatal and infant mortality, and life expectancy. 94% of births are attended by trained personnel and, generally, initiation of breastfeeding is good — 70% within six hours and 99% within 24 hours.[3] The low birth weight rate though remains high at 25%.

Perinatal Health Indicators

The gradual reduction in the neonatal mortality rate during the post independence era is shown in Table 21.

Table 21 Neonatal mortality trends in Sri Lanka, 1950–1989.

Year	Neonatal mortality rate
1950	49.2
1960	34.2
1970	29.7
1980	22.4
1989	13.0

Many factors have contributed to the reduction of neonatal mortality rates in Sri Lanka:

- A strong political priority given to health.
- The establishment of a network of primary health care facilities with a strong emphasis on maternal and child health.
- Universal adult franchise in post-independent Sri Lanka.
- Free education at primary and secondary levels for both boys and girls.
- Food subsidisation.
- High levels of female literacy.
- Subsidised public transport.
- A very active basic and in-service training programme in maternal and child health for health personnel.

In spite of Sri Lanka's achievements in reducing neonatal mortality, there are still areas of concern in relation to perinatal care:

- A high prevalence of maternal malnutrition and anaemia.
- A high prevalence of low birth weight.
- High rates of birth asphyxia and neonatal sepsis.
- Geographical pockets with high neonatal mortality rate (e.g. 29 per 1,000 in Nuwara Eliya district).
- Poor enthusiasm among mothers and health staff for intrauterine transfer.
- Non availability of appropriate transport services for sick newborn infants.
- Relatively poor facilities for tertiary care of neonates.

Training programmes run by the Ministry of Health encourage the provision of facilities and preventive measures to reduce maternal malnutrition, anaemia, low birth weight, birth asphyxia and neonatal sepsis, and antenatal detection of infants at risk and their transfer *in utero*.

Perinatal Care Services

A good infrastructure has been in existence since before Sri Lanka's independence in 1948. The main changes in recent years have been an increasing involvement of private medical institutions and non-government organisations (NGOs) in maternal and child health services, and the virtual elimination of untrained birth attendants in the government health care providing institutions of the country.

Health services for mothers and newborn infants are currently provided by

- The Ministry of Health of the central government through its 215 preventive health units, manned by qualified medical officers and family health workers, and tertiary care hospitals made up of the national hospital, seven teaching hospitals and eight provincial hospitals.
- The provincial ministries through their 22 base hospitals, 244 district hospitals and 356 primary care hospitals.
- Private hospitals and NGOs.
- Estate hospitals.

Health care is given free to all of Sri Lanka's citizens except in the private hospitals. All tertiary care centres and the 22 base hospitals have paediatricians (48 in total) and obstetricians who have been provided with post-graduate training in neonatology and obstetrics, while the 244 district hospitals are managed by medical officers with basic training in MCH, including neonatal care. The 356 primary care hospitals have either medical officers and/or midwives trained in MCH and basic neonatal care.

Most private hospitals have visiting paediatricians and obstetricians, and most deliveries are under the supervision of trained staff. Estate hospitals still possess a few untrained midwives but this issue is being addressed by the government.

All tertiary and secondary care units and most primary care hospitals have ambulances. The others have access to ambulances at the closest hospital. However, these ambulances lack the facilities for the safe transfer of sick neonates and often transferred neonates arrive in tertiary care hospitals in a poor state.

An audit in a tertiary care unit (*Teaching Hospital, Peradeniya*)

The Teaching Hospital in Peradeniya is one of seven teaching hospitals which together with the national hospital provides care for the neonate at all three levels: primary, secondary and tertiary. It provides care for about 4,000 infants born within the hospital and about 300 infants transferred from the primary and secondary care units in the region.

Approximately 27% of the infants cared for are less than 2,500 g (low birth weight) which is slightly higher than the national average of 25%, as might be expected of a tertiary care unit. Low birth weight is a major challenge for Sri Lanka and LBW infants are a major drain on hospital and community health resources due to their immediate postnatal problems and later chronic incapacitating illnesses.

Mortality and resuscitation

There is a progressive increase in mortality with decreasing birth weight (Table 22). It is particularly high in the < 2,000 g birth weight range. Birth asphyxia, neonatal sepsis and intracranial haemorrhage account for a very large proportion of these deaths.

LBW infants also have difficulty in initiating spontaneous breathing. The need for resuscitation is a proxy for the condition at birth. Up to 50% of infants under 1,500 g at birth require resuscitation compared with 6–9% of infants above 2,000 g. A progressive increase in the need for resuscitation is seen particularly in the < 2,000 g group except in the < 1,250 g category. This exception may be explained by a less enthusiastic attitude towards resuscitation of infants with the poorest prognosis. Resuscitated infants have a higher risk of morbidity and mortality due to the invasive procedures that are sometimes required during resuscitation and due to the underlying cause of poor initiation of respiration.

Table 22 Trends in neonatal mortalitry in relation to birth weight.

Birth weight (g)	Neonatal mortality (%)
< 1,000	100
1,000–< 1,250	78
1,250–< 1,500	68
1,500–< 1,750	51
1,750–< 2,000	21
2,000–< 2,500	5
≥ 2,500	1

Neurological sequelae in low birth weight survivors

Mental subnormality, cerebral palsy and other neurological deficits are commoner in the LBW infant. The presence of meningitis, convulsions, intraventricular haemorrhage grade III or IV, ultrasonic evidence of structural lesions in the brain or ventricular space, or focal neurological signs before discharge were considered as markers of possible chronic neurological sequelae. The presence of such markers against birth weight is shown in Table 23 from data collected at Peradeniya Teaching Hospital.[4] Amongst the survivors very high rates of such markers were seen for LBW infants particularly those less than 2,000 g. The cumulative sum of deaths and markers of possible chronic neurological sequelae in relation to birth weight are also shown.

Table 23 Percentage of newborns with 'markers' of neurological sequelae or 'good quality survival'.

Birth weight (g)	Markers of neurological sequelae (%)	Either died or had markers of neurological sequelae (%)	Infants with 'good quality survival' (%)
< 1,000	–	100	0
1,000–< 1,250	75	94	6
1,250–< 1,500	71	91	9
1,500–< 1,750	26	64	36
1,750–< 2,000	12	31	69
2,000–< 2,500	2	7	93
≥ 2,500	1	3	97

Ensuring good quality survival and allocation of resources

On the basis of these figures we consider our priority in neonatal care is to improve the quality of survivors in the > 1,500 g birth weight category. As a corollary we could estimate the expected survivors with a good quality in relation to birth weight in this population, as shown in the final column of Table 23. The 1,500–2,000 g infants yield a very low percentage of expected good quality survivors, compared with industrialised countries and their heavier counterparts, so the immediate challenge for Sri Lankan perinatologists is to improve the quality of survivors of those with a birth weight above 1,500 g. In my own unit the scarce resources available are reserved for those in this category and heroic measures are withheld in the lower weight groups, except under special circumstances.

The status of transferred infants

A major concern in Sri Lanka is the poor condition of neonates transferred after birth from primary and secondary care units. Most transferred premature, LBW or sick infants are either severely hypothermic or in an advanced state of sepsis or neurological illness. Apart from promoting proper antenatal screening, there is an urgent need to promote intrauterine transfer of the at-risk neonate and, where these measures fail, to promote the safe transfer of these neonates after initially stabilising the infant. Good facilities for communication, transport, the availability of mobile life support systems and well-trained staff are absolute prerequisites for the improvement of mortality and morbidity of such transferred neonates.

Conclusion

The aim of neonatal care should not simply be the reduction of mortality but the improvement of the quality of survivors. Training of health personnel in antenatal and perinatal care; resuscitation methods; the prevention and treatment of sepsis; the awareness of conditions that necessitate early intervention; stabilisation of the sick neonate and safe transportation; coupled with the political will to provide the necessary infrastructure to realise these goals will continue hopefully to improve both survival rates and the quality of survivors.

References

1. UNICEF, *State of the World's Children*, Oxford University Press (1995).
2. Ministry of Health, Sri Lanka. *Annual Health Bulletin, 1991 and 1994.*
3. Wijekoon A *et al.* "First trimester feeding in a rural Sri Lankan population," *Social Science and Medicine* **40**(4) (1995): 443– 449.
4. Wijekoon A *et al.* "Morbidity and mortality in a tertiary care unit in Peradeniya, Sri Lanka," (in press).

Section 2:

Social, Economic and Cultural Aspects of Motherhood in South Asia

Chapter 3

SOCIAL AND DEVELOPMENTAL ISSUES AFFECTING THE PERINATAL HEALTH OF MOTHERS AND THEIR INFANTS

Hilary Standing
Senior Lecturer in Social Anthropology, University of Sussex

and

Anthony Costello
Reader in International Child Health, Institute of Child Health

How is Women's Health Affected by the General Socio-Economic Context?

Demographic and health indicators

Most South Asian countries rank low, not only on general development indicators, but also — as Table 1 makes clear — on many gender-related indicators. For the UNDP Gender-Related Development Index, which takes into account a range of demographic and "quality of life" indicators, the South Asia countries fare badly with the exception of Sri Lanka. The country rankings are Sri Lanka (62), India (103), Pakistan (107) Bangladesh (116) and Nepal (124). In much of South Asia, poverty interacts with gender discrimination to produce particularly poor health outcomes for women. Table 2 compares indicators across the countries of South Asia.

Gender bias is variously manifested in social, political, economic, nutritional, and health status. Of particular significance for perinatal health are low female literacy rates, poor calorie intake and the high proportion of low birth weight babies. These interactions are most clearly shown in the adverse demographic regimes found in India, Nepal, Pakistan and Bangladesh, where imbalanced sex ratios and higher female mortality and morbidity rates are found. For instance, in India, the female-to-male ratio (FMR) is 935/1,000. This is the reverse of the general demographic pattern, where females tend to have higher life expectancies and lower morbidities than males. In India, the very high mortality rate of female children under five largely accounts for the imbalanced sex ratio, but female mortality during the reproductive years is also up to 50% higher than male mortality.[1,2]

Socio-economic interactions

While the overall picture suggests persisting high levels of gender disadvantage, the national level data disguise important regional differences. Pakistan, North India, Nepal and Bangladesh show broad similarities in their demographic and socio-economic regimes, while South India and Sri Lanka have regimes much less adverse to women's health and socio-economic status.[1] There are also major rural-urban differences across South Asia which are reflected in women's access to health care and education. The picture is also a dynamic one, with significant changes taking place in contraceptive prevalence rates and in the capacity of institutional and NGO programmes to reach women.

Two important variables may be noted. First, women's health status is noticeably better in those areas where substantial long-term investment has taken place in primary health care and MCH services, as in Sri Lanka and some parts of South India, such as Kerala. Second, there is a general correlation between women's economic activity rates and their socio-economic status. Although poverty is an important predisposing factor to poor health, there is some evidence that females survive better in poor families where they are actual or potential economic actors. For example, Dyson and Moore[3] found higher survival rates for females in rice producing areas of India than

Table 1 Gender-related development indicators: South Asia compared with the rest of the world.

Indicator	World	Industrial countries	Developing countries	Least developed countries	South Asia
Population (millions) by year 2000	6,120	1,244	4,876	671	1,466
GNP per capita (US$)	4,570	16,394	970	210	309
Female share of earned income (%)	32	37	31	33	24
Female life expectancy, 1993 (in years)	65	78	63	52	61
Infant mortality rate, 1993	na	na	70	110	84
Maternal mortality rate	307	28	384	1,015	576
Female literacy rate	69.6	98.5	59.8	36.1	35
Total number of illiterate females (age 15 and above, millions), 1995	nk	nk	544	92	257
Combined primary, secondary and tertiary enrolment (as % of the relevant age group)	60	82	55	35	52
Public expenditure on education as % of GNP	5.1	5.4	3.9	3.0	3.8
Daily calorie supply (as % of north)	–	100	81	65	76
Total fertility rate, 1992	3.1	1.8	3.5	5.8	4.2
Births attended by trained personnel	69	99	63	29	33
Contraceptive prevalence rate	58	73	55	19	41
LBW infants (%)	18	6	19	23	32
Gender-related development index	0.600	0.868	0.530	0.318	0.410

Source: Human Development Report 1996. Published for the United Nations Development Programme, Oxford University Press. (nk = not known)

Table 2 Selected gender-related development indicators: comparison of the five South Asian countries (source UNDP).

Indicator	Bangladesh	India	Nepal	Pakistan	Sri Lanka
Population (millions) by year 2000	134.4	1,022	24.8	161.8	19.5
GNP per capita (US$), 1993	220	300	190	430	600
Female share of earned income (%)	23	25	32	19	33
Female life expectancy, 1993 (in years)	55.9	60.7	53.3	62.9	74.3
Infant mortality rate, 1993	106	81	98	89	17
Maternal mortality rate, 1993 (per 100,000 live births)	850	570	1,500	340	140
Female literacy rate, 1993	25	36	13	23	86.2
Total number of illiterate females (age 15 and above, millions), 1995	45.1	290.7	9.1	48.7	0.8
Combined primary, secondary and tertiary enrolment (as % of the relevant age group), 1993	40	55	57	37	66
Public expenditure on health as % of GDP, 1990	1.4	1.3	2.2	1.8	1.8
Public expenditure on education as % of GNP, 1992	2.3	3.7	2.9	2.7	3.3
Military expenditure as % of combined health and education expenditure, 1990–1991	41	65	35	125	107
Daily calorie supply as % of north, 1992	65	77	63	74	73
Total fertility rate, 1992	4.4	3.8	5.4	6.2	2.5
Births attended by trained personnel	10	33	6	35	94
Population per nurse, 1988–1991	20,000	3,333	33,333	3,448	1754

Table 2 (*Continued*)

Indicator	Bangladesh	India	Nepal	Pakistan	Sri Lanka
Contraceptive prevalence rate, any method (%), 1986–1993	40	43	23	15	62
LBW infants (% less than 2,500 g)	50	33	na	25	25
Gender-related development index (GDI) rank	116	103	124	107	62
Human development index rank	143	135	151	134	89

Source: Human Development Report 1996. Published for the United Nations Development Programme, Oxford University Press.

in wheat producing ones. Miller[4] examined juvenile sex ratios in South Asia and found either less biased or female favourable ones in southern districts of India and in Sri Lanka. Female favourable ratios occurred where the labour force participation rate was high among 15–34 year olds. Cultural variables also intervene. In eastern India, labour force participation is low, yet women's health and demographic indicators are not as poor as in the northern belt.

Miller associates high dowry and marriage costs with adverse juvenile sex ratios, and low costs with less adverse ratios. Low literacy and low school enrolment are also prevalent in areas where "female survival and labour force participation are low, marriage costs high and early marriage and childbearing the norms."[4]

The life cycle

There is an important life cycle element in this. Nearly all women marry — do so early — and share a household with in-laws. Their ability to take decisions is limited. Decisions regarding access to health care are mostly made by senior kin. However, where females have higher mortality rates than males, this trend changes after the age of 35 years. This reflects the improved social and economic valuation of women after they pass the reproductive stage. They acquire more social status as mothers-in-law and may also contribute financially to the household. This change through the life cycle points to mothers-in-law as a potentially important focus for intervention in relation to the reproductive health of young married women.

Empowerment

Women's poorer socio-economic status continues to be reflected in their absence of political voice. Manandhar[5] found that Village Development Committees and Health Post Support Committees in Nepal had almost no female representation, yet much of primary health care concerns the health of women and children. Women of reproductive age are particularly unlikely to be actively involved in community decision making because of their subordinate position in the household.

Historical evidence shows generally that variables which improve women's position in society are decisive in improving mortality and morbidity rates. Excess female mortality in Sri Lanka declined as female education increased and fertility fell.[1] However, it persisted longest in women in their prime childbearing years (age 20–24). It is likely that a similar pattern will be followed in other South Asian countries.

What is clear is that there is a very important link between women's economic and social status and their reproductive status. Women's health during the perinatal period, together with the health of their newborn infants, are products of multiple, interacting and reinforcing factors *occurring together and through time*. Factors such as the social valuation of women interact with factors such as access to and utilisation of health services to produce particular medical outcomes. Through time, and particularly through the reproductive life cycle, there is a strong reinforcement effect. This means that, for instance, poverty and discrimination against girl children translates eventually into poorer pregnancy and perinatal outcomes, which in turn perpetuate disadvantage into the next generation of girls. In the following sections, this cyclical process of socio-economic disadvantage in relation to reproductive health is considered in more detail.

Table 3 Key factors affecting women's health before conception.

Health issues	Social-economic factors
Nutritional status/malnutrition	Poverty, gender bias in food allocation
Morbidities affecting general health, e.g. parasite infections, malaria	Poor public health and sanitation infrastructure
Occupational health risks	The sexual division of labour in household, agricultural and paid work
Access to health care	Gender bias in access/utilisation; cost and availability
Access to knowledge about reproductive processes and basic health	Cultural and economic constraints on women's knowledge acquisition
Access to family planning to delay/control first conception	Control over young women's fertility and education opportunities in the hands of parents, husbands, in-laws

Before Conception

It is now well understood that women's health in the reproductive years depends importantly on their health status as children and adolescents. This, in turn, is closely linked to the socio-economic environment in which they develop. Table 3 summarises some key factors.

Nutritional status

In both India and Bangladesh, a number of micro-level studies have shown that males receive more calories and protein than females at all ages.[1] Food intake is generally a matter of household status rather than nutritional requirement, although there is regional variation. While some macro-level data do not reflect these findings (see Chapter 4) this is likely to be because they are too highly aggregated to detect the links between poverty and nutritional discrimination. Micro-level studies have tended to focus on poorer populations.

A study in Uttar Pradesh found that girls are less likely to be given milk, eggs and ghee than boys, and tend also, along with their mothers, to eat after men and boys. Boys spent more time out of the house which gave them access to raw vegetables and fruits not available to girls. Girls were deliberately fed less in some cases in order to delay their adolescence and, hence, to give more time to collect resources for their dowry.[6]

A comparison by Das *et al.* of "privileged" and "underprivileged" children in Indian Punjab found 24% of females malnourished in the privileged group, compared with 14% of boys; and 74% of girls malnourished in the underprivileged group compared to 67% of boys.[1] These findings suggest that gender bias persists into higher status socio-economic groups.[7] Female children are not only more likely to suffer from malnutrition, but the severity of their malnutrition is also usually greater.[1]

Women's and girls' paid and unpaid work produce an energy deficit if combined with low calorie intake. Girls tend to work longer hours than boys on household and economically productive work but are less well remunerated than boys, whose contribution is valued more highly. Micronutrient deficiencies, particularly vitamin A, calcium and iron, are prevalent among preschool and adolescent girls.[1]

Morbidity

The interactive and synergistic effects of illnesses such as respiratory infections, parasites, anaemia and malaria are also important for reproductive health outcomes. Poor public health infrastructure affects women and girls in particular ways, as they are responsible for household work. For example, wood smoke inhalation from cooking fires is a major health hazard for poor girls and women, who may spend long periods in unventilated kitchens. Chatterjee[1] quotes a study of four villages in Gujarat, where women were exposed to six times the amount of smoke compared with other household members, and fifteen times that of residents of heavily polluted New Delhi. Exposure to such pollutants has been linked to impaired foetal development and low birth weight, and increased risk of perinatal mortality.

Occupational health risks

Women in much of South Asia carry a large share of the burden of field labour as well as working in family based enterprises. This work is largely unremunerated or low value-added, and not valued either economically or culturally. The division of labour determines the particular health hazards that girls and women face.

Important occupational health hazards include transplanting and weeding in rice producing areas, which increase the risk of various infectious and chronic diseases; and sweated labour requiring long periods adopting an abnormal posture. Girls often carry heavy work burdens of household and field labour before they are fully developed (see Chapter 5).

Access to health care

Evidence suggests that where gender discrimination seriously affects women's health, disadvantage in access to health care is a major determinant of poor health status.[8] Micro-level studies have shown that girls are less likely to be taken to qualified doctors than boys, and that household medical expenditure on boys is greater than on girls. Health facilities report lower attendances and admissions by girls and women than by boys and men. Where girls and women are taken for treatment it is usually later in the illness than for boys and men.[1] Traditional remedies and local indigenous practitioners are generally used more by females.

Numerous barriers to access exist: distance, the opportunity costs of women's time, the need for a chaperone, the higher economic and social valuation placed on males than females when resources are scarce, and cultural views about appropriate behaviour.[9,10]

Knowledge about health and reproductive processes

Literacy rates are lower among women than men in most of South Asia. Girls, particularly in poor families, are not only less likely to go to school, but leave school earlier than boys. Adolescence is a crucial time for girls.

Cultural pressures to control girls' sexuality begin to bear down most heavily at this time. At the same time, adolescents generally have poor access to information on reproductive health in particular. Those not in formal schooling have little opportunity to learn about basic health. Gupta *et al.*[11] note that when sexual and gynaecological matters were discussed with local women participating in a Women and Development Programme in Rajasthan, many were surprised to find out that urine and menstrual flow pass out through different orifices.

Access to family planning

Most girls have little control over their life choices, such as right to schooling and delayed marriage. Both poverty and culture combine to circumscribe their futures. The low mean age of marriage leads to prolonged childbearing. Nearly 40% of rural Indian girls in the 15–19 age group are married . The average age of marriage for women in Nepal is still less than 16 years. Risks of maternal death are much higher in this age group and in their offspring.

Again, several factors combine to prevent young women from delaying first conception and using family planning services. Young married women are under pressure from their in-laws to demonstrate their fertility. Male preference remains strong. In more traditional rural areas, fertility decisions are under the control of the senior generation rather than the couple themselves.

Schooling, especially secondary schooling, has a profound impact on fertility. Educated women usually marry educated men, and often make their own fertility decisions. As Jeffery and Basu point out, "the demographic variable most strongly, universally and linearly associated with female schooling is child mortality" (p. 34).[12] Conditions which reduce infant and child mortality are also likely to reduce foetal mortality.

Pregnancy

The extent to which a pregnancy develops "normally" is partly an outcome of antecedent factors in a woman's life. Factors influencing the progress of pregnancy are summarised in Table 4.

Table 4 Key factors affecting women's health during pregnancy.

Health issues	*Social-economic factors*
Anaemia	Poverty/gender bias induced inadequacy of nutrition
Malaria	Lack of awareness of seriousness in pregnancy
Other diseases affecting pregnancy, e.g. STDs/RTIs	Economically and culturally produced neglect of women's health needs
Size of mother	Nutritional bias/inadequacy in childhood and adolescence
Age and parity of mother	Cultural pressures to high fertility, low age at marriage
Pregnancies too close together	Lack of control by women of fertility decisions
Dietary intake	Poverty/lack of awareness of need for increased intake
Energy levels	Women rarely able to rest or reduce workloads due to poverty/lack of awareness of needs in pregnancy
Antenatal care	Take up may require permission and chaperoning. Pregnancy not defined as a "medical" state

Anaemia, malaria and other infectious diseases

Anaemia affects many women in South Asia (see Chapter 4), resulting in increased complications of pregnancy, maternal deaths, low birth weights, and reduced child survival. A study by the Indian Council of Medical Research found that 95% of girls aged 6–14 years around Calcutta were anaemic, 70% around Delhi and Hyderabad, and 20% around Madras. 50–60% of

Indian women are estimated to be anaemic at the time of pregnancy. A high percentage of deaths among women during pregnancy and childbirth are attributed to anaemia, often caused by early malnutrition.[1] A recent survey in Punjab, India, found 86% of pregnant women showing some degree of anaemia, with 56% suffering from severe anaemia.[1]

Exposure to malaria and other infectious diseases, such as viral hepatitis is again determined in part by the extent to which the sexual division of labour gives exposure to higher risk environments,[13] and reduces access to appropriate antenatal care. Those in the household responsible for health care decisions, need to gain awareness of the seriousness of conditions such as malaria in pregnancy. Treatment delays are more common for females, and pregnancy is not customarily treated as a special condition which requires medical intervention.

High levels of gynaecological and sexually transmitted infections have been found in some recent studies in rural India.[14,15] These cause multiple, interrelated complications of conception, pregnancy and delivery. A study of 650 women in Maharashtra found that 92% suffered from a gynaecological or sexually transmitted infection, and less than 8% had ever had a gynaecological examination.[14] Again, these conditions are rarely acknowledged or treated. In part, this reflects the lack of STD services and routine gynaecological screening, as well as the often "silent" nature of STDs in women. It also reflects a common cultural neglect of women's health needs.

Status of the mother

Early motherhood brings about inadequate growth, poor nutrition and anaemia. In northern India, most women become pregnant before reaching full maturity.[16]

Poor nutrition in childhood and adolescence, aggravated by poverty, produces stunting, which increases the risk of obstetric complications and low birth weight babies. A study of 15-year olds in Kerala in the mid-1980s found that half were under-height and two thirds were underweight for their age.[1] Yet Kerala is a southern Indian state with substantially better health and demographic indicators.

Age at first and last pregnancies, and the spacing of pregnancies are largely culturally determined. They are linked to pressures on women's fertility behaviour exerted by the senior generation, the local fertility "culture", and the extent to which the woman herself is able to influence decisions about her education and marriage. In India, more than one-third of births occur within two years of the last birth. Spacing is also influenced by whether a son has been born. Until this happens, many women are under additional pressure to conceive quickly.

Dietary intake and energy levels

Due to both poverty and lack of awareness of the need, food intake rarely increases during pregnancy.[17] Indeed, it may be restricted. In many parts of South Asia, there are cultural taboos on eating certain foods during pregnancy. These may be foods of particular value to a pregnant woman, such as eggs. Food restriction, so-called "eating down", can also be due to fear of producing a large foetus which would cause a difficult labour. In India, the calorie gap in pregnancy is estimated to average 500–600 per day. Nutritional discrimination, especially against women doing physical labour, has serious implications for pregnancy and lactation. More pregnancies only exacerbate maternal nutritional depletion.[1]

Similarly, pregnancy is rarely considered a reason to rest or refrain from normal daily household and economic activities. Poverty and the unavailability of household substitutes also prevent modification of workloads (see Chapters 4 and 5).

Antenatal care

Even when available, antenatal care utilisation is uneven. In urban areas of India, 77% of pregnant women receive an antenatal check from a health professional, compared to only 41% of rural women. Pregnancy is often perceived as a normal state not needing intervention, but there are also cultural constraints to the use of services.

Table 5 Key factors affecting women's health during delivery.

Health issues	*Social-economic factors*
High risk pregnancies	Cultural pressures to continue child-bearing
Access to routine and emergency obstetric services	Distance, cost and lack of basic infra-structure to expedite emergency referrals
Utilisation of safe obstetric services, including trained paramedics or TBAs	Preference for customary modes of delivery, control of delivery by senior relatives, perceived poor quality of services
Unsafe abortion and its sequelae	Poverty a cause of high rates of unsafe abortion. No infrastructure to manage it

Women generally prefer female doctors, but these are in short supply, particularly in less accessible or rural areas. They (or their relatives) may refuse internal examination by a male doctor.

The quality of government health services is often poor — with a lack of privacy, and rude and dismissive staff — especially where there is a major status difference between the woman and the service provider. Women's gynaecological complaints are not always taken seriously.[11] There can be important opportunity costs of using health services, such as loss of income and lack of substitutable care for other children.

Delivery

Interlinked factors affecting delivery outcomes are summarised in Table 5.

High risk pregnancies

An important social factor in the occurrence of high risk pregnancies is the pressure to continue fertility, especially where no sons have been born.

Bhatia, in a WHO-sponsored retrospective field study of deaths among females of reproductive age in Anantapur District, Andhra Pradesh, India, in 1984–85 (described in World Bank Report: 27–8[1]), found significant demographic differences between those who died and matched survivor controls. The women who survived had more living children and more living sons than those who died (55% of those who died did not have a living son, compared to 25% in the control group). Yet the women who died had much poorer health and obstetric histories than the survivors, which indicates heavy pressure on women to bear sons.

Access to routine and emergency obstetric services

Women's access to services is determined, first and foremost, by their availability. There is an absolute lack of availability of obstetrically trained personnel in, for example, most remote areas of Nepal. In other areas, services are a long distance away, and lack of transport is a major deterrent. The critical link between community level and referral services able to deal with obstetric emergencies is often weak or lacking. Lack of institutional and organisational support to front line female health workers also makes it difficult for them to reach women in need.[1]

These difficulties are compounded by "demand side" barriers, such as lack of awareness by household decision makers of warning signs during labour.

Utilisation of safe obstetric services

As pregnancy is not necessarily seen as a condition requiring medical intervention, established patterns of behaviour around delivery change quite slowly. In South Asia, except Sri Lanka, most deliveries are at home (Table 2). Mothers generally lack control of health seeking behaviour and decisions about the place and mode of delivery. Poverty renders home environments unavoidably unhygienic through lack of clean water and sanitation.

Dutta *et al.*[18] found that even in semi-urban areas with good access to obstetric services, over a quarter of high risk pregnant women did not use them. Service quality was an important factor implicated in non-utilisation. As for antenatal care, facilities often have poor infrastructure, non-availability of suitable personnel and weak interpersonal skills among health staff.

Unsafe abortion

High rates of unsafe abortion, often procured locally from unskilled village women, are reported in several studies.[1] Families cannot afford additional children, or — where it is legally available — the costs involved in access to formal services. The actual toll of mortality and morbidity from abortion (including infertility) is difficult to quantify but is thought to be high. As with emergency obstetric services, access to services able to manage the sequelae of unsafe terminations is uneven.

Table 6 Key factors affecting women's health during the postnatal period.

Health issues	*Social-economic factors*
Low birth weight	Poverty, antecedent nutritional factors
Postnatal hygiene and preventable diseases	Poverty and conditions of delivery. Concepts of birth pollution can compromise this
Maternal rest and recuperation	Availability of female kin to take on the extra workload
Lactation/Breastfeeding	Availability of food to maintain it, bias against female infants, decline of breastfeeding in urban areas
Prevention of early conception	Locus of control of fertility, access to user friendly family planning services.

The Postnatal Period

The period immediately following birth is vital both to the survival of the infant and the full recovery of the mother. Table 6 summarises the interlinked factors affected these.

Low birth weight

In South Asia, low birth weight rates are high and are correlated with poor socio-economic conditions, maternal nutritional status early pregnancy, and short birth intervals (see Chapter 4 for a more detailed discussion).

Postnatal hygiene and maternal recuperation

Most births in rural South Asia take place at home. The common belief that childbirth is associated with "pollution" means that postpartum care is perfunctory and often left to low status women.[19] While this association can help women by giving them time to recover, rest time is conditioned by the availability of others to share work burdens. Older women without senior female kin to run the household may be particularly disadvantaged.[12]

The World Bank study suggested that the concept of postpartum care is not well understood even by trained health staff, and contact visits are more likely to concentrate on family planning or immunisation than on care for the mother.[1]

Lactation/breastfeeding

Lactation, like pregnancy, requires increased calorie and nutritional intake and puts additional demands on poorer mothers with marginal nutritional intakes.

Breastfeeding has important interactions with two socio-economic variables: bias against female infants and the re-establishment of fertility. First, some evidence suggests that female infants receive less breast milk less frequently and for a shorter period than boys. For example, a study by

McNeill in Tamil Nadu, India, found male children were breastfed on average five months more than female children, and a male child in a landed family nearly ten months more than a female child in a labourers' family.[1] Short breastfeeding of girls also reduces the anovulatory period and hastens further conception. A study by Basu in two Delhi slum populations in 1989 found that only 50–65% of female infants under one year received adequate nourishment.[1]

Girls of high birth order suffer particularly. Das Gupta found that in Ludhiana, a district of Punjab, the death rate among children aged 0–4 was higher for second born females than males and this bias became more prominent with each successive birth. If there was already a living girl, a subsequent female was also less likely to survive than if the firstborn was a male (cited in World Bank *op.cit.*). Second, breastfeeding affects subsequent fertility. While there are positive relationships between female schooling and age at marriage, and schooling and child mortality, there is a negative relationship between breastfeeding and length of schooling, which also affects the length of postpartum abstinence.[12] Both educational level and urbanisation are associated with a decline in breastfeeding.

Preventing early conception/family planning

In India in 1992, 37% of births occurred within two years of the previous live birth, and infant mortality is more than twice as high for these children as for infants born after 48 months. Enabling women to plan their pregnancies requires both social interventions (increasing access to education for girls) and improving the quality and accessibility of family planning services.

While use of family planning services is partly determined by demand, it is also influenced by quality. Family planning services are often unfriendly and offer poor choice of alternatives. For instance, sterilisation accounts for 85% of total modern contraceptive use in India of which 90% is female sterilisation (World Bank *op.cit.*).

References

1. Chatterjee M, "Indian women: Their health and economic productivity," *World Bank Discussion Paper 109*, Washington DC: The World Bank (1990).
2. Kynch J and Sen A, "Indian women, well-being and survival," *Cambridge Journal of Economics* **7** (1983): 363–380.
3. Dyson T and Moore M, "On kinship structure, female autonomy and demographic behaviour," *Population and Development Review* **9**(1) (1983): 35–60.
4. Miller B, *The Endangered Sex Neglect of Female Children in Rural North India*, Ithaca, Cornell University Press (1981).
5. Manandhar M, "Exploratory Study of Local Health Committees in Three Countries: A Case Study of Nepal Consultancy Report," London, Centre for International Child Health (1996).
6. Ghosh S, "Women's role in health and development," *Health for the Millions* **XIII**(1 & 2) (1987): 2–7.
7. Sen AK and Sen GS, "Malnutrition of rural children and the sex bias," *Economic and Political Weekly* **28** (1983): 855–862.
8. Timisan J, "Access to care: More than a problem of distance," In: The Health of Women: A Global Perspective, Koblinsky M, Timisan J and Gay J. eds, 1993 Oxford Westview Press (1993).
9. Gilson L, "Government health care charges: Is equity being abandoned?" *EPC discussion paper number 15*, London School of Hygiene and Tropical Medicine (1988).
10. Duggal R and Amin S, "Cost of health care: A household survey in an Indian district," Foundation for Research in Community Health, India (1989).
11. Gupta N *et al.*, "Health of women and children in Rajasthan," *Economic and Political Weekly* **22**(42) (1992).
12. Jeffery R and Basu A, *Girls' Schooling, Women's Autonomy and Fertility Change in South Asia New Delhi*, Sage Publications (1996).
13. Standing H, Consultancy report on Gender/Women and Development Issues. The World Bank Malaria Control Project, India. Report of a Preparation Mission. London, Malaria Consortium (1996).
14. Dharmaraj D, "Reproductive tract infections — The issues and priorities for India," In: *Women and Health Report*, Voluntary Health Association of India, New Delhi (1994).
15. Bang RA, "High prevalence of gynaecological diseases in rural Indian women," In: *Gynaecological disorders*, New Delhi, Voluntary Health Association of India (1990).

16. Rohde J, "Adolescence — The forgotten and neglected opportunity," *Indian Journal of Paediatrics* **60** (1993): 321–326.
17. Bhatia BD, "Dietary intakes of urban and rural pregnant, lactating and non-pregnant non-lactating vegetarian women of Varanasi," *Indian Journal of Medical Research* (1981): p. 74.
18. Dutta PK *et al.*, "Utilisation of health services by "high risk" pregnant women in a semi urban community of Pune — An analytical study," *Indian Journal of Maternal and Child Health* **1**(1) (1993): 15–19.
19. Jeffery R *et al.*, *Labour Pains and Labour Power: Women and Childbearing in India*, New Delhi, Manohar (1989).

Chapter 4

EPIDEMIOLOGICAL TRENDS IN NUTRITIONAL STATUS OF CHILDREN AND WOMEN IN INDIA

H. P. S. Sachdev

*Professor and Incharge, Division of Clinical Epidemiology,
Department of Pediatrics, Maulana Azad Medical College,
New Delhi, India*

Introduction

Over the past three decades, there has been a slow but definite improvement in the under-five, infant and neonatal mortality rates in the country.[1] It is therefore logical to direct increasing attention to nutritional status, an important index of the "quality" of survivors. The direct relationship between neonatal morbidity or mortality on one hand and maternal or neonatal nutritional status on the other, is well documented. For a meaningful dialogue on "improving newborn health in developing countries", it is imperative to address pertinent issues in relation to maternal and neonatal nutritional status. This chapter focusses on recent epidemiological trends and the current scenario in relation to the nutritional status of children and women in India with particular emphasis on the neonatal and maternal periods, wherever relevant information is available.

Data on trends in the nutritional profile of neonates and mothers (pregnant and lactating) in India is lacking in several areas of interest. However, valid indirect inferences may be possible by scrutiny of available data in relation to under-fives and women because

1. Epidemiologic transitions in nutrition generally occur in the same direction in proximate age groups;
2. The nutritional status of under-fives is partially determined by their earlier profile in the neonatal period;
3. Pre-pregnant nutritional status in eligible women is also an important determinant of neonatal outcome.[2]

Adolescence, the immediate precursor of adulthood, assumes particular significance in the Indian context as marriage and pregnancy during this period are still prevalent.

Data collection methods

It was essential to have access to published information of recent changes in the nutritional status in similar geographic and socio-economic profiles, preferably at the national level. Micro-level research was also sought although clearly such inferences may not be generalisable. A computerised Medlar search proved disappointing, yielding only a few micro-level studies. This was not surprising since a large proportion of relevant data was in the form of non-indexed publications including reports, chapters in books, and other periodicals. Subsequently, institutions and workers known to be engaged in such research were contacted on a personal basis. It is realised that the data collected in this manner may not be complete but, nevertheless, substantial information became available to draw some valid inferences.

The chapter is organised under four main headings:

1. protein energy malnutrition
2. intrauterine growth
3. micronutrients
4. nutrient intake

Protein Energy Malnutrition

Clinical assessment

The most outstanding achievement on the national nutrition front during the last four decades has been the virtual "banishment" of acute large-scale famines, of the type that used to decimate sizable sections of the country's population with distressing regularity (once in seven years) for centuries.[3] The Bengal famine of the early 1940s was the last great tragedy of its kind in the country. This is not to deny that pockets of acute hunger still exist in some parts of the nation in some seasons and in times of disasters like droughts and floods, but these are now dealt with more efficiently.[3]

Kwashiorkor and Marasmus

Personal experience of pediatricians throughout the country indicates that in the past three decades there has been a significant decline in severe protein energy malnutrition (classical Kwashiorkor and extreme forms of Marasmus) in hospitalised children. The decline has been particularly dramatic in relation to classical Kwashiorkor, which has virtually disappeared from numerous regions. This change in the spectrum has been quantified.[4] Reliable community based data generated by the National Nutrition Monitoring Bureau (NNMB) from eight central and southern states (Andhra Pradesh, Gujarat, Karnataka, Kerala, Madhya Pradesh, Maharashtra, Orissa, and Tamil Nadu) also confirms a decline in clinical deficiency signs in rural preschool children (one to five years old) between 1975–79 and 1988–90.[5] The overall prevalence of Marasmus decreased from 1.3 to 0.6% and Kwashiorkor from 0.4 to 0.1%. Amongst the 12,000 children evaluated in the "Repeat Surveys", Gujarat showed the highest prevalence of both forms (1.1% Kwashiorkor and 4.9% Marasmus), while in the other states, their prevalence was below 1%. In the NNMB and National Council for Applied Economic Research (NCAER) linked survey conducted in 1994 in the same eight states but in differently sampled rural areas,[6] among 1,828 preschool children the overall prevalences of Kwashiorkor and Marasmus were 0.2%

and 0.4% respectively. In fact, cases of Kwashiorkor were seen only in Madhya Pradesh, where the prevalence was about 1.4%. However, Marasmus was observed in four states — the prevalences ranging from 0.4% in Tamil Nadu and Andhra Pradesh to about 1.4% in Madhya Pradesh and Orissa. Fortunately, a similar declining trend was documented in the underprivileged urban slums[7] of these six states (cities included Ahmedabad, Bangalore, Bhubenashwar, Cuttack, Hyderabad, Nagpur, and Trivandrum). The overall prevalence of Marasmus diminished from 3.7% in 1975–79 (n = 519) to 0.2% in 1993–94 (n = 334). No case of Kwashiorkor was observed.

Nutritional anthropometry

Children

In developing countries, anthropometry, despite its inherent limitations, still remains the most practical tool for assessing the nutritional status of children in the community.[8] In India, there have been many small-scale surveys, but the data may not be representative of the country as a whole. The two major national surveys, which provide data related to nutrition and cover large segments of India's population are:

1. the periodic surveys carried out by the NNMB[5–7,9] of the National Institute of Nutrition, Hyderabad, and
2. the recent National Family Health Survey (NFHS) initiated by the Ministry of Health and Family Welfare, Government of India.[10]

The data derived from these surveys have their limitations and are not strictly comparable.

Before attempting any valid comparisons, it is important to be aware of several factors, notably the sampling framework, which can potentially influence the estimates of malnutrition prevalence from these surveys.[11] The NFHS covered 24 states, as well as Delhi, and was designed to be representative of 99% of the young child population (0–4 years). However, the focus was on reproductive health and data related to nutrition was secondary and somewhat limited. For first phase states (Andhra Pradesh,

Himachal Pradesh, Madhya Pradesh, Tamil Nadu, and West Bengal), only weight was measured. It was felt[10] that the lack of height measurements for these states would not substantially bias the national estimates of height for age and weight for height since these five states clustered closely around the national estimate of underweight children. In comparison, the NNMB surveys covered only eight states (detailed above) with a primary focus on the rural population, and the preschool age data relates to the 1–5 year age group. The repeat (1988–90) surveys[5] are particularly valuable as these were conducted in the areas evaluated[9] earlier (1975–79) with a specific purpose of eliciting nutritional trends. The latest (1994) NNMB–NCAER survey had covered dissimilar rural areas with a smaller sample size in the same eight states. Some information on trends in the underprivileged urban slum population, albeit on a smaller sample, is available from six of these eight states.[7]

Table 1 compares the estimated prevalences of various indices of malnutrition in these surveys as per the current international recommendation and nomenclature.[8,11] A distinct improvement in the prevalences of underweight and stunting (including severe category, namely, below 3 SD) is evident from the NNMB data at an average rate of 1% per annum. The NFHS estimates[10,12,13] were still lower than the NNMB–NCAER[6] prevalences at comparable time periods. This could be primarily due to differences in sampling design, areas surveyed (whole country versus eight states, and urban plus rural versus rural), and the age groups analysed (0–4 vs. 1–5 years). Malnutrition in these two indices is lower in the first year of life,[14] urban areas[13] and the northern part of the country.[12,13,15,16] Fortunately, a similar overall declining trend was documented in the underprivileged urban slums[7] of six states between the periods 1975–79 to 1993–94 for weight for age (Gomez classification based on National Center for Health Statistics reference).

It must be carefully noted that there is virtually no change in the profile of wasting in this period and the NNMB and NFHS estimates are also identical (Table 1), indicating that the improvement in weight-for-age index is predominantly due to an increase in height.

Despite the observed decline, malnutrition is still a significant problem in the country. In the NFHS data, the prevalence of underweight ranged

Table 1 Changes in prevalence (%) of childhood malnutrition.

Malnutrition Index	Survey			
	NNMB[5] 1975–79 (n = 6,428)	NNMB[5] 1988–90 (n = 13,422)	NNMB[6] 1994 (n = 1,832)	NFHS[10] 1992–93 (n = 25,578)*
Weight for age underweight				
< 2 SD	77.5	68.6	63.6	53.4
< 3 SD severe	38.0	26.6	24.7	20.6
Height for age stunting				
< 2 SD	78.6	65.1	63.0	52.0
< 3 SD severe	53.3	36.8	35.8	28.9
Weight for height wasting				
< 2 SD	18.1	19.9	16.7	17.5
< 3 SD severe	2.9	2.4	2.6	3.2

*For weight for age assessment only. The sample size for other two indices was lower (for details refer to related text).

from 28% in Mizoram and Kerala to 59% in Uttar Pradesh and 63% in Bihar; severe malnutrition likewise ranged from around 5% in Mizoram and 6% in Kerala to 31% — again in Bihar. Regional variations were also observed for stunting and wasting. In comparison to the urban areas, in rural areas the overall prevalences of underweight (45.2% vs. 55.9%) and stunting (44.8% vs. 54.1%) were higher while interestingly wasting (15.8% vs. 18%) was comparable.[10] Overall, there was no gender differential — in approximately half the states, girls had higher underweight prevalences, while boys fared worse in the other half. However, on examining severe malnutrition only, a gender differential became apparent with a higher proportion of girls being severely malnourished in 11 of the 14 large states.[13]

Women

A few studies have attempted to quantify secular trends in height by comparison of mothers and daughters.[17-22] No positive trend was discerned in women from poor socio-economic strata[19-22] whereas a significant increase, even up to a mean value of 5 cm,[18] was documented in well-to-do communities.[17,18]

An analysis of the NNMB "Repeat Survey"[5] aggregate data (pooled for all the states) on heights, weights, and body mass index over the period show a definite improvement. The average values of measurements, in general, for almost all the age groups in both sexes show an increase; height increments tended to be more in children with weight increments more visible in adults and adolescents. Statewise data clearly indicate that the heights of children and adolescents, and weights of adults and adolescents in the state of Kerala and to some extent in Maharashtra and Gujarat were distinctly better compared with the 1970s.[23]

The time trends in NNMB data[5,6,9] for weight and triceps fat fold thickness in females between the ages of 12 to 47 years are depicted in Figure 1. The adolescent age group (12 to 18 years), of particular interest in the Indian setting, has also been analysed. A positive trend in all anthropometric parameters is evident at virtually all the ages examined, with each successive survey recording higher mean values than the preceding one.

The differences in *height* (not shown in the figure) between the NNMB 1988–90 and NNMB 1994 surveys were negligible at several ages. The positive time trends in height in the "Repeat Surveys" (1988–90) were more marked in the age group 12 to 14 years (mean differences between 1.7 to 3.0 cm) than later (mean differences between 0.3 to 1.4 cm). The mean increase in adult stature between 1975–79 and 1988–90 was calculated to be 1.2 cm.[24] The quantum of difference (marginal) in height may be related to the relatively short inter-observation period (average 12 years) for documenting secular trends in this parameter.

The differences in mean *weight* ranged from 0.7 to 2.2 kg between the 1975–79 and 1994 surveys, and the corresponding figures for mean *triceps fat fold thickness* were 1.5 to 2.5 mm. These differences too were not striking

Secular Trend in Weights of Women

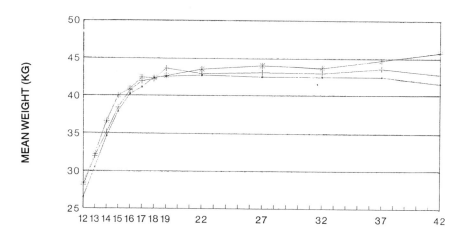

Trend in Fat Fold of Women

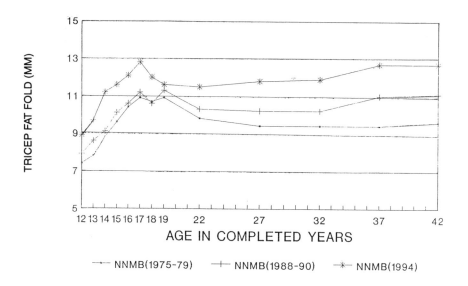

Figure 1 Times trends in NNMB data[5,6,9] for weight and triceps fat fold thickness in females between the ages of 12 to 47 years.

for an average inter-observation period of 17 years, but they do represent the initiation of a positive nutritional trend in the relatively poor rural population. A similar analysis was not feasible for the urban poor as the published report[7] did not provide comparative figures for this purpose.

In the NNMB 1994 survey in rural areas,[6] the mean heights of reproductive women (15–44 years) ranged from 151 to 152 cm while the corresponding figures for weight were 40 to 43.5 kg from 15 to 25 years and 44 to 45.8 kg thereafter. Major inter-state differences were not apparent.[6] The "Repeat Survey" (1988–90) data[5] indicates that 33% of 18-year old women have body weights below 40 kg and 15% have heights less than 145 cm, the conventional cut-off points for defining obstetric high risk.[23] Similar data on ever-married eligible women in the reproductive age period of 13–49 years is available from urban slums from a multicentric study conducted by the Indian Council of Medical Research (ICMR) in the early 1980s.[25] A total of 12,577 subjects were surveyed from three centres (Calcutta, Delhi and Madras). The mean heights ranged between 148.5 to 150.3 cm and 16 to 23% were less than 145 cm tall. The mean weights ranged from 43.3 to 46.4 kg. The percentage of women in the weight categories less than 40 kg and 41–45 kg ranged from 25 to 32% and 26 to 35% respectively. The mean skinfold thickness was 12 mm. Delhi centre had the best nutritional profile and Calcutta the worst. Thus, the nutritional status of women in underprivileged urban slum populations in 1983–85 was largely comparable to the NNMB rural estimates of 1994.

Body Mass Index (BMI) is being increasingly used as a measure of nutritional adequacy in adults and is considered to be a better indicator of chronic energy deficiency (CED).[23] The time trends in BMI of adult women from the NNMB data are summarised in Table 2. A distinct shift of the distribution to the right is evident in the rural population. Interestingly, the underprivileged urban slum population had the best values. However, CED is prevalent in 37–47% of the women with the severe variety being documented in 10%. Obesity is also beginning to emerge (7 to 12%). In the rural population, regional differences were apparent and a positive relationship was observed between adult BMI (both sexes) and proxies for economic status such as possession of agricultural land, major occupation, and income.[23,24]

Table 2 Trends in Body Mass Index in adult women.

*Body Mass Index** *Definition* *(value)*	*Survey (values in %)*			
	NNMB[5] *1975–79* *(n = 6,428)*	*NNMB[5]* *1988–90* *(n = 13,422)*	*NNMB[6]* *1994* *(n = 1,832)*	*NNMB* *Slum[7]* *1993–94* *(n = 1,319)*
Chronic energy deficiency				
Third < 16	12.7	11.3	10.4	9.5
Second 16–17	13.2	12.9	11.2	9.2
First 17–18.5	25.9	25.1	25.5	18.0
All < 18.5	51.8	49.3	47.1	36.7
Normal 18.5–2.5	44.8	46.6	46.3	51.7
Obese > 25	3.4	4.1	6.6	11.6

*Body Mass Index (BMI) is defined as weight (kg)/height^2 (m). The percentages for NNMB surveys 1975–79 and 1988–90 for the various categories were taken from Reference 24. The percentages for different categories for BMI < 18.5 for NNMB survey (1994) were recalculated from the total adult sample.

Intrauterine Growth

Pregnancy weight gain

Studies of weight gain during pregnancy indicate that the average value is 6 kg in urban women of low-income groups and 11 kg in high-income groups, which is similar to developed countries.[23,26]

Birth weight

Trends

In developing countries, intrauterine growth has been invariably assessed by birth weight. In India, even today a majority of the deliveries are conducted in the community. Logistic difficulties in recording birth weight at home precludes accurate national estimates of the magnitude and trends of low birth weight (LBW). A large volume of data on birth weight from the 1950s is available from individual studies, mostly hospital based, and this information has been exhaustively compiled and reviewed.[22,27-30] Regional, urban-rural and socio-economic differentials are evident, generally in the same direction as nutritional anthropometry. The usual estimates of mean birth weight and LBW have ranged between 2.5 to 3 kg and 22.4 to 40%, respectively. In the community based ICMR multicentric study,[25] the urban slum computations of LBW were 27% for Madras, 38% for Delhi, and 56% for Calcutta. The often cited nationally representative figure for LBW is 30%.[23]

National reviews suggest no differences in mean birth weights and LBW rates between the 1960s and the 1980s.[22,23] These inferences were based on comparison of data from disparate settings at various time points. Given the expected marginal magnitude of change in birth weight in two to three decades in a nation commencing epidemiologic transition, inferences from such a research design are not surprising. It would be more valid to analyse data from the same area at different time points.

On analysis of this nature (Table 3), a positive time trend for birth weight is evident in most hospital based data and the solitary community study.[31-37] The mean improvement in birth weight is marginal (52 to 126 g), but this produces a greater reduction of LBW prevalence (by 8 to 12% usually and 22% in one report). These calculated mean improvements in birth weight are probably underestimates[35] since concomitant changes in other important associates have been ignored. With time, the mean birth order has also decreased and correction for this factor alone[35] (because first born infants have lower weights than later births) enhanced the magnitude of change in the community study (rural and urban areas combined) from 70 to 100 g. The absent time trend in the two Delhi hospitals may be related to the relatively short gap in one report[37] and the fact that these institutions primarily provide care to the underprivileged population in whom the transition is expected to commence last of all.

Table 3 Trends in intrauterine growth.

| Area | Setting | Comparison period (Mean gap in yrs) | Observed changes | | |
			Weight	Gestation	IUGC
Rourkela, Orissa[31]	Industrial hospital	1962 and 1986 (23)	MBW +74 g LBW −34 to 25%	NA	NA
Delhi[32]	Hospital poor	1969 and 1989 (20)	NA	Term +*	0
Delhi[33]	Hospital better off	73−74 and 85−87 (12.5)	NA	NA	+
North Arcot, Tamil Nadu[34]	Rural	69−73 and 89−93 (20)	MBW +78 g LBW −27 to 16%	M +0.7 wk PT −21 to 16%	+P
	Urban	69−73 and 89−93 (20)	MBW +52 g LBW −19 to 11%	M +0.8 wk PT −20 to 15%	
Vellore[35]	Hospital	1969 and 1994 (25)	MBW +126 g LBW −27 to 15%	Me +0.3 wk PT −14 to 10%	NA
Mumbai[36]	Hospital poor	1988 and 1995 (8)	LBW −60 to 38%	0	NA
Delhi[37]	Hospital poor	1986 and 1996 (11)	0	0	NA

+Indicates significant increase; +P indicates significant at some gestations; − indicates significant decline; 0 indicates no significant change.

IUGC — Intrauterine growth curves; M — Mean; Me — Median; MBW — Mean birth weight; NA — Not available; wk — Gestation in weeks;

*Calculated by comparison with earlier study values cited in Reference 29.

The slender improvement in birth weight is probably contributed to by increases in both gestation and birth weight at different gestations (intrauterine growth curves). The mean improvement in gestation was again marginal (0.3 to 0.8 weeks) and was not uniformly observed. However, these marginal changes in mean gestations resulted in an improvement in prematurity rates (by 4–5%).

The NNF institutional data for 1995

Recently, efforts have been made to collect nationally representative estimates of birth weights from institutional[38] and community[39] settings. The reliable institution based National Neonatology Forum (NNF) data[38] for the year 1995 on 30,632 births (0.1% births in the country) from 14 participating centres (Ahmedabad, Bangalore (3 centres), Baroda, Calcutta, Chandigarh, Delhi, Indore, Ludhiana, Madras, Mumbai, Pondicherry, and Shimla) yielded a LBW prevalence of 31.2% among 29,412 live births.[38] Only 35% of the LBW infants were preterm.

The Child Survival Safe Motherhood (CSSM) Programme linked District based data (health facility based delivery in 14 Districts in ten states — Assam, Gujarat, Madhya Pradesh, Karnataka, Maharashtra, Orissa, Punjab, Rajasthan, Tamil Nadu, and West Bengal) on 27,069 births estimated the LBW prevalence to be much lower at 18.4%.[39] Wide regional variations were apparent with values ranging from a low of 2.7% (Madhya Pradesh) and 5.1% (Assam) to a high of 24.7% (Tamil Nadu) and 40% (Orissa). The strikingly low figures in comparison to earlier published literature, especially for the poor performing states (Madhya Pradesh — 2.7% and Rajasthan — 12.8%) in other nutritional parameters, including protein energy malnutrition, questions the reliability of the integrated data.

Gestation

In contrast to developed countries, labour appears to be initiated at an earlier gestation in a larger proportion of pregnant women. The incidence of premature birth (< 37 weeks gestation) ranges from 7.1 to 22.3% in contrast to about 5% in the developed countries. The latest NNF data provides a national estimate of 12.8%. Only 2% of births occur at 36 weeks in western countries, while 3 to 12% of infants are born at this gestational age in India. In the Indian setting, the maximum number of births occur at 39–40 weeks gestation, whereas in the West the corresponding figure is 40–41 weeks.[29]

Apart from inter-regional differences, there is a marked variation in the gestational distribution in privileged versus underprivileged segments of population in the same area. The contrast from developed countries is very striking in the low socio-economic population of India, but the difference is considerably narrowed and even disappears in the privileged class.[29]

Birth weight and gestation

A two-way distribution of birth weight and gestation shows that in the birth weight group of 1,501 to 2,000 g, only 30 to 45% of infants are preterm, the majority being full-term or post-term. For the birth weight group 2,001 to 2,500 g, 85% or more are term or post-term and only 13 to 15% are preterm. These findings are consistent for hospital and community births[25] and have a bearing on the identification of high risk neonates and defining criteria for LBW infants in the Indian setting.[29]

Intrauterine foetal growth curves

A comparison of foetal growth curves shows disparity between regions and socio-economic classes. The economically privileged population has higher mean birth weights at different gestations, the difference becoming pronounced after 34 weeks.[29]

A classification for infants at birth based on the hospital-derived intrauterine growth curves has been proposed.[40] The suggested definitions for any gestation are

- large-for-date (LFD): birth weight above +2 SD;
- appropriate for gestational age (AGA): birth weight between −1 SD and +2 SD;
- intrauterine growth retarded (IUGR): birth weight between −1 SD and − 2 SD;
- small-for-date (SFD): birth weight below −2 SD.

This classification has support from observations on the distribution of live births, morbidity and mortality in different groups.[29] The percentage distribution for all gestations for LFD, AGA, IUGR and SFD in the same hospital and draining urban cohort births were 3, 85, 10.5 and 1.5% respectively. The distribution of AGA, IUGR and SFD in term infants with birth weight of 2,001 to 2,500 g was 13, 85 and 1–2% respectively. This observation needs to be investigated further as this is the group which contributes maximally to LBW infants in India.[29]

Micronutrients

Vitamin A deficiency

This micronutrient deficiency has generated considerable interest and controversy[30,41,42] recently because of pressure by international agencies for periodic massive dose vitamin A prophylaxis as a cost-effective strategy for improving child survival. The possibility of utilising massive dose vitamin A prophylaxis in lactating mothers to simultaneously benefit the woman and augment the vitamin A status of newborns[43] has added fuel to the fire. Since preschool children bear the brunt of the deficiency, nationally representative surveys have primarily focussed on this age group.

Keratomalacia

A nationwide survey conducted by the ICMR during 1971–74 showed that 2% cases of blindness were attributable to corneal disease caused by vitamin A deficiency.[23] In the subsequent (1985) national survey of blindness, carried out under the auspices of the Government of India and the World Health Organization (WHO), this figure declined to 0.04%.[23,30] Data from the School of Tropical Medicine, Calcutta, once the hot-bed of keratomalacia, and from the Christian Medical College, Vellore,[30] are also suggestive of a sharp reduction in the documentation of keratomalacia (0 to 0.008% in late 1980s). A careful scrutiny of the hospital data from Calcutta in fact suggests that the decline in the incidence of keratomalacia started before the massive dosage prophylaxis programme had been instituted.[30]

Bitot spots and night blindness

Reported prevalence rates of Bitot spots in preschool children from macro surveys[5-7,44,45] show an overall marked decline between the 1960s and 1990s, especially in the NNMB "Repeat Survey".[5] The slight apparent increase in later surveys is probably related to the different sampling areas. Wide regional variations are evident and in some areas no child with Bitot spots was seen. In the NNMB 1994[6] rural survey, none of the children in Kerala, Andhra Pradesh and Gujarat had Bitot spots while the prevalence ranged from 0.4% in Karnataka and Orissa to 5.6% in Madhya Pradesh. The prevalence was more than 0.5% — a level suggestive of public health problem, according to WHO criterion — in the States of Tamil Nadu (0.8%), Maharashtra (1.5%) and Madhya Pradesh (5.6%).

The NNMB 1992–93 rural survey in ten states was conducted on a much larger sample size of 26,760 preschool children to specifically address the issue of linking periodic dosing of vitamin A with universal immunisation programmes.[45] The prevalence of Bitot spots ranged from 0.3% in Kerala and 0.4% in Tamil Nadu to 3.2% in Gujarat and 3.6% in Madhya Pradesh. The prevalence was above 0.5% in eight of the ten states. Interestingly, and paradoxically, the overall prevalence of night blindness (1.1%) was lower than Bitot spots (1.9%) in 1–5 year old children. A noteworthy observation was the absence of Bitot spots in infancy, even in slums, in the surveys conducted in the 1990s. In the baseline survey,[45] it was reported that only 22.8% of children 0.5 to five years of age had received at least one dose of vitamin A during the preceding one year. While 13.1% of children had received one dose, 9.7% had received two doses. There was a wide variation in the coverage of children in different states. The figures for one dose ranged from 1.9% in Gujarat and Uttar Pradesh to 55.2% in Karnataka. The coverage was below 25% in Kerala, Orissa and Uttar Pradesh.

Adolescent girls

In the NNMB 1994 rural survey,[6] overall 0.9% of adolescent girls (12–18 years old) had Bitot spots; the range being 0.6 to 2.7%. In four states no case of Bitot spot was observed in this age group. The overall prevalence in adult females was 0.7% (range 0% in Gujarat to 3.3% in Tamil Nadu). Only in two States (Tamil Nadu 3.3% and Madhya Pradesh 1%) were values above 0.3% documented.

Iron deficiency

Anaemia rates

Anaemia has been the most common parameter employed to determine iron deficiency. Over four decades ago, "primary" iron deficiency was heavily compounded by "secondary" iron deficiency induced by chronic malaria and hookworm infestation,[30] but these problems have been considerably mitigated since.[30] This is probably partly responsible for the personal experience of older Indian paediatricians and obstetricians who describe a dramatic decline of severe anaemia with oedema in children and women (pregnant and non-pregnant). A limited comparison of studies conducted in similar areas on comparable age and physiological groups at different time periods yielded two such series.[46–48] In Vadodra, there was a significant (p = 0.014) decline in the prevalence of anaemia (haemoglobin < 11 g/dl) from 71% (n = 500) to 65% (n = 610) between 1982–84 and 1993–94 in urban low-income preschool children.[48] In pregnant women from Hyderabad, possibly from different settings,[46,47] the prevalence of anaemia (haemoglobin less than 11 g/dl) significantly declined from 48.5% to 33.2%.

There is considerable information on haemoglobin levels in various age groups from hospital based studies, but this does not provide reliable estimates for populations. In most studies, women of childbearing age had the highest prevalence of anaemia, followed by preschool children, school children, and adult men.

Nationally representative estimates for the neonatal age group are not available. The generally cited figures for preschool children (53%) relate to the ICMR multicentric study[44] published in 1977. Children below the age of three years had a higher prevalence compared to older peers (63% vs. 44%). A later collaborative study (published in 1982) involving large numbers of rural children (1–6 years old) in Delhi, Calcutta and Hyderabad documented a prevalence of 64.8% with a staggering figure of 90% for Calcutta.[49] Similarly, estimates suggest that a great majority (nearly two-thirds, according to some data) of young adolescent girls aged 6–14 years are anaemic; and in a considerable proportion the anaemia is of a moderate or severe degree.[50] The ICMR multicentric "High Risk" study[25] on ever-married eligible women (13–49 years) recorded an anaemia (haemoglobin < 12 g/dl) prevalence of 82% in rural areas (n = 5,929) and 85% in urban slums (n = 7,371).

Available data from several large-scale surveys on urban and rural pregnant women from low-income groups in the early 1980s suggest the prevalence of anaemia in pregnancy (haemoglobin < 11 g/dl) was high with estimates of 40–50% in some urban areas, 50–70% in rural areas, to almost 90% in rural areas where hookworm infestation is endemic.[26] Estimates based on the ICMR evaluation in 1984–85 of the National Nutritional Anaemia Prophylaxis Programme indicate that 88% of pregnant women are anaemic with 47% having haemoglobin values below 9 g/dl.[51] The latest estimates pertaining to the ICMR multicentric field supplementation trial (published in 1992) on 1968 pregnant women have lowered these estimates to 62 and 17% respectively.[47] Anaemia prevalence figures above 90% were recorded in two of the six centres.

Iron supplementation

The National Nutritional Anaemia Prophylaxis Programme evaluation study[51] revealed a poor performance in all the states. The coverage of pregnant women with iron supplementation ranged from 3 to 26%. The number of children covered was negligible.

Iodine deficiency

Goiter has been recognised as an endemic problem in the Himalayan and sub-Himalayan region for the past century.[23] Surveys between 1945–53 in the sub-Himalayan belt, stretching from Kashmir in the north west to Nagaland in the east indicated a prevalence of goiter ranging from 26 to 90%.[52] Subsequent surveys conducted by several agencies and investigators indicated that not a single State or Union Territory was free from the problem of iodine deficiency disorders (IDD).[53] A variety of indicators have been recommended recently by international agencies[54] to quantify the magnitude of IDD including goiter, thyroid volume by ultrasound, iodine excretion, and thyroid stimulating hormone (TSH) in newborn blood. Children in the age group of 8–10 years (excluding TSH) are the recommended target population because of their combined high vulnerability, representativeness of the community, and easy accessibility.[54] However, nationally representative information in the country is primarily based on goiter prevalence surveys in the entire population, and occasionally on clinical evidence of cretinism which may be unreliable.

The effects of salt iodisation

An early intervention study initiated in 1954 showed an appreciable decline in the goiter prevalence rate following six years of iodisation of salt in Kangra Valley, Himachal Pradesh.[55] In Delhi, the goiter prevalence rate in school children declined from 55% in 1980[56] to 9% in 1996;[57] the salt iodisation programme was implemented in 1989. The routine surveys conducted by the Directorate General of Health Services[58] indicate a significant decline in total goiter prevalence rate in 17 out of 21 Districts from different states in which repeat information was available. The magnitude of decline ranged from 6 to 35% (values above 30% in the Himalayan region and Uttar Pradesh) for repeat surveys performed six to 40 years later. Time series data revealed a marked reduction in the incidence of neonatal chemical hypothyroidism (NCH) in highly endemic areas of Uttar Pradesh following salt iodisation.[59,60] The observed NCH rates in 1992–96 following salt iodisation are much lower than earlier projections in other areas also.[60]

The commonly cited[23,24] IDD prevalence figures pertain to the ICMR survey in 14 districts[61] which documented an overall goiter prevalence rate of 21% (range 12% in plains to 66% in the Himalayan region) and a cretinism prevalence rate of 0.7% (range 0.1% to 6.1%).

Universal salt iodisation has recently gained considerable momentum. In the NNMB 1994 rural survey,[6] the goiter prevalence rate (mostly grade 1) in adolescent girls was only 3.9% (documented in only three out of eight states). The corresponding figure for adult females was 2.8% and goiter was mostly seen in the States of Kerala, Karnataka, Madhya Pradesh and Orissa. The latest estimates from sample surveys conducted by the Directorate General of Health Services show 228 of the 367 surveyed districts in the country are IDD endemic (goiter prevalence > 10%). The reported rates of NCH from the few available studies prior to salt iodisation ranged from six to 133 per thousand births (Uttar Pradesh, Delhi, Mumbai, and Vishakapatnam). There was a strong correlation with goiter prevalence rates.[59]

Nutrient Intake

Feeding practices play a pivotal role in determining the nutritional status, morbidity and survival of infants, particularly in the neonatal period. Additionally, they influence maternal nutrition and fertility regulation. Traditionally, Indian society has practised prolonged breastfeeding, but recent reports indicate an erosion of this practice, especially in urban settings.[62–64]

Breastfeeding and supplementation

The recently (1992–93) conducted NFHS data provides nationally representative estimates on breastfeeding and supplementation based on 50,001 children born in the four years preceding the survey.[10] Fortunately, breastfeeding is still nearly universal in India, with 95% (92–99%) of all children having been breastfed. However, only 10% began breastfeeding within one hour of birth and a quarter within one day of birth (Table 4). A majority of women squeezed the first milk from the breast before commencing breastfeeding.[10]

Exclusive breastfeeding was quite common for very young children, but even at age 0–1 month more than one-third of babies were given water or other supplements. Overall, 51% of infants under four months were given only breastmilk, while 73% received predominant breastfeeding (only

Table 4 Breastfeeding and supplementation indicators.

Indicator	Percentage	Range (%)
Breastfeeding within one hour of birth*	10	3–64
Breastfeeding within one day of birth*	26	12–84
Discarding first milk#	64	44–93
Breastfed (any amount) at ages (months)		
12	88	–
24	57	–
36	28	–
47	14	–
Solid/mushy food in breastfed children at ages (months)		
12	68	–
24	89	–
36	89	–
47	97	–
Internationally recommended feeding indicators		
Children 0–3 months exclusively breastfed	51	3–74
Children 6–9 months receiving breastmilk and solid/mushy food	31	9–69
Children 12–15 months breastfed	88	53–98
Children 20–23 months breastfed	67	36–84
Last born children < 12 months bottle fed	14	7–67

*Among last born children only, (n = 38,457).

#Among last born children only; excludes Andhra Pradesh, Himachal Pradesh, Madhya Pradesh, Tamil Nadu and West Bengal, (n = 26,657).

The Table is based on NFHS data.[10]

additional plain water allowed). The overall median durations of exclusive and predominant breastfeeding were 1.4 months (range 0.4–4) and 4.7 months (range 0.5–7.5).

Use of formula milk

The use of infant formula was fortunately rare (less than 1% below two months; maximum 11% at nine months; and overall 6% of breastfeeding subjects under four years). Similarly, the use of bottles with nipples was relatively rare for breastfeeding children, increasing from 4% in the first month after birth to a high of 15% for children aged five to six months, after which it declined slowly to near zero for children approaching four years.

Weaning

Unfortunately, supplementation by solid or mushy food was grossly inadequate, showing a rise from only 17% at six months of age to 79% by age 15 months and a slower rise thereafter to more than 90% for children who were four years old. Even though 95% of infants aged six to nine months were breastfed, less than one-third received complementary semi-solid foods as recommended. Supplementation of breastmilk by other milk rose steadily with age to 46% at age eight months and remained fairly constant (at 45–55%) in most older age groups. Breastfeeding typically continued for long durations (Table 4). The overall median length of breastfeeding was slightly over two years (24.4 months; range 16.5–33.8 months).[10]

Regional variation

Interesting regional differentials emerged. Goa had extraordinarily high usage of feeding bottles (almost twice as high as any other region) and very poor achievement of the goals for duration and exclusivity of breastfeeding. Punjab, Jammu and Meghalya also had an exceptionally low proportion of children under the age of four months who were exclusively breastfed. Rajasthan, Bihar and Uttar Pradesh were the poorest performers for receiving complementary foods at the appropriate age. Some feeding problems were universal, however. No state came even close to achieving the recommendations for exclusive breastfeeding of children under four months or the supplementation of breastmilk with semi-solids at age six to nine months.[10] Both these factors, particularly the latter, are believed to be important factors contributing to the high prevalence of malnutrition.

General dietary intake

Comparative data is available from the NNMB 1975–79 and 1998–90 surveys[5] in which the nutrient intake was quantified in a proportion of sampled households by 24 hour recall and weighing. During this period, the household food security situation had hardly changed.[23] Similarly, there was little alteration in the overall intake of quantified nutrients during these 10–15 years.[24] However, the disaggregated data revealed that the energy intake of landless labourers belonging to the lowest income bracket had increased by 1.36 kcal per consumption unit (CPU) during this period. Further, the diets of preschool children also showed some improvement, resulting in enhanced energy intake: about 75 kcal in children from one to three years (from 834 to 908 kcal; RDI 1,240 kcal) and 140 kcal in the case of children in the four to six years age group (from 1,118 to 1,260; RDI 1,690 kcal).

According to the latest estimates, the diets provided adequate amounts of prostein (62 vs. 60 g/CU/day), calcium, iron, and thiamine, but the intake of other quantified nutrients (energy, vitamins A and C, and riboflavin) was below the recommended dietary intake (RDI) as laid out by the ICMR. Energy intake (2,280 kcal/CU) showed a marginal deficit while the maximum deficit was seen in vitamin A (350 vs. 600 mcg/CU).[23,24] There was a direct relationship between the level of energy consumption and protein consumption. This was expected considering that the main source of calories and of protein in the habitual diets of the poor is nearly the same — consisting of a single staple cereal with insignificant amount of fat (calorie-rich) and protein-rich food like pulses or meat.[12] Wide regional and socio-economic variations in nutrient intake are found. The urban poor have the least intake followed by rural and urban better-off populations respectively.[5,24]

Poor association between consumption and malnutrition

A striking finding was the lack of association in a given state between the average household calorie and protein consumption, and the prevalence of undernutrition in its children. Thus, the state which showed the best record (lowest prevalence) with respect to undernutrition in children, namely Kerala, was the poorest with respect to household food consumption. The state with a fairly poor record (Madhya Pradesh) showed the best figures for household food consumption (figures for household food consumption for Orissa were not available). This would suggest that either intra-family distribution of food was more unfavourable with respect to children in Madhya Pradesh, compared with Kerala, or that infections which contribute to malnutrition are more promptly and efficiently combated in Kerala.[12]

Intra-family distribution

Analysis of dietary data to assess intra-family distribution of food revealed that in 50% of the households surveyed, levels of energy adequacy did not differ between preschool children, adult men, and women. Either all of them were consuming adequate amounts (31% of households) or inadequate amounts (19% of households). In a quarter of households, the intake was adequate in adults but inadequate in children. Calorie inadequacy was documented in a greater proportion of children (60%) than adults (44%).[24]

No obvious gender bias was documented. When the intakes were corrected for requirements, the average calorie intake levels of women were close to 94% of their RDI as against 85% in men. This is contrary to the general belief that women get the least.[23]

Conclusion

Overall, the recent trend in nutritional outcomes of women, children, and newborn infants in India has been positive but modest, manifesting itself predominantly in a reduction of the more severe varieties of malnutrition. A favourable transition appears to have been initiated also in the less severe varieties of undernutrition, illustrated by slender improvements in anthropometry and birth weight, even amongst the poor. These encouraging observations in poor women and children, despite a steep increase in population and continued social and economic inequity, are indications that, at long last, India may be at the turning point with respect to nutrition.

A disconcerting aspect is the current magnitude of deficiencies in virtually all nutritional public health indicators, as assessed by conventional international definitions. The sub-optimal infant feeding practices, particularly in relation to exclusive breastfeeding and complementary feeding, also warrant urgent consideration.

The near total disappearance, within the last four decades, of florid nutritional deficiency diseases which were once major public health problems, and the initiation of a positive trend in the less severe forms of undernutrition, have important managerial implications. With the possible exception of iodine deficiency disorders, none of these changes can be credited to any effectively instituted specific nutritional intervention. These observations argue for an integrated rather than an isolated approach towards combating undernutrition. Before planning a vertical approach, evaluation of secular trends in the absence of any intervention and cost-effectiveness analysis for achieving additional benefit should be made.

References

1. Puri RK and Sachdev HPS, "Secular trends and determinants of under five mortality components in India: Implications for child survival strategies," Report Submitted to the Ministry of Health and Family Welfare under USAID Child Survival Programmes, September 1991.
2. Sethi GR, Sachdev HPS and Puri RK, "Women's health and fetal outcome," *Indian Pediatrics* **28** (1991): 1379–1393.
3. Gopalan C, "The changing profile of undernutrition in India," *Nutrition Foundation of India Bulletin* **12**(1) (1991): 1–5.
4. Bhattacharya AK, Chattopadhyay PS, Roy Paladhi PK, Ganguli S and Bhattacharyya N, "Kwashiorkor and Marasmus: Changing hospital incidence of syndromic presentation (1957–88)," *Indian Pediatrics* **27** (1990): 1191–1198.

5. National Nutrition Monitoring Bureau. Report of Repeat Surveys (1988–90). Hyderabad, National Institute of Nutrition (1991).
6. Nutritional Status of Rural Population: Report of NNMB Surveys. Hyderabad, National Nutrition Monitoring Bureau, National Institute of Nutrition (1996).
7. National Nutrition Monitoring Bureau. Report of Urban Survey — Slums (1993–94). Hyderabad, National Institute of Nutrition (1994).
8. WHO Working Group, "Use and interpretation of anthropometric indicators of nutritional status," *Bulletin of the World Health Organization* **64** (1986): 929–941.
9. National Nutrition Monitoring Bureau. Report for the Year 1979. Hyderabad, National Institute of Nutrition (1980).
10. National Family Health Survey: MCH and Family Planning. India 1992–93. Bombay, International Institute for Population Sciences (1995): 269–287.
11. Sachdev HPS, "Assessing child malnutrition: Some basic issues," *Nutrition Foundation of India Bulletin* **16**(4) (1995): 1–5.
12. Rai MK and Vailaya J, "The national nutrition scene: An analysis of the results of two national surveys," *Indian Pediatrics* **33** (1996): 305–312.
13. Gillespie S, "Child nutrition in India: Findings from the National Family Health Survey (1992–93)," *Nutrition Foundation of India Bulletin* **17**(1) (1996): 6–8.
14. Carlson BA and Wardlaw TM, "A global, regional and country assessment of child malnutrition," United Nations Children's Fund Staff Working Papers Number 7. New York, UNICEF (1990).
15. Agarwal DK and Agarwal KN, "Physical growth in Indian affluent children (birth–six years)," *Indian Pediatrics* **31** (1994): 377–413.
16. Kumar R, Aggarwal AK and Iyengar SD, "Nutritional status of children: Validity of mid-upper arm circumference for screening undernutrition," *Indian Pediatrics* **33** (1996): 189–196.
17. Kapoor S, Kapoor AK, Bhalla R and Singh IP, "Parent off-spring correlation for body measurements and subcutaneous fat distribution," *Human Biology* **57** (1985): 141–150.
18. Visweswara Rao K, Balakrishna N and Shatrugna V, "Secular trends in height of well to do adults and the associated factors," *Man in India* **73** (1993): 267–273.
19. Shatrugna V and Viswesvara Rao K, "Secular trends in heights of women from the urban poor community," *Annals of Human Biology* **14** (1987): 375–377.
20. National Institute of Nutrition, Annual Report 1986–87. Secular changes in heights of daughters as compared to their mothers. Hyderabad, National Institute of Nutrition (1987): p. 84.

21. National Institute of Nutrition, Annual Report 1987–88. Studies on adolescent girls. Hyderabad, National Institute of Nutrition (1988): p. 35.

22. Srikantia SG, "Pattern of growth and development of Indian girls and body size of adult Indian women," In: *Women and Nutrition in India*, eds. Gopalan C and Kaur S, New Delhi, Nutrition Foundation of India, Special Publication Series 5 (1989): 108–152.

23. Reddy V, Shekar M, Rao P and Gillespie S, "Nutrition in India," Hyderabad, National Institute of Nutrition (1992).

24. Reddy V, Pralhad Rao N, Gowrinath Sastry J and Kashinath K, "Nutrition trends in India," Hyderabad, National Institute of Nutrition (1993).

25. Bhargava SK, Singh KK and Saxena BN, "A national collaborative study of identification of high risk families, mothers and outcome of their offsprings with particular reference to the problem of maternal nutrition, low birth weight, perinatal and infant morbidity and mortality in rural and urban slum communities," A Task Force Study. New Delhi, Indian Council of Medical Research (1990).

26. Ramachandran P, "Nutrition in p regnancy," In: *Women and Nutrition in India*, eds. Gopalan C and Kaur S, New Delhi, Nutrition Foundation of India, Special Publication Series 5 (1989): 153–193.

27. Gopalan C and Vijayaraghavan K, "Nutrition atlas of India," Hyderabad, National Institute of Nutrition (1969).

28. Gopalan C and Vijayaraghavan K, "Nutrition atlas of India, "Hyderabad, National Institute of Nutrition (1971).

29. Bhargava SK, Sachdev HPS, Iyer PU and Ramji S, "Current status of infant growth measurements in the perinatal period in India," *Acta Paediatrica Scandinavia* **319**(Suppl) (1985): 103–110.

30. Gopalan C, "Nutrition research in South-East Asia: The emerging agenda for the future," New Delhi, World Health Organization — Regional Office for South East Asia (1994).

31. Satpathy R, Das DB, Bhuyan BK, Pant KC and Santhanam S, "Secular trend in birth weight in an industrial hospital in India," *Annals of Tropical Paediatrics* **10** (1990): 21–25.

32. Man M, Shiv Prasad SR, Chellani HK and Kapani V, "Intrauterine growth curves in north Indian babies: Weight, length, head circumference and ponderal index," *Indian Pediatrics* **27** (1990): 43–51.

33. Singhal PK, Paul VK, Deorari AK, Singh M and Sundaram KR, "Changing trends in intrauterine growth curves," *Indian Pediatrics* **28** (1991): 281–283.

34. "Trends in intrauterine growth of single live borns during 1969–73 and 1989–93 among rural and urban communities of North Arcot Ambedkar District, Tamil Nadu, India. Longitudinal Studies in Growth and Development," Monograph No. 21. Department of Biostatistics, Christian Medical College, Vellore.

35. Mathai M, "Changes in health status and birthweight in Vellore over 25 years (1969–1994)," Paper presented at Workshop on "Health in Transition" in Norway, May 1995. *Personal communication* (1995).

36. Fernandez AR, "Changes in birthweight and gestation patterns in Sion, Mumbai," *Personal communication* (1996).

37. Ramji S, "Changes in birthweight and gestation patterns in Delhi," *Personal communication* (1997).

38. National Neonatal Perinatal Data Base: Report for the Year 1995. National Neonatology Forum Secretariat and National Neonatal Perinatal Database Nodal Centre, Department of Pediatrics, All India Institute of Medical Sciences, New Delhi (1996).

39. Ramji S, "Birth weight in Child Survival and Safe Motherhood Programme Districts," *Personal communication* (1997).

40. Bhargava SK and Ghosh S, "Nomenclature for newborns," *Indian Pediatrics* **11** (1974): 445–447.

41. Gopalan C, "Vitamin A and child mortality — Now the Nepal study," *Nutrition Foundation of India Bulletin* **13**(1) (1992): 6–7.

42. Gopalan C, "Vitamin A and vaccination," *Nutrition Foundation of India Bulletin* **16**(4) (1995): 6–8.

43. Underwood BA, "Maternal vitamin A status and its importance in infancy and early childhood," *American Journal of Clinical Nutrition* **59**(Suppl) (1994): 517S–524S.

44. Studies on Preschool Children. Report of the Working Group of Indian Council of Medical Research. New Delhi, ICMR Technical Report Series No. 26 (1977).

45. Vijayaraghavan K, Brahmam GNV, Reddy G and Reddy V, "Linking periodic dosing of vitamin A with universal immunization programme — An evaluation," Hyderabad, National Institute of Nutrition (1996).

46. Prema K, Neelakumari S and Ramalakshmi BA, "Anemia and adverse obstetric outcome," *Nutrition Report International* **23** (1981): 637–648.

47. "Field supplementation trial in pregnant women with 60 mg, 120 mg and 180 mg of iron with 500 mcg of folic acid," Indian Council of Medical Research Task Force Study, New Delhi, ICMR (1992).

48. Seshadri S, "Change in prevalence of anemia in urban low income preschool children in Vadodra," *Personal communication* (1997).

49. Report of the Working Group on Fortification of Salt With Iron, "Use of common salt fortified with iron in the control and prevention of anemia — A collaborative study," *American Journal of Clinical Nutrition* **35** (1982): 1442–1451.

50. Gopalan C, "Nutrition in developmental transition in South East Asia," World Health Organization, Regional Office for South East Asia, Regional Health Paper, SEARO, No. 21 (1992).

51. "Evaluation of National Nutritional Anemia Prophylaxis Programme," New Delhi, Indian Council of Medical Research (1989).

52. "Epidemiological study of endemic goiter and endemic cretinism: An ICMR Task Force study," New Delhi, Indian Council of Medical Research (1981).

53. Gopalan C, "The National Goiter Control Programme — A sad story, In: *Combating Undernutrition: Basic Issues and Practical Approaches*, Nutrition Foundation of India Special Publication Series 3. ed. Gopalan C, New Delhi, Nutrition Foundation of India (1989): 329–333.

54. "Indicators for Assessing Iodine Deficiency Disorders and their Control Through Salt Iodisation," WHO-UNICEF-ICCIDD, Geneva, World Health Organization (1994).

55. Sooch SS, Deo MG, Karmarkar MG, Kochupillai N, Ramachandran K and Ramalingaswami V, "Prevention of endemic goiter with iodised salt," *Bulletin of the World Health Organization* **49** (1993): 307–312.

56. Pandav CS, Kochupillai N, Karmarkar MG, Ramachandran K, Gopinath PG and Nath LM, "Endemic goiter in Delhi," *Indian Journal of Medical Research* **72** (1980): 81–82.

57. Kapil U, Saxena N, Ramachandran S, Balamurugan A, Nayar D and Prakash S, "Assessment of iodine deficiency disorders using the 30 cluster approach in the National Capital Territory of Delhi," *Indian Pediatrics* **33** (1996): 1013–1017.

58. Unpublished reports of the All India Goiter Prevalence Surveys conducted by the Directorate General of Health Services, Ministry of Health and Family Welfare, Government of India (1956–1996).

59. Kochupillai N, "Neonatal chemical hypothyroidism of nutritional origin: A major public health problem that impairs growth in developing countries," In: *Recent Trends in Nutrition*, ed. Gopalan C, Oxford University Press (1993): 181–193.

60. Kochupillai N, "Micronutrient deficiency and human health and development," Srikantia Memorial Lecture at the XXIX Annual Meeting of the Nutrition Society of India, Hyderabad November 21–22, 1996 (unpublished data).

61. Indian Council of Medical Research, "Epidemiological survey of endemic goiter and cretinism: An ICMR Task Force study," New Delhi, Indian Council of Medical Research (1989).
62. Walia BNS, Gambhir SK, Sroa SR and Choudhary S, "Decline in breastfeeding in urban population of Chandigarh during a decade," *Indian Pediatrics* **24** (1987): 879–887.
63. Gopalan C, "Infant feeding practices," Nutrition Foundation of India, Scientific Report No. 4. New Delhi, Nutrition Foundation of India (1984): 31–38.
64. Kapil U, Sachdev HPS, Verma D, Narula S, Shah AD, Nayar D and Gnanasekaran N, "Study of breastfeeding and weaning practices with special reference to use of commercial weaning foods and nutritional status of children amongst scheduled caste communities in Haryana," Report submitted to the Indian Council of Medical Research (1993).

Commentary

MATERNAL NUTRITION AND HEALTH OF THE NEWBORN

Ramesh K. Adhikari
Reader in Paediatrics and Child Health,
Institute of Medicine, Tribhuvan University, Kathmandu

Foetal Growth

Various genetic and environmental factors determine foetal growth. Persistent deficiency of nutrients during intrauterine life will limit the ability of the foetus to reach the growth potential and severe, prolonged deficiency will threaten its survival.[1] According to Winick,[2] there are three phases of foetal growth: a phase of cellular hyperplasia followed by a phase of cellular hyperplasia combined with cellular hypertrophy, and the final phase of cellular hypertrophy alone. A deficiency of nutrients in the early phase of pregnancy will result in decreased numbers of cells whereas a late nutritional insult will result in reduction of cell size with normal number of cells. This explains the occurrence of symmetrically and asymmetrically growth-retarded neonates in chronically and acutely undernourished mothers respectively.

Many women in developing countries, particularly in South-East Asia suffer from chronic undernutrition. This is reflected in their low postpartum weights and heights (Table 1).

The poor nutritional status of the mothers also shows a direct relationship with a high incidence of low birth weight (LBW) babies in these countries (Table 1). In short, growth-retarded mothers deliver growth retarded babies.[3]

Table 1 Weights, heights and LBW rates of postpartum mothers in South East Asian countries.

Country	Weight in kg (SD)	Height in cm (SD)	LBW (%)
India	42.1 (4)	150 (5)	28.2 (n = 4,307)
Indonesia	46.0 (6)	149 (4)	10.5 (n = 1,647)
Myanmar	46.9 (8)	151 (5)	17.8 (n = 3,582)
Nepal (rural)	43.0 (5)	150 (5)	14.3 (n = 2,529)
Nepal (urban)	44.6 (6)	150 (5)	22.3 (n = 3,629)
Sri Lanka	43.5 (7)	150 (5)	18.4 (n = 1,851)
Thailand	49.9 (7)	153 (5)	9.6 (n = 4,124)

Source: Report of the WHO expert committee on the anthropometry for women during the reproductive cycle and the newborn infant, 1993. (NB: More recent data suggests the LBW estimates for Nepal in this Table to be too low. See Chapter 2.)

Interventions to Reduce LBW?

Is there a place for intervention? Does supplemental feeding of pregnant mothers improve birth weight? Different studies have shown conflicting results. Venkatachalam, Gopalan, Srikantia and Leela Iyengar, and Bhatnagar (all from India), and Krasid Tontisirin from Thailand[4] have reported a significant positive impact of nutritional supplementation on birth weight. However, Kradjati *et al.* from Indonesia, Blackwell from Taiwan, and Adams *et al.* and Rush *et al.* from USA have shown no difference in the maternal weight gain during pregnancy or any improvement in the birth weight in the populations they studied.[4]

One explanation of this difference is the variation in the habitual food intake in the different groups: the study population in India and Thailand were malnourished with dietary intakes lower than the recommended daily allowances, whereas other groups studied were well nourished and had a habitually better dietary intake.

Most studies provide extra food to increase the energy and protein intake. However, in a separate study Leela Iyengar from India[4] has shown that while iron supplementation alone during pregnancy did not show significant improvement in the birth weight of infants, iron and folate supplementation did bring about a significant increase of 200 g. We might conclude therefore that food supplementation during pregnancy is beneficial only in those mothers whose diets are poor or marginally adequate, and iron and folate supplementation alone may also be helpful in lowering the prevalence of LBW infants in poorly nourished communities.

Adaptive mechanisms

It appears that adaptive mechanisms like a reduction in maternal basal metabolic rate (BMR) and increased efficiency of nutrient utilisation in pregnancy maximise essential substrates for foetal growth in well nourished mothers if they face a short period of food scarcity. However, these mechanisms do *not* operate if

- the mother is already malnourished;
- there is reduction in the dietary intake from the prepregnancy level;
- the energy expenditure is above the habitual level;
- the pregnancy has occurred during adolescence;
- pregnancy has occurred during lactation; or
- the interpregnancy interval is less than two years.

Apparently, a threshold level exists for maternal nutrition below which foetal size and nutrition are affected but above which no beneficial effect of food supplementation can be expected.[6]

In the context of South Asian countries, issues in relation to maternal nutrition go beyond food intake and encompass broader socio-economic disadvantage (see Chapter 3).

The Effect of Adolescent Pregnancy

Various studies have shown that adolescence provides women with a second opportunity to grow to reach their ultimate potential.[7] However, the puberty-induced growth can be interfered with by early marriage and teenage pregnancy. In South Asian countries like Nepal and India the average age for marriage is 15.8 and 16.7 years respectively. The prevalence of teenage pregnancy is also high: data from the main maternity hospital in Kathmandu showed that 18% of mothers admitted for delivery were below 19 years of age. Another important factor is excessive burden of work on women (see Chapter 5). Many studies in Nepal have shown that women in all age groups work more than men, their work burden increases with age and the work burden is highest in the mountains, followed by the midhills and the plains.[7]

Future Policy Interventions

What are the options for future intervention? Stunting in the present generation of mothers cannot be corrected but future generations might be protected by improving the dietary intake combined with a decreased workload during pregnancy. The stunting of mothers might be improved with better nutritional status of adolescent girls: important steps in that direction would be to delay adolescent marriages and to improve opportunities for female education, but these are policies which are slow to get into practice. The strategies to lower the incidence of LBW babies, to improve childhood stunting, and to improve the status of female children will need a multisectoral approach for a long time. In the short term, strategies to improve dietary intake (at least in the last trimester of pregnancy) and to decrease the work burden need to be stressed. Leela Iyengar's study showing a positive impact of supplementation with iron and folates probably shows a less difficult approach for dietary intervention.

Further research

There are a large number of unanswered questions to be addressed:

- Why are there differences in the prevalence of LBW infants in countries with a similar socio-economic situation?
- What is the relationship between folate intake and the incidence of LBW?

- Which strategies will improve dietary intake during pregnancy cost effectively?
- How can the growth of adolescent girls be improved by increasing food intake, reducing work burden, or delaying marriages?
- How can comprehensive policies under existing government programmes be implemented more effectively and sustainably?

References

1. Arias F, "Fetal growth retardation," In: *Practical Guide to High Risk Pregnancy and Delivery*. 2nd ed. Mosby Year Book, St.Louis (1991): p. 301.
2. Wiwick M, "Cellular changes during placental and fetal growth," *American Journal of Obstetrics and Gynecology* **109** (1971): p. 166.
3. Luke B, "Nutritional influences of foetal growth," *Clinical Obstetrics and Gynecology* **37**(3): p. 1004, 538–545.
4. Gopalan C, "Nutrition research in South East Asia," *WHO Regional Publ.* No. 23, South East Asia Regional Office, New Delhi (1994).
5. Kardjati S, "Energy supplementation in last trimester of pregnancy in East Java: I. Effect on birth weight," *British Journal of Obstetrics and Gynaecology* **95** (1988): 783–794.
6. Soundararaghavan S, "Effects of maternal nutrition on the foetus," *Souvenir 16th Annual Convention of National Neonatology Forum of India*, Chandigarh, India (1996).
7. Regmi S and Adhikari R, "A study of factors influencing the nutritional status of adolescent girls in Nepal," International Centre for Research on Women, Washington DC, May 1994.

Chapter 5

WOMEN'S WORK AND MATERNAL–CHILD HEALTH: ANTHROPOLOGICAL VIEWS ON INTERVENTION

Catherine Panter-Brick
Reader in Anthropology, Durham University, UK

Introduction

An important health issue: Women's work during the childbearing period

In many societies of the developing world, women continue to work throughout pregnancy and soon after delivery. Jimenez and Newton made this point forcefully using data from an ethnographic survey of 202 societies, showing that mothers usually resumed their habitual tasks at two weeks postpartum.[1] Few of us need to be convinced that heavy workloads during the childbearing period constitute an important health issue for women in many parts of the world. But how much work do women actually do, what opportunity exists for a significant reduction of physical activity during pregnancy or lactation, and what health outcomes are observed for women and their newborn children? This chapter addresses questions which centre on the relationships between women's work and the nutritional status of mothers and young infants.

135

Physical activity levels and energy requirements

Gathering data on physical activity levels is particularly important as this crucially affects officially accepted notions of extra nutritional requirements for women during the childbearing period. There is general agreement that the energy costs of pregnancy are set to an additional 1,300 kJ/day (300 kcal), if a woman gains the 10–12 kg deemed compatible with a favourable pregnancy outcome, while the costs of lactation are an extra 2,100 kJ/day (500 kcal), if she produces 850 ml/d of breastmilk in the first three months postpartum.[2,3] Additional requirements for protein (30 g/day during pregnancy on top of the 0.8 g per kg body weight baseline) and micronutrients have also been recommended. The FAO/WHO/UNU,[3] however, noted that the notion of extra energy requirements during pregnancy and lactation would be negated if a woman substantially reduced her physical activity.

General awareness that many poor women in the developing world undertake substantial work during their lifetime, even while childbearing, led to a call for more precise quantitative data to document both actual levels of women's physical activity and their specific impact on maternal–child health.[4] Indeed, poor women in the developing world present a challenge to the official view based on calculations of extra nutritional requirements. Rarely do they consume extra or better food, and hardly ever do they gain much weight during pregnancy (usually less than 8 kg, although women may even lose weight when pregnant during a rainy season, as in rural Gambia.[5] Often they lactate for two or three years postpartum without adopting significantly improved diets or reduced activity. In brief, pregnant and lactating women subsist on inadequate intakes, and yet manage reasonably successful reproductive outcomes.

In the words of Rajalakshmi, "the poor woman in India and in many similar countries lives on a diet providing 1,600 kcal/day or less and does not appreciably increase her intake during pregnancy and lactation… In spite of this she achieves a satisfactory weight gain of about 7 kg during pregnancy, produces a reasonably healthy infant weighing on an average 2.6–3 kg and nurses the infant with remarkable success for at least four to five months of life producing on average 700–750 ml of milk. The composition of this milk compares with that of upper class and western women... She often manages all this through several successive parities without a decline of her performance and without losing weight in the process. In fact, the birth weight of the infant is found to increase slightly till the fifth or sixth parity in a number of studies" (Ref. 6, pp. 187–188). While this statement reflects concern with undernutrition rather than heavy physical activity, and food intakes are notoriously prone to be underestimated, the capacity for women to reproduce "against the odds" — as appropriately phased by Prentice and Prentice[7] — is nothing short of remarkable. While this is indicative of the human ability to cope with nutritional stress, it nonetheless calls for efforts to improve the lives of women faced with these difficult situations.

It is widely believed that a reduction in habitual activity is the major means of meeting the "extra" costs of pregnancy and lactation.[8] The issue of how much work women actually do during the childbearing period is thus clearly important, given the expectation that, whenever possible, they will minimise their workloads. But given powerful environmental and socio-economic constraints, are mothers always able to significantly curtail their economic activities? Here I wish to focus attention on poor subsistence societies where women cannot afford to cut back their work outside the home whilst childbearing.

An anthropological contribution

I present here the results of anthropological research on the lives of women, rather than clinical evidence obtained from maternity centres. Anthropology focusses on field situations, rather than clinical settings, to document "what really happens out there", namely the importance of environmental constraints, the nature of coping strategies, and the range of health outcomes. It also presents an integrated perspective on women's lives, bridging demographic, nutritional and epidemiological information with detailed observation on actual behaviour in a local setting. Last but not least, anthropologists also make room for people's "voices", showing how "inside" perspectives on work, health and childbearing may impact on the success or failure of possible "outside" interventions.

Women's Work in Rural Areas

Levels of work and seasonality

This section focusses on agrarian subsistence communities, paying particular attention to how levels of physical activity vary with seasonality. Monsoon seasonality is particularly important for South Asia, generating variation in food variety, quality and intake, time for meal preparation, economic work and childcare, as well as energy spent in habitual tasks. There are also changes in body weight and composition, timing of births, wage rates, and employment opportunities that profoundly affect the lifestyles of local populations.

Women in rural areas of developing countries generally sustain moderate to very heavy workloads. A number of studies can be quoted to illustrate this point.[48] Over the last 15 years, for instance, I have conducted research in a relatively isolated Himalayan village, without health post, roads, or electricity. The community is characterised by demanding workloads rather than limited food availability: each year, people plant and harvest five main crops on fields terraced from 1,350 to 2,500 m. Women are actively involved in all aspects of the economy. The monsoon rains (July–September receive three-quarters of a staggering 4 m/year rainfall) trigger an increase in workloads to plant rain-fed millet and irrigated paddy rice, and this periodic seasonal stress helps to draw a contrast between times of very hard work and times of respite from intense activity. A detailed time-allocation study (assembling a total of 5,280 hours of minute-by-minute observation on work patterns over a calendar year) was coupled with measures of energy intake and expenditure. I also appraised variation in health and well-being with anthropometric data on child growth and adult nutritional status, records of mortality and morbidity, blood and saliva samples to estimate physiological status and stress reactivity, and steroid hormones to measure reproductive ability.[9–12]

In this community, women spend 6.4 hours in the winter in outdoor subsistence activities and 8.2 hours in the monsoon, devoting 41% and 62% of this time to agricultural work in the respective seasons. In terms of total energy expenditure (TEE), women achieve a work output of 9.1 MJ/d in the winter and 10.5 MJ/d in the monsoon (an increase of 15% above the already high winter baseline). By comparison, men expend 11.8 MJ/d and 13.9 MJ/d in the two seasons. These TEE values are among the highest reported for rural populations in the developing world. In a rural farming community of South India, TEE were reported as 8.3 MJ/d for non-pregnant, non-lactating and lactating women and 12.0 MJ/d for men;[13] seasonal variation in TEE was not tabulated, and activity measurements were based on 24-hour recall — not direct observation. Other studies in South India have not tabulated data (e.g. Bangladesh[14]) or have not included women (e.g. Burma[15]).

Physical activity levels

Current international conventions[3] broadly classify physical activity levels (PAL) into three categories: light (office clerk), moderate (susbsistence farmer), and heavy (not specified). They recommend expressing PAL as a ratio of energy (for undertaking activity) over basal metabolic rate (energy for sustaining life, as predicted from sex, age, and body weight). The conventions specify sex-specific cut-off points (for reasons which remain obscure[12]) — for women: PAL of 1.56, 1.64 1.82, and for men: PAL of 1.55, 1.78 and 2.1 denote light, moderate and heavy work respectively.

Figure 1 shows examples of studies which have graded subsistence workloads in terms of PAL, following international conventions, for the year overall or for contrasting seasons, and for both men and women. The impact of seasonality is clearly important. Thus, in Nepal, women sustain moderately heavy (1.77) workloads in winter and very heavy (2.01) workloads in the monsoon. In South India, seasonal variation was especially marked for women between post-harvest (winter) and pre-harvest (summer) times, and furthermore dependent on socio-economic status: over the year as a whole, PAL was heavy (1.96) for men and moderate (1.69) for women.[16]

Interestingly, the workload of women is actually less than men's in Nepal and India, in contrast with the situation often reported for Africa (here illustrated by the Gambia). There are communities in South or South-East Asia in which women work more than men — Nag *et al.*[17] reported that rural Javanese women worked an average 11 hours a day, almost 2.5 hours

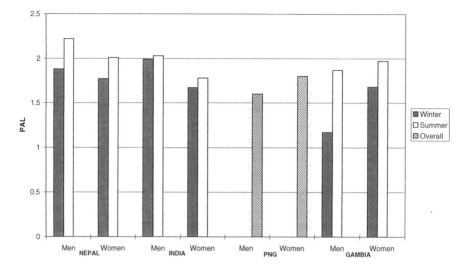

Figure 1 Seasonal variation in physical activity levels for men and women in rural Nepal,[11] South India,[16] highland Papua New Guinea and the Gambia.[19]

more than men. Often however, women sustain heavy workloads not because they alone shoulder the most important agricultural tasks, but because the whole household eeks a living at subsistence level.

It is also important to note, as I have shown elsewhere in the case of the Nepali community,[12] that the back-breaking work of farming rather marginal land results from working very long hours in subsistence activity, rather than shouldering tasks that entail particularly heavy energy expenditure. Thus, when travelling on uneven terrain, farming and carrying heavy loads (up to 130% body weight), men and women pace themselves in order to sustain a work schedule that demands endurance rather than intense speed, avoiding fatigue rather than maximising short-term productivity. Gender differences and seasonal increases in workloads also result from the length of time spent in food production, rather than the heavy nature of work *per se*. This has implication for intervention programmes which aim to reduce overall workload: it is wise to alleviate those tasks which require not just intense effort, but substantial time investments.

Working behaviour during the childbearing period

To what extent do women reduce their workloads when pregnant or lactating? In general, women will decrease optional tasks but not essential subsistence activity. In Nepal, I found that seasonality profoundly constrained modifications of behaviour during the childbearing period. While in winter months pregnant and lactating mothers did reduce their workload, no significant differences of time and energy investments were observed during the monsoon, when urgent agricultural work must take place.[9] Physical activity levels averaged 1.89 for non-pregnant, non-lactating women, 1.72 for (third-trimester) pregnant, and 1.58 for lactating (1–35 months) women in late winter months; 2.01, 1.90 and 1.94 for women respectively in the monsoon (Figure 2). In the winter, PAL are significantly reduced by 9% for pregnant women, and by 16% for lactating women, relative to the NPNL baseline. In the monsoon, the differences are minimal (4–5%).

These mothers carried their infants to the workplace, and absorbed normal childcare responsibilities in the time normally allocated for rest during the work schedule. While other women stood or sat to rest and smoke in the fields, lactating women settled to breastfeed: nursing accounted for only ten

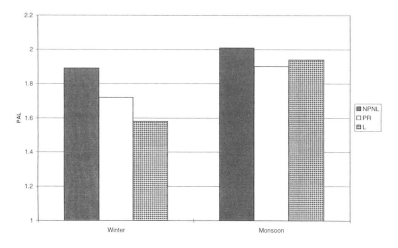

Figure 2 Physical activity levels of non-pregnant, non-lactating (NPNL), pregnant (PR) and lactating (L) rural Nepali women at two contrasting times of the year.[9]

minutes extra rest time per working hour, representing the degree of a child's interference during monsoon agricultural work.[12] Reductions in physical activity levels will obviously depend upon the stage of pregnancy and lactation. In rural Gambia, for example, women reduce physical activity by 25% in the last term of pregnancy. Again, this is achieved through curtailing time for non-essential housework and leisure, and a tendency to go less often to the fields, not through curtailing time actually working in the fields.[18] Maternal workloads are also reduced immediately after postpartum, but by three months women return to very heavy levels habitually sustained.[19]

Changes in activity may well also be modulated by household composition and parity, according to the availability of alternative caretakers. While few quantitative data document this point, in highland Papua New Guinea a reduction in energy expenditure was reported in the last three months of pregnancy and in the first six months of lactation, especially in the case of the first child.[20-25] In Nepal, seasonality was a much more powerful constraint on levels of physical activity than a woman's age, household composition, socio-economic status, or for that matter, current childbearing experience. While in South India, where more pronounced wealth stratification existed, PAL did vary with socio-economic status, interactions between socio-economic and childbearing status were not reported.[16]

In brief, decreased levels of physical activity during late pregnancy and early lactation may result in energy savings of about 15%,[5] as reported in rural South India,[21] Nepal[9] and the Gambia.[19] McNeill and Payne[21] seemed satisfied with changes of this magnitude, but in my opinion, this achieves a rather modest reduction in workload, which generally occurs for a limited period immediately before and after birth, and which does not benefit women during the season of peak workload.

Work and Maternal Nutritional Status

It is reasonable, therefore, to expect that the relationship between work output and maternal nutritional status might be modulated by seasonality. Possibly the most comprehensive investigation of such relationships was undertaken in rural Gambia. It was shown that women were faced with tight energy constraints, and that seasonality profoundly affected their nutritional status and reproductive performance, as well as birth weights and subsequent childhood morbidity and mortality.[5,7,22] In rural Bangladesh also, significant seasonal variations in women's workload (indexed by self-reported participation in crop-processing) and maternal–child anthropometric status were noted, particularly among landless families.[14] By contrast, in South India, climatic and workload seasonality made no actual impact on changes in body weight or body fat changes for either men or women.[16]

Changes in body weight

A recent overview of the literature on nutritional seasonality in the rural developing world noted rather modest changes in adult body weight (within a 5% margin), generally less pronounced for women than for men, and less marked for thinner than heavier individuals.[23] In Nepal, I also recorded rather suprisingly small changes in body weight, given the mismatch of peak workloads (July–August) and energy intakes (December). Seasonally, women lost only 0.2 kg (0.3% of initial weight) while men lost about one kg (2% of initial weight), over the four years of anthropometric measurements.[12] But these averages mask large individual variation: thin men and women could gain weight throughout the year, while heavy individuals show marked weight fluctuations before and after the monsoon. These observations could be related to work patterns: workload seasonality is more pronounced for men than for women, and thin individuals maintain high workloads throughout the year, while the activity of heavy individuals fluctuates by 23%. Here, behavioural options at times of relative leisure are particularly important: in the winter, people could undertake low-cost activities such as herding cattle, thereby having access to nutritious milk and an opportunity for weight gain (at least until the urgent agricultural work during the monsoon).

By implication, one should perhaps focus on the lifestyle of communities at times of relative leisure, rather than on nutritional vulnerabilities at times of intense workloads. One is perhaps neglecting scope for interventions at less constraining times of the year, which would help make nutritional stress a seasonally transient rather than chronic phenomenon.

Reproductive ability

Even very modest changes in body weight, however, have significant impact on women's reproductive ability.[48] In the Nepali community, there was a strong association between seasonal weight change and suppression of ovulation for healthy, normally menstruating women. A loss of just 1 kg (2% of inital weight) entailed suppressed ovulation in the monsoon relative to winter, as measured by a drop in progesterone levels, assayed from saliva samples collected through-out a menstrual month. Changes in body weight, not thinness *per se*, governed this striking relationship, corroborating recent findings for Western women undergoing even moderate physical exercise.[5,24,25] These are modest and reversible changes in female reproductive function, which help space births in condition of negative energy balance.[9] Fecundity is thus sensitive to seasonality, and in particular to small losses of maternal body weight that signal unfavourable conditions and potentially poor reproductive outcome. In Nepal, the impact of temporary infecundability was detected on actual fertility: conception rates dipped in the month of August, following weight loss at the beginning of the monsoon season.

As noted by Palmer,[26] seasonal changes in women's workloads may well produce "a seasonality in advanced pregnancy and birth dates which is irrational from the point of view of women's health and infant survival" (Ref. 26, p. 41). The impact of workload can be mediated either through losses of body weight, as detailed above, or through early weaning of nursing infants, as documented for Bangladesh — but not Nepal. In Bangladesh, births peak at times of heavy workloads. In Nepal, more women become pregnant immediately after the monsoon, and births peak at the next monsoon, when women experience very heavy workloads also.[27]

Dimensions of vulnerability

Obviously, women who suffer from chronic energy deficiency are thought to be at greater risk of unfavourable health outcomes. A simple index of vulnerability, now adopted by international organisations, is low Body Mass Index (BMI = weight/height^2), defined for women as 18.5 kg/m^2. Significant mortality, morbidity, and low work capacity are associated with low BMI or large weight losses (10% of inital values) *per se*. Individuals with low BMI (e.g. in South Asia, a woman whose weight is 38 kg and height 1.44 m) are considered especially vulnerable to seasonal stress.[28,29] In a study of foetal outcome for poor and well nourished rural Indian women, however, a maternal pre-pregnancy weight less than 40 kg, a pregnancy gain less than 5 kg, and mid-upper arm circumference under 23 cm, were found to predict the risk of low birthweight better than simple BMI.[30]

Severe anaemia, which is so prevalent for women in South Asia, has an important impact on work productivity, as well as on birth weights and newborn immunity.[31] Blood haemoglobin less than 9–10 g/dl was identified as one of the "disturbing features" in the reproductive performance of poor Indian women, along with poor pregnancy weight gain.[6] In Nepal, I found women with haemoglobin less than 6 g/dl undertaking habitual subsistence tasks, including load-bearing. It is the moderate pace of work which ensures that anaemic individuals can undertake even moderately heavy tasks, frequent pauses allowing time for recovery from elevated heart rates.

Work and Newborn Infant Nutritional Health

Newborn infant prospects

While one might reasonably expect a direct relationship between maternal levels of physical activity and newborn health (particularly birth weights), few studies have addressed this question with necessary rigour: there are a host of potentially confounding factors, such as poor maternal nutrition, which couple with high workloads. Barnes *et al.*[32] reviewed the available literature (mostly of working women in the developed world), listing six studies which found that physical activity prejudiced birth weight and/or gestational age, and four other studies which found no such effect (p. 163). The authors go on to clarify the pathways through which specific components of physical activity might affect pregnancy outcomes (Figure 3), namely posture, energy expenditure, and physical exertion. These three dimensions of physical activity, and their impact on newborn health, were recorded for

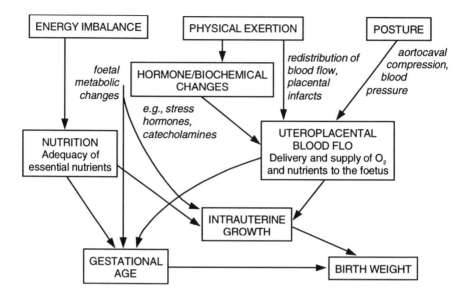

Figure 3 Pathways through which components of physical activity may affect the outcomes of pregnancy. Reprinted with permission, Barnes *et al.* (1991).

three groups of urban Filipino women, who were waged outside the home, generated an income at home, or were economically inactive. There were no differences in birth weight among all three groups, yet among housewives, posture did negatively affect birth weight (by 121 g) for those who completed upright more than half their domestic tasks. As well as standing, these women were frequently squatting, which is thought to restrict blood flow to the placenta. Somewhat unexpectedly, the study also found a strong, positive relationship between total energy expenditure and birth weights, possibly indicating that the hard-working mothers were in fact the most healthy, physically fit women.

One of the rare studies focussing on women in the developing world to determine whether strenuous work during pregnancy affected foetal growth was undertaken in Ethiopia.[33] This was a clinic based study, where women were simply asked to report on levels of physical activity (hard work or light) and whether or not they had access to domestic help. Hard-working pregnant women had smaller pregnancy weight gains, irrespective of final birth weights.

Undernourished women, who kept to lower levels of physical activity, did not show foetal growth retardation. The study concluded that the effects of a poor diet, known to affect foetal growth, were compounded by heavy physical work during pregnancy, possibly via nutrient utilisation and oxygen debt.

Another study was undertaken in a maternity centre in Senegal.[34,35] Two separate indicators, newborn stunting (body size/head circumference) and foetal wasting (weight/body length), were examined in relation to maternal nutritional status, as measured by maternal mid upper arm circumference. Here, maternal nutritional status was not responsible for foetal growth retardation, as indexed by stunting. The author suggested that since women worked extremely hard throughout pregnancy, long hours spent upright restricted placental blood flow, entailing insufficient supply of nutrients to the growing foetus.

There are no corresponding studies of rural women undertaken in "the field", rather than maternity centres, that examine workload *per se* and pregnancy outcome. In a study of high altitude Ladhakis in India, birth weights were significantly related to maternal characteristics, such as parity, age and weight.[36] In this study, activity patterns (self-reported changes in activity relative to pre-pregnancy) also seemed to play an important role, in that women who worked more than usual had substantially smaller infants than those who worked less (independently of maternal weight). Here again an interaction between energy expenditure and inadequate nutrition was noted. However, all these variables explained only a small proportion of the observed variance in birth weights. While maternal age, parity and anthropometric status (weight, height, fat stores) have a positive impact on birth weight, these factors generally explain less than 18% of variation in birth weights.[37]

Early breastfeeding patterns

Another important issue concerns the impact of women's physical activity, not just on the newborn, but also on nutrition in the child's early life. In the case of Nepal, for example, does work away from home involve curtailed time for infant care? For young infants, I found no detrimental effects of maternal activity, as mothers carried along infants everywhere. Nursing times showed no seasonality, despite the increase in workload during the monsoon, as women nursed frequently during the times normally allocated for rest. Only when children became too cumbersome to carry — in their third year of life — was this strategy abandoned. Thus, women's outdoor activities affected the health of older children, but not that of young infants.[38] Similarly, Gubhaju,[39] on the strength of mortality data showing comparable infant death rates between farm-working and house-working women in the hill regions of Nepal, concluded that "farmwork probably does not interfere with their caring for an infant", but may prejudice older children.

In contrast, seasonal variation of nursing time was reported in rural Bangladesh, as women nursed less for their children (initially 18 months of age) during the harvest season, due to demands on women's time for processing the rice crop.[40] Because women adapt breastfeeding patterns around the work schedule, or conversely reduce workload to breastfeed, I have called the nursing behaviour of working mothers "opportunity feeds" rather than the better-known term "on-demand".

Mediating behaviours

It is important to draw attention to particular local behaviours which help to minimise the impact of heavy workloads on maternal–child health. I have discussed elsewhere these mediating behaviours,[38] such as the importance of work pace, flexible work organisation, and long birth intervals for rural working women. In Nepal, a moderate pace of work, offering opportunity time for childcare or recovery from exertion, ensures that pregnant/lactating mothers or anaemic individuals could complete the daily work schedule. Explicitly egalitarian work patterns, fostered in order to meet multiple and seasonally urgent labour demands in a subsistence economy, ensure that ill or weak individuals, as well as mothers encumbered with children, were not excluded or discriminated against in the workforce. Long birth-spacing, the result of frequent breastfeeding even though mothers work away from home and suppressed fecundity triggered by seasonally small but significant losses of body weight, is also instrumental in helping women integrate infant care and subsistence activity. Given this delicate complex of work-related factors, outside interventions aimed at reducing levels of poverty should not unwittingly undermine, but strengthen, the coping strategies already in evidence in local communities.

Scope of Interventions

Work reduction vs. food supplementation

Interventions targeted at improving maternal–child health in developing countries have generally focussed on supplementation of maternal food intake, rather than reduction of workloads. This approach neglects two important facts. First, energy stress may occur in relation to increased physical exertion, rather than mere shortage of food, especially where climatic seasonality correlates with pronounced changes in subsistence workloads. Second, women involved in dual subsistence and childbearing responsibilities face important constraints upon their time: a reduction of workload fulfills a double function by introducing savings of time as well as energy.

Moreover, dietary intervention *per se* has met with limited success. An instructive example is provided by Gambia.[22] Introduced with the explicit aim of increasing birth weight and milk production, the intervention consisted in giving mothers a high-energy biscuit, providing an extra 3,000 kJ/d. Supplementation did result in increased birth weight for third-trimester pregnant women in the wet season, but had no impact on birth weight if given earlier in pregnancy, or at other times of the year. Furthermore, birth weights increased by no more than 10%, despite the mothers' poor nutritional status. Supplementation also had very little impact on breastmilk output, because other factors than nutrition, such as disease suppressing the appetite of infants, were responsible for depressed milk production. However, as a direct result of the supplementation study, women resumed ovulation more rapidly postpartum, and became pregnant sooner than controls, an inadvertent outcome of the intervention. The programme had minimal impact on maternal body weight and composition (extra energy was possibly used for increased physical activity), but had large unwanted effect on fertility.[22]

The use of "appropriate technologies" and introduction of labour-saving devices for reducing women's workload is an obvious means for intervention. However, their actual impact made on women's lives is not always straight-forward. Such programmes, as in the case of dietary supplementation, have rarely met expectations.[41] Here, I detail a few examples of programmes for workload reduction, the impact of which has been appropriately evaluated.

In South Asia, new technologies, such as small mechanical mills, have been introduced to alleviate the intensive work of women in crop-processing activities. However, because the mills were owned and run by men, they resulted in a net loss of income to poor women who previously offered their labour for processing grain.[41] In rural Bangladesh where female seclusion is the rule, processing rice in household compounds before the advent of rice mills had represented the "single most important source of socially-acceptable employment".[26] The impact of many new technologies introduced in many rural areas of South and South-East Asia has been to change gender roles and social relations of production and seriously threaten the income-gaining opportunity of landless women, while the impact of agricultural intensification programmes has been to increase the seasonal work and time constraints of women.[42]

In Upper Volta, a project aimed at increasing women's participation in non-formal education was begun in 1965 and evaluated a decade later.[43] Three main labour-saving technologies to reduce women's workloads and thereby create "free time" for education were introduced: mechanical grain mills to reduce grinding and pounding activities, which took women 1.75 hours a day; water wells, to cut down on a 4-km trip to muddy swamps, particularly in the dry season; and carts, to help with fuel transport. Available technology did not, however, significantly lighten women's workloads. "Rather than create free time, the time saved was used for other household tasks, such as the preparation of meals or spinning of cotton (Ref. 43, p. 137). The authors concurred with Szalai[44] who opposed the argument that technological development *per se* will soon liberate women from household chores. Nonetheless, while the intervention did not create leisure time, the preparation of more frequent and better meals might well have improved nutritional health.

Policy implications

Hamilton *et al.*[45] drew the following policy implication from such examples: "Designers of any programme targeted at women in developing countries must take into consideration (...) that women face heavy constraints on their time. Any programme which puts further demands on women's time is likely to have limited success, especially in terms of reaching the neediest women who are often those with the least free time available. This situation suggests delivering services (or interventions) at or near women's work locations" (Ref. 45, p. 82)... and during the season or time of year that women are relatively free of other responsibilities! In particular, seasonality used to be "grossly overlooked by programme planners." (Ref. 45, p. 83)[45] Thus, one lesson of anthropological field studies is to pay close attention to the demands on women's time, not just focus on energy stress incured by subsistence life in constraining environments.

Hamilton *et al.*[45] also warn that "while it is clear that introducing appropriate labour-saving technology may indeed reduce women's time constraints, it is not clear that women will spend that extra time on home food production and preparation" (Ref. 45, p. 82) which might result in a substantial improvement in their nutritional status. They note that intervention programmes "often demand time investments from women rather than helping them 'make time' (Ref. 45, p. 41). Thus, in a number of cases, for instance by generating income-generating employment, development programmes have *increased* women's time spent in subsistence and their levels of physical activity.

Cautionary remarks

Another simple but important point is that interventions must be geared to introduce changes that are actually desired by the community. In highland Papua New Guinea, a water pump was provided to reduce the considerable time and effort spent by women to carry water from distant sources. However, it transpired that women had welcomed the opportunity to leave their homes and husbands and socialise with other women; when the water pump broke down, it was left in disrepair as the women claimed they did not need it (GA Harrison, *personal communication*). Here, an anthropologist's in-depth knowledge of local communities can here be invaluable to understand reasons underlying the success of failure of such interventions.

Poor rural women may actually resist interventions which are explicitly aimed at increasing birth weights, through reduction of workloads, as they realise that large infants will entail more difficult childbirth and risks of maternal death. Nepali mothers explicitly told me that they smoked cigarettes and worked hard during pregnancy to keep birth weights down and facilitate delivery. Similarly in India, the low level of participation of pregnant women in an intervention project was attributed to the twin beliefs that one's pregnancy should not be publicly declared and that a large foetus made delivery more difficult[45] (p. 63).[46] Again in Ethiopia, most women "greatly feared that a large baby would lead to an obstructed labour" (Ref. 33, p. 224).[33] While women may welcome an easier working life, those who have no regular access to formal medical care may voice other fears ruling health and reproductive behaviour.

Conclusion

The literature which explores the relationships between women's work and maternal–child health is enormous, but deals mostly with women in formal wage employment, and its consequences on the older child.[47] Evidence for the direct effects of women's subsistence work on newborn infant health is rather limited, although most studies suggest a strong association that will be mediated by maternal nutritional status.

It is not surprising to find contradictory or inconsistent conclusions in the literature to-date, as relationships between workloads, general maternal health during pregnancy, and newborn nutritional health are bound to be mediated by complex factors such as time, income, energy balance, and environmental constraints such as seasonality.

In this chapter, I have tried to emphasise a comprehensive, contextual approach to examine maternal–child health, and in particular some aspects and consequences of working behaviour. With reference to the scope for successful interventions aimed at reducing women's workloads, particular efforts must be made to hear local voices; respect any existing integration of labour and childcare strategies; and generally anticipate unwanted and inadvertent consequences of change. Lunn,[19] for example, concludes that because of doubts regarding the validity of many food consumption surveys in third world countries, which most often yield underestimated intakes, it seems likely that "in many populations, nutritional stress occurs primarily as a result of heavy workloads rather than dietary inadequacy" (Ref. 19, p. 210). But he also warns that "either a better diet or a reduction in maternal workload during lactation can be expected to shorten the duration of lactational infecundity" (p. 211), with possible unwanted consequences in terms of increased fertility.

References

1. Jimenez MH and Newton N, "Activity and work during pregnancy and the postpartum period: A cross-cultural study of 202 societies," *American Journal of Obstetrics and Gynecology* 135(2) (1979): 171–176.
2. National Research Council. Committee on Maternal Nutrition, "Maternal Nutrition and the Course of Pregnancy: Summary Report," Washington, DC, National Academy of Sciences (1980).
3. FAO/WHO/UNU Expert Consultation, "Energy and protein requirements," Technical Report Series 724, World Health Organization, Geneva (1985).
4. Durnin JVGA, "Food consumption and energy balance during pregnancy and lactation in New Guinea," In: *Maternal Nutrition During Pregnancy and Lactation*, Aebi H and Whitehead RG, eds., Hans Huber Publishers, Bern (1980): 86–95.
5. Ulijaszek SJ, "Human energetics in biological anthropology," Cambridge: Cambridge University Press (1995).
6. Rajalaksmi R, "Gestation and lactation performance in relation to the plane of maternal nutrition," In: *Maternal Nutrition During Pregnancy and Lactation*, Aebi H and Whitehead RG, eds., Hans Huber Publishers, Bern (1980): 184–202.
7. Prentice A and Prentice A, "Reproduction against the odds," *New Scientist* 118 (1988): 42–46.

8. Ferro-Luzzi A, "Work capacity and productivity in long-term adaptation to low energy intakes," In: *Nutritional Adaptation in Man*, Blaxter K and Waterlow JC, eds., London & Paris, John Libbey (1985): 61–67.

9. Panter-Brick C, "Seasonality and levels of energy expenditure during pregnancy and lactation for rural Nepali women," *American Journal of Clinical Nutrition* **57** (1993): 620–628.

10. Panter-Brick C, Lotstein DS and Ellison PT, "Seasonality of reproductive function and weight loss in rural Nepali women," *Human Reproduction* **8**(5) (1993): 684–690.

11. Panter-Brick C, "Seasonal and sex variation in physical activity levels of agro-pastoralists in Nepal," *American Journal of Physical Anthropology* **100** (1996): 7–21.

12. Panter-Brick C, "Physical activity, energy stores, and seasonal energy balance among men and women in Nepali households," *American Journal of Human Biology* **8**(2) (1996): 263–274.

13. Gillespie S and McNeill G, "Food, health and survival in India and developing countries," Delhi, Oxford University Press (1992).

14. Chen LC, Chowdhury AKMA and Huffman SL, "Seasonal dimensions of energy protein malnutrition in rural Bangladesh: The role of agriculture, dietary practices, and infection," *Ecology of Food and Nutrition* **8** (1979):175–187.

15. Tin-May-Than and Ba-Aye, "Energy intake and energy output of Burmese farmers at different seasons," *Human Nutrition: Clinical Nutrition* **39C** (1985): 7–15.

16. McNeill G, Payne PR, Rivers JPW, Enos AMT, de Britto JJ and Mukarji DS, "Socio-economic and seasonal patterns of adult energy nutrition in a South Indian village," *Ecology of Food and Nutrition* **22** (1988): 85–95.

17. Nag M, White B and Peet RC, "An anthropological approach to the study of the economic value of children in Java and Nepal," *Current Anthropology* **19** (1978): 292–306.

18. Roberts SB, Paul AA, Cole TJ and Whitehead RG, "Seasonal changes in activity, birth weight and lactational performance in rural Gambian women," *Transactions of the Royal Society of Tropical Medicine and Hygiene* **76** (1982): 668–678.

19. Lawrence M and Whitehead RG, "Physical activity and total energy expenditure of child-bearing Gambian village women," *European Journal of Clinical Nutrition* **42** (1988): 145–160.

20. Greenfield H and Clark J, "Energy compensation in childbearing in young Lufa women," *Papua New Guinea Medical Journal Proceedings 10th Annual Symposium*, Papua New Guinea Medical Society (1975).

21. McNeill G and Payne PR, "Energy expenditure of pregnant and lactating women," *Lancet* **ii** (1985):1237–1238.

22. Lunn PG, "Breast-feeding practices and other metabolic loads affecting human reproduction," In: *Variability in Human Fertility*, Rosetta L and Mascie-Taylor GGN, eds., Cambridge: Cambridge University Press (1996): 195–216.

23. Ferro-Luzzi A and Branca F, "Nutritional seasonality: The dimensions of the problem," In: *Seasonality and Human Ecology*, Ulijaszek SJ and Strickland S, eds., Cambridge: Cambridge University Press (1993): 149–165.

24. Ellison PT and Lager C, "Moderate recreational running is associated with lowered salivary progesterone profiles in women," *American Journal of Obstetrics and Gynaecology* **154**(5) (1986): 1000–1003.

25. Rosetta L, "Aetiological approach of female reproductive physiology in lactational amenorrhoea," *Journal of Biosocial Sciences* **24** (1992): 301–315.

26. Palmer I, "Women in rural development," *International Development Review* **22**(2–3): 39–45.

27. Panter-Brick C, "Proximate determinants of birth seasonality and conception failure in Nepal," *Population Studies* **50**(2) (1996): 203–220.

28. Ferro-Luzzi A, Branca F and Pastore G, "Body Mass Index defines the risk of seasonal energy stress in the Third World," *European Journal of Clinical Nutrition* **48** (1994): S165–S178.

29. Shetty PS and James WPT, "Body Mass Index: A measure of chronic energy deficiency in adults," FAO Food and Nutrition Paper 56, Rome: FAO (1994).

30. Tripathi AM, Agarwal DK, Devi RR and Cherian S, "Nutritional status of rural pregnant women and fetal outcome," *Indian Pediatrics* **34** (1987): 703–712.

31. Fleming AF, "Anaemia as a world health problem," In: Weatherall DJ, Ledingham JGG and Warrell DA, eds., Oxford Textbook of Medicine **II** (1987): 19.72–19.79.

32. Barnes DL, Adair LS and Popkin BM, "Women's physical activity and pregnancy outcome: A longitudinal analysis from the Philippines," *International Journal of Epidemiology* **20**(1) (1991): 162–172.

33. Tafari N, Naeye RL and Gobezie A, "Effects of maternal undernutrition and heavy physical work during pregnancy on birth weight," *British Journal of Obstetrics and Gynaecology* **87** (1980): 222–226.

34. Briend A, "Foetal malnutrition — The price of upright posture?" *British Medical Journal* **2** (1979): 317–319.

35. Briend A, "Foetal Stunting, foetal wasting and maternal nutritional status," In: *Maternal Nutrition During Pregnancy and Lactation*, Aebi H and Whitehead RG, eds., Hans Huber Publishers, Bern (1980): 150–159.

36. Wiley AS, "Neonatal and maternal anthropometric characteristics in a high altitude population of the Western Himalaya," *American Journal of Human Biology* **6**(4) (1994): 499–510.

37. Habicht JP, Lechtig A, Yarbrought C and Klein RE, "Maternal nutrition, birth weight and infant mortality," In: *Size at Birth*, Elliott K and Knight J, eds., Ciba Foundation Symposium No. 27 (N.S.), New York: American Elsevier (1974): 353–370.

38. Panter-Brick C, "Women's working behaviour and maternal–child health in rural Nepal," In: *Physical Activity and Health*, Norgan N, ed., Cambridge: Cambridge University Press (1992): 190–206.

39. Gubhaju BB, "Regional and socio-economic differentials in infant and child mortality in rural Nepal," *Contributions to Nepalese Studies* **13**(1) (1985): 33–44.

40. Huffman SL, Chowdhury AKMA, Chakraborty J and Simpson NK, "Breastfeeding patterns in rural Bangladesh," *American Journal of Clinical Nutrition* **33** (1980): 144–154.

41. McGuire JS and Popkin BM, "Helping women improve nutrition in the developing world: Beating the zero sum game," *World Bank Technical Paper* No.114, Washington, DC, The World Bank (1990).

42. Palmer I, "Women in rural development," *International Development Review* **22**(2–3) (1980): 39–45.

43. McSweeney BG and Freedman M, "Lack of time as an obstacle to women's education: The case of Upper Volta," *Comparative Education Review* **24**(2, pt 2) (1980): S124–S139.

44. Szalai A, "The situation of women in the light of contemporary time-budget research," E/CONF.66/BP/6, New York, United Nations (1975): 8–10.

45. Hamilton S, Popkin B and Spicer D, *Women and Nutrition in Third World Countries*, Bergin & Garvey Publishers (1984).

46. Nichter M, "The ethrophysiology and folk dieretics of pregnancy: a case study from South India," In: *Anthropology and International Health-Asian Case Studies*. Tucson: Gordon and Breach Publishers (1996): 35–69.

47. Leslie J and Paolisso M, eds., *Women, Work, and Child Welfare in the Third World*, Boulder, CO: Westview Press (1989).

48. Panter-Brick C and Pollard TM, "Work and hormonal variation in subsistence and industrial contexts," In: *Hormones, Health, and Behavior — A Socio-ecological and Ligespan Perspective*. Cambridge: Cambridge University Press (1999): 139–183.

Chapter 6

PERINATAL MORTALITY IN NEPAL: IMPLICATIONS FOR BEHAVIOUR MODIFICATION

Shyam Thapa

Senior Scientist, Family Health International, North Carolina

At present: Technical Advisor, Family Health Division,
Ministry of Health, and Population Division,
Ministry of Population and Environment, Kathmandu, Nepal

Very little is known about the levels and differentials (demographic, social and biological) of perinatal mortality in Nepal. This may be largely due to the unavailability of reliable data. This chapter presents levels and differentials of perinatal mortality based on a 1996 national survey, and draws implications for behaviour modification that could contribute to reducing perinatal mortality in Nepal.

Data and Methods

The data presented in this chapter come from a national health survey, the Nepal Family Health Survey. This survey was part of the World Demographic and Health Surveys. The primary objective of the survey was to provide national level estimates of fertility, child mortality, and contraceptive practice.

The sample was designed to provide estimates of fertility, child mortality and contraceptive practice for the country as a whole and for urban and rural areas separately. The eligible respondents for this survey were ever-married women in the reproductive ages (15–49 years) at the time of the survey. Of the total number of 8,580 ever-married women eligible for the survey, 8,429 or 98% were successfully interviewed.[1] Data were collected from January through June 1996. The "pregnancy history" approach was used to collect data on all pregnancies that women have had in their lifetime. The pregnancies included information on all the respondents' children born alive or dead, whether or not still living, and all the pregnancies that did not end in a live birth.

The perinatal mortality rate is calculated by summing all stillbirths and deaths of infants within the first week of life and dividing by the sum of all stillbirths and live births. The perinatal mortality rate thus includes stillbirths and early neonatal deaths among all the live births and stillbirths during a specific time period. Information on perinatal mortality is obtained from reports of pregnancy losses and pregnancy duration (which defines stillbirths for pregnancies of at least 28 weeks), and deaths of infants within the first week of life.

The events of stillbirths and early neonatal deaths are highly susceptible to omission and/or misreporting. Preliminary evaluation of the data on fertility and mortality (infant and child) indicated that there are "no serious biases" in reporting of trends and levels, and hence the data may be considered fairly good quality.[1]

The survey recorded a total of 23,458 live births and 5,343 dead children (or a total of 28,801 births) among all the respondents. The differentials of perinatal mortality presented in this chapter refer to a period of 120 months or ten years immediately preceding the survey date. The ten years data (mid-1986 to mid-1996) are used to minimise sampling errors in the estimated rates. The survey was not designed to ascertain clinical or other underlying causes of perinatal deaths. Hence, only the non-clinical factors associated with higher and lower perinatal mortality rates are examined.

Results

Estimates based on the survey indicate that perinatal mortality has been declining gradually over the years in Nepal (Table 1). The data indicates that between 1984 (mid-point of the period, 1981–86) and 1994 (mid-point of the period, 1991–96), perinatal mortality declined by just 1.1 points per year.

Estimates based on the data for the 1986–96 period found the national perinatal mortality rate of 56.9 (Table 2). The table also shows the differentials by background characteristics of the mothers, and the relative difference ratio (RDR) which refers to the difference in perinatal mortality rates between the categories of a given variable. The reference category refers to the category with the lowest mortality rate within a given variable. RDR is obtained by dividing the perinatal rate of a particular category by the reference category.

There are differences in rates between and among the categories within each of the variables. The largest differential is between the three ecological sub-regions. The mothers in the Terai have 1.4 times higher perinatal mortality than those in the hill region. Similarly, those in the mountain region have 1.3 times higher mortality than those in the hill region. Mothers in the rural areas have 1.2 times higher perinatal mortality than those in the urban areas. Mothers in the central and western regions have about the same perinatal

Table 1 Trends in perinatal mortality rate, Nepal.

Time period	Rate
1981–1986	63
1986–1991	58
1991–1996	52

Source: Nepal Family Health Survey, 1996.
Notes: Perinatal mortality rate is defined as the number of still and early neonatal deaths (live births dying before day seven) per 1,000 stillbirths and live births. The rate for 1986–91 is based on a linear interpolation. The time period refers to approximately the mid-month of each calendar year.

Table 2 Perinatal mortality rates and relative difference ratios (RDR) during the 1986–96 period, by residence, ecological and development regions, and educational characteristics of mothers (15–49 years old), Nepal.

Background Characteristic	Mortality Rate	RDR
Residence		
Urban	47.7	ref
Rural	57.6	1.2
Ecological region		
Mountain	60.8	1.3
Hill	45.8	ref
Terai	65.8	1.4
Development region		
Eastern	62.2	1.2
Central	52.9	ref
Western	52.9	1.0
Mid-western	62.0	1.2
Far-western	57.6	1.1
Education		
No education	57.8	1.1
Primary	52.6	ref
Secondary and higher	58.7	1.1
All Nepal	56.9	

Source: Nepal Family Health Survey, 1996.
ref = Reference category
Note: Relative difference ratio refers to risks of perinatal mortality compared to the lowest risk (reference) category of a given variable. The time period refers to approximately the mid-month of each calendar year.

mortality levels. Eastern and mid-western regions have 1.2 times higher mortality than those in the central or western regions.

The perinatal mortality rates do not vary considerably by mothers' education. This is surprising as more educated mothers are generally found to have lower infant mortality than less educated mothers.[2]

Table 3 Perinatal mortality rates and relative difference ratios (RDR) during 1986–96 period, by maternal age, number of pregnancies, and pregnancy interval, Nepal.

Background Characteristic	Mortality Rate	RDR
Age group (yrs)		
15–20	60.9	1.2
20–29	56.2	1.1
30–39	51.5	ref
40–49	76.5	1.5
No. of pregnancies at event		
1	70.7	1.5
2–3	47.4	ref
4–5	49.7	1.1
> 5	68.1	1.4
Previous pregnancy interval		
< 2 years	77.2	2.5
2–3 years	44.0	1.4
> 3 years	31.3	ref
All Nepal	56.9	

Source: Nepal Family Health Survey, 1996.
ref = Reference category
Note: RDR refers to the risk of perinatal mortality compared to the lowest risk (reference) category of a given variable. The time period refers to approximately the mid-month of each calendar year.

In Table 3 we present perinatal mortality rates by the mothers' age groups, number of pregnancies at event, and previous pregnancy intervals. As with the previous table, we also present relative difference ratios (RDR). There is a J-shape relationship between the lowest and highest age groups. Mothers in the age group 30–39 have the lowest perinatal mortality. Those in the age group 40–49 have 1.5 times higher mortality rate than those in the reference age group (30–39). There is a U-shape relationship with the number of pregnancies. Those with either the first pregnancy or more than five pregnancies experience the highest perinatal mortality. The mothers who have two to three pregnancies have the lowest perinatal mortality.

Of the seven variables considered in the analysis (Tables 2 and 3), the largest differential in perinatal mortality is found by the birth interval. The absolute difference between the highest and lowest rates is 46 points (77–31). Children born within less than two years of birth interval have 2.5 times higher risk of perinatal deaths than those with more than three years of birth interval. Those with two to three years of interval have 1.4 times higher mortality than those with more than three years of interval.

Implications for Behaviour Modification

There are two main approaches to reducing perinatal mortality: preventive and curative. The latter focusses on interventions designed to enhance the survival of the children already born, while the former aims at identifying high risk pregnancies that may be avoided in order to achieve lower mortality. Some of the initiatives adopted in the curative sector in the largest women's hospital in Nepal have been described by Manandhar and Costello.[3] This chapter has focussed on identifying high risk perinatal pregnancies for preventive interventions. Analysis of differentials in the mortality rates help identify which particular sub-groups have lower and higher experience of perinatal mortality and draw implications for ways toward further reduction in perinatal mortality.

The importance of pregnancy interval

The results presented here indicate that the most significant factor producing the largest differentials in perinatal mortality is pregnancy interval. Children born within two years of the previous pregnancy interval are at the highest risk of resulting in stillbirths or deaths (within the first seven days of delivery). Conversely, the higher birth interval, the better the chances of survival. The implication of the findings seems clear: birth spacing saves perinatal lives.

In Nepal, fully one-quarter of all births take place with a pregnancy interval of less than two years.[1] This implies that a large proportion of these children are at particularly high risk. Slightly over one-third (36.4%) of all the births take place in an interval of two to three years, and the remaining

(39.6%) are born after three years of the previous birth interval. The national perinatal mortality could even be higher if a larger percentage of the children were born within two years of interval. Conversely, perinatal mortality could be considerably lower if all births took place in an interval of at least two years. The challenge therefore lies in encouraging women (and their spouses) to modify their reproductive behaviour in order to avoid having births in short intervals (less than two years).

The components of a birth interval

Figure 1 shows the events determining the reproductive lifespan and the components of a birth interval (with or without intrauterine death). Among married and fecund women, reproduction takes place at a rate inversely related to the average duration of birth interval. Short birth intervals are associated with high fertility and vice versa. In the absence of intrauterine mortality, the length of a birth interval is determined by three factors: (1) the postpartum infecundable period, (2) waiting time to conception, and (3) full-term pregnancy. In case a pregnancy ends prematurely in a spontaneous or induced intrauterine death, the birth interval is lengthened by the following additional components: a shortened pregnancy, a brief infecundable period, and a conception delay.

Bongaarts and Potter[4] have shown that if no breastfeeding and postpartum abstinence are practiced in a population, the birth interval averages about 20 months comprising of:

1. minimum postpartum anovulation	1.5	months
2. waiting time to conception	7.5	months
3. time added by spontaneous intrauterine mortality	2	months
4. full-term gestation	9	months

They have also found that the effects of intrauterine mortality and the average waiting time to conception varies within a narrow range (5–10) across populations. The duration of full-term pregnancy is known to be about the same across populations. Thus, the 18.5 months (7.5 + 2 + 9) of a birth interval may be considered a standard (model) duration.

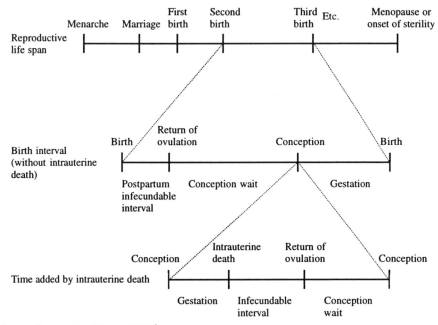

Source: Bongaarts and Potter (1983)[4]

Figure 1 Events determining the reproductive life span and the rate of childbearing.

The duration of postpartum infecundability is the only factor that varies considerably across populations. In populations in which the practice of contraception or induced abortion is non-existent or negligible (which are referred to as "natural fertility" populations in the demographic literature), the duration of infecundability is only about 1.5 months. It may vary significantly either due to breastfeeding, postpartum abstinence, use of contraception, or to some extent by induced abortion. An induced abortion averts less than one birth because allowance must be made for

- the chance that the terminated pregnancy might have ended in a late miscarriage or stillbirth,
- the shorter period before which ovulation resumes following an abortion compared to a live birth, and
- the briefer period of gestation for abortions than the live births.

The effects of perinatal death and early marriage

Among couples who do not practice contraception, a woman who loses her newborn infant through death returns to fertility more quickly. This biological factor leads her to be pregnant soon.[5] Hence, these women are most likely to have a particularly short birth interval. In Nepal, the mothers who have short birth intervals are mainly those whose last child was dead or those in the 15–19 age group.[1] This suggests that the primary reason for the short intervals are intrauterine mortality and stillbirth. This suggests that women should be encouraged to delay their marriage or first birth until they are at least 20 years old. In Nepal, 50% of women are married by 16.2 years of age[1] and 50% of the married women have their first child by the age of 20.[1]

Breastfeeding and the use of contraception

Full breastfeeding has been determined to provide nearly 100% protection against pregnancy in the first 4–6 months.[6] Beyond breastfeeding and postpartum abstinence, the only other factor that could contribute to lengthening the birth interval is the use of contraception. The practice of contraception can play a critical role in lengthening the pregnancy interval, hence reducing perinatal mortality. It may be the most effective preventive strategy in reducing perinatal mortality among the younger and older women (those under 20 and over 39 years of age) whose pregnancies are found to be particularly at high risk of resulting in perinatal deaths.

In Nepal, the spacing methods of contraception available through the public as well as private sectors include the pill, three-monthly injectables, condoms, implants (Norplant), IUDs, and female barriers. Of these, injectables have been the most popular[1] and their use has been increasing over the years.[7] The Ministry of Health has recently updated and revised the guidelines for the provision of family planning services.[8] Several of the existing "medical barriers" to access and use of contraception have been removed. The national standards and the training curricula[9–12] represent the most comprehensive reference materials for family planning service delivery. They not only fill a long-existing gap, but also aim at changing many outdated and unnecessary practices that have existed over the last 25 years in family planning programmes in Nepal. Further, policy dialogue on "emergency contraception"[13] is just beginning in the country. It may be prudent to recommend emergency contraception for women with especially short birth intervals.

Underlying mechanisms for the effect of birth interval on perinatal mortality

As mentioned earlier, the survey data analysed here do not permit us to explore the underlying reasons for high risk of perinatal mortality. Among the several possible reasons, an important one might be that the mothers with short birth intervals between children are unable to provide care to both the previous child and the current pregnancy due to competing demands. Another factor may be that a pregnancy in a short interval adversely affects the mother's physiological and nutritional conditions and lead to underweight birth which is known to be an important factor in perinatal deaths. It is also possible that mothers who have high perinatal mortality are biologically and socio-economically selected to continue to experience successive perinatal deaths.

While the underlying reasons and specific mechanisms remain unclear, the specific reasons for high risk of perinatal deaths, it is obvious from the data reviewed here that the health care advocates and providers should ascertain the birth interval status of the women of childbearing age and use it as a sensitive indicator for the survival chances of the future births. Women who have very short interval should be encouraged to use contraception to lengthen the next birth interval. A significant achievement in this behaviour modification alone will go a long way towards reducing perinatal mortality. Birth spacing of at least two years would mean higher child survival throughout the first year of life.[14] An effective preventive health programme will also lessen the burden on the curative sector of perinatal and infant survival care.

Conclusion

Children born within an interval of less than two years have the highest risk of perinatal deaths and those born after three years of interval have the lowest risk in Nepal. These findings imply that health care advocates should encourage women and their families to avoid short birth spacing (less than two years). Similarly, preventive health care counsellors and service providers should ascertain the birth interval status and use it as a indicator towards minimising perinatal mortality. Those mothers whose last birth was less than two years should be advised and encouraged to practice effective spacing methods of contraception. This intervention alone could contribute to substantial reduction in perinatal mortality in Nepal and most probably in similar settings elsewhere.

Acknowledgements

The perinatal mortality rates presented here are taken from the 1996 Nepal Family Health Survey report cited in the chapter. The data tabulations were carried out at Macro International, Maryland, USA. The author thanks the contributors of the report, but does not implicate them for the interpretation of the data and views expressed in this chapter. Thanks are also due to Jason Smith for reviewing an earlier draft. Support for the preparation of this chapter was provided by the United States Agency for International Development as part of its policy research support to Family Health International. The usual disclaimer applies.

References

1. MOH (Ministry of Health), *Nepal Family Health Survey 1996*. Kathmandu, Ministry of Health (1997).
2. Thapa S, "Infant mortality and its correlates and determinants in Nepal," *Journal of the Nepal Medical Association* **34**(118 & 119) (1996): 94–109.
3. Manandhar DS and de L. Costello AM, "A low-cost special care baby unit at the Maternity Hospital in Nepal," *Journal of the Nepal Medical Association* **34**(118 & 119) (1996): 172–176.

4. Bongaarts J and Potter RG, *Fertility, Biology, and Behavior: An Analysis of the Proximate Determinants*, New York, Academic Press (1983).
5. Taylor CE, Newman JS and Kelly NU, "The child survival hypothesis," *Population Studies* **30**(2) (1976): 263–278.
6. FHI (Family Health International), "Consensus statement: Breastfeeding as a family planning method," *Lancet* **2** (1988): 1204–1205.
7. Pandey KR and Thapa S, "Family planning in Nepal: An update," *Journal of the Nepal Medical Association* **32** (1994): 131–143.
8. MOH (Ministry of Health), National Medical Standards for Reproductive Health, Vol. 1, Contraceptive Series. Kathmandu: Family Health Division, Ministry of Health (1995).
9. MOH (Ministry of Health), *Comprehensive Family Planning (COFP) Course: Reference Manual*, Kathmandu, National Health Training Center, Ministry of Health (1995).
10. MOH (Ministry of Health), *Comprehensive Family Planning (COFP) Course: Trainer's Handbook*, Kathmandu, National Health Training Center, Ministry of Health (1995).
11. MOH (Ministry of Health), *Comprehensive Family Planning (COFP) Course: Participant's Handbook*, Kathmandu, National Health Training Center, Ministry of Health (1995).
12. MOH (Ministry of Health), *Audiovisual and Training Materials in Family Planning Services*, Kathmandu, National Health Training Center, Ministry of Health (1995).
13. SSC (South-to-South Cooperation), "Consensus statement on emergency contraception," *Contraception* **52** (1995): 211–213.
14. Hobcraft J, "Does family planning save children's lives?" Technical background paper prepared for the International Conference on Better Health for Women and Children through Family Planning, Nairobi, Kenya (1985).

Chapter 7

TRADITIONAL AND CULTURAL ASPECTS OF NEONATAL CARE IN DEVELOPING COUNTRIES

Shashi N. Vani

Professor of Paediatrics, Ahmedabad, Gujarat, India

Introduction

The study of traditional and cultural practices in neonatal care (TPNC) has a special place amongst efforts aimed at improving neonatal care in developing countries for a number of reasons.

Home delivery

In most countries, routine institutional care of mothers during pregnancy, delivery and neonatal care is only a few decades old. Even today, in India the majority of deliveries are conducted at home by women who may be professional traditional birth attendants from the locality, or elderly women from the family or neighbourhood. The same women offer advice on care for the newborn infants. This situation is not only prevalent in remote rural areas where modern medical services are not easily available, it is also the norm in crowded and poor urban slums, despite the fact that free medical services are available close by at large hospitals and maternity homes provided by the government and local municipal corporations.

Institutional delivery

The available neonatal care services remain under-used for many socio-cultural reasons. Equally, the training of the family physicians who offer primary care is by and large poor, even in basic neonatal care. Even though various national programmes exist aimed at the reduction of morbidity and mortality of mothers and children, they do not include any system of regular neonatal care and follow-up. The highly trained neonatologists and obstetricians generally offer care only to critically ill or sick newborns. This care is often based on the principles used in developed countries, and is very expensive, requires sophisticated equipment, and is often not relevant in a local context. Unnecessary investigations are carried out and strong medicines prescribed even for common, minor complaints. This escalates the cost of care and makes patients fearful. Even among those few who opt to deliver in public or private hospitals, very few have their newborn infants cared for by a neonatologist, and all remaining care is influenced by the family environment and traditions. Lack of available services, underutilisation, and little community demand for better neonatal care services all help to perpetuate the influence of traditional and cultural practices and beliefs on the well-being of newborn infants in developing countries.

The origins of traditional infant care

Many developing countries have a valuable heritage from ancient civilisation and a rich culture. For thousands of years, they have been rearing their newborn infants fairly successfully. They have evolved neonatal care practices, handed down through generations, which are unique and usually relevant to their environment, resources and socio-cultural needs. On close scrutiny, these local traditions appear to have a basic core of knowledge and ancestral wisdom. Some may be intuitive and some superstitious, but many seem to have some scientific basis and logic and are closely related to local ancient systems of medicine, e.g. Ayurveda, Siddha, and Unani in India. Whilst some practices are clearly beneficial, others have either lost their relevance or become unacceptable in the way they are currently practised in the community.

All TPNC in developing countries require careful study and evaluation in order to discover their positive and negative effect on neonatal care in the community; to tap the potentially valuable store of knowledge which they contain to improve neonatal care using locally relevant, acceptable and low-cost methods; and to improve neonatal care by discouraging harmful practices. It must be borne in mind that even when practices are clearly found to be harmful, they may be difficult to eradicate.

Why Continue Traditional Practices?

Many practices have evolved on the basis of core wisdom, common sense, scientific observations made in the distant past, and the experience of generations. TPNC are affordable, culturally acceptable, relevant to the local environment and needs of the people, and can be used by most of the population. Traditional practices and home remedies are promoted by midwives, village healers, physicians practising native systems of medicine, wise people in the community, and of course charlatans and quacks. They may have more or less relevance depending on the context of a tradition-bound society, the cultural background of the family, the educational level of family members — especially the mother — and the proximity and availability of modern medical care. Practitioners of so-called modern medicine should be careful not to reject traditional practices of neonatal care out of hand, and to guard against giving advice based on simple imitation of foreign practices without taking the context into account.

The need for an evidence based approach to TPNC

What is needed is a scientific analysis of currently prevalent TPNC and recommendations for classification into the categories: good practices worth promoting; harmful practices that should be discontinued; harmless practices which may be ignored; and practices that need further research. Some modern practices which have the potential to be considered 'traditional' in the near future (e.g. bottle feeding, use of pacifiers, early separation of newborn infant from his/her mother, etc.) should also be considered. Once beneficial and harmful practices have been identified, suitable communication strategies should be developed for individual and community education. A special effort should be made to study home remedies for simple problems and to promote those that are effective.

Before an attempt is made to classify specific local practices and incorporate them into health education messages it is necessary to know the type and extent of TPNC prevalent in a local community. Published reports are few and incomplete, and mostly only anecdotal or descriptive. There are hardly any reports based on observations of actions actually taking place. Comprehensive studies of TPNC are much needed.

Guidelines for the Classification of Traditional Practices

With so many diverse cultures and ethnic groups, it is difficult to develop globally relevant classification systems and recommendations on TPNC. However, some broad guidelines can be laid down based on accepted norms of essential newborn care. Recommendations with reference to TPNC should start with maternal care, from the care of the girl child, minimum basic antenatal care including proper nutrition, prevention of anaemia, tetanus toxoid vaccination, early detection and suitable management of high risk situations, early and emergency management of severe life-threatening complications of pregnancy, and measures to ensure delivery of a mature healthy newborn infant weighing more than 2.5 kg.

TPNC related to immediate care of the newborn at delivery should ensure proper prevention and management of neonatal asphyxia and hypothermia; and after delivery, promotion of early breastfeeding, continued management of prevention of hypothermia and infections, and early detection of risk factors including severe/lethal congenital malformations. Management of simple, common neonatal problems and rational use and limitations of home remedies are further important considerations. Provision of psychological support, security, and early stimulating activities for the newborn infant also play a significant role in various TPNCs.

Classifying TPNC as useful or harmful

In the following paragraphs, the common traditional and cultural practices of neonatal care currently prevalent in many areas of India have been classified as useful, harmful, harmless, or needing further research. The same approach can be used in different countries to develop locally relevant guidelines for further action. The type and extent of TPNC still in use needs to be evaluated from time to time and suitable modifications made to the recommendations.

As already emphasised, this approach is relative. For example, routine administration of prelacteal feeds to mature healthy newborns is not considered good practice as it may interfere with successful breastfeeding and even introduce infections and diarrhoea, but arguably, it may be justified for very low birth weight newborn infants in remote rural homes to prevent hypo-glycaemia and supply calories and fluids until breastfeeding is established. Similarly, use of simple home remedies and ghutties may be justified for treating minor gastrointestinal discomfort in newborns in remote areas where medical advice is not readily available, but prolonged use of such methods or routine use of gripe water or janamghutties (herbal concoctions used in newborn infants) is not appropriate. In general, special preparations should only be used under the proper guidance of an experienced person or a well qualified professional healer in the local system of medicine. Blatant advertisements and over-the-counter sales of so-called herbal remedies need to be controlled vigilantly.

TPNC in India that are Worth Promoting

- Giving proper emotional support to a pregnant woman, especially during the first pregnancy. In India, premarital sex education is a taboo. Girls are married young, pregnancy occurs early, and these young mothers-to-be may have fears and anxiety about the processes of pregnancy and delivery. A number of socio-cultural rituals aimed at giving psychological support to such mothers are celebrated among women in the family. A variety of nutritious food preparations are brought for the pregnant woman; songs, dances and festivities are held. All these help to allay her fears and keep her in a positive mood.

- Feeding of pregnant woman with a special calorie-rich nutritious diet (mostly middle- and upper-income groups).
- Pregnant woman going to the mother's home for confinement so that she can rest and relax.
- Postnatal isolation and rooming together of mother and newborn infant for at least the first 40 days. This encourages breastfeeding and emotional bonding, and minimises exposure to infection.
- Keeping the newborn infant well-covered with washed and sun-dried cotton clothes and caps in a room which is kept warm.
- Breastfeeding and proper guidance and support from elderly women from the family and neighbourhood.
- Instillation of colostrum into the newborn infant's eyes.
- Use of traditional feeding aids like a "Paladey" (a beak-shaped feeder) or cup and spoon for top-up feeding.
- Use of simple herbal preparations for care of newborn infant skin during bathing.
- Body massage of the newborn infant with oil.
- Bathing of newborn infants by holding them on the attendant's feet and not using bathtubs. (May minimise cross-infections and choking.)
- Use of simple home remedies for the treatment of minor discomforts of the newborn infant like regurgitation, coughs, and colds.
- Good nutritious diet for lactating mothers.
- Use of cradles.

TPNC in India that are Harmful and should be Discouraged

- Neglect of a girl child both emotionally and nutritionally.
- Rare episodes of selective female infanticide.
- Specific restriction of caloric-rich nutritious diet in pregnancy especially in the last few months. This practice is found in many rural areas where it is thought to reduce the size of the newborn infant and facilitate easy delivery.

- Undue physical exercise during pregnancy.
- Considering delivery as a physiological process and not taking even minimum routine antenatal care. No registration of pregnancy with health workers.
- Allowing delivery by untrained, ill-equipped and illiterate people.
- Not adopting the 'three cleans of delivery', i.e.:
  — conducting delivery on a dirty surface;
  — not washing the hands properly before conducting delivery, using unsterile instruments for cutting and tying cord; and
  — using unclean substances like kumkum, cow dung, ghee, etc. for cord dressing.
- Bathing all newborn infants immediately after birth, even low birth weight and preterm newborn infants.
- Bad feeding habits, e.g. throwing away colostrum, unnecessary use of prelacteal feeds, delayed start of breastfeeding, giving water in between breast feeds.
- Food taboos for lactating mothers (e.g. pulses, legumes, and certain fruits are not given for fear that they may affect the newborn infant, and the mother is deprived of good nutrition).
- Instillation of oil drops, and blowing into ears, eyes and nostrils of newborn infant during bathing.
- Feeding of unhygienically prepared herbal preparations (ghutti) and application of sooty preparations to the eyes (kajal).
- Routine administration of opium and brandy to newborn infants.
- Use of unclean pacifiers. These can promote infection and interfere with breastfeeding, and are often the starting point for malnutrition.

TPNC in India which are Harmless and may Continue

At present, these practices are not thought to be harmful so they should be allowed to continue for the time being. Even so, some apparently harmless practices may lead to delay in seeking medical aid with a resultant deterioration in the state of an infant:

- Notional use of prelacteal feeds in the form of a few drops of clean honey, ass's milk, or even cow's urine.
- Ear piercing, circumcision, etc., provided they are done with care and using fully aseptic precautions. (This might need to be reviewed if HIV infection is widely prevalent in a community.)
- Use of amulets, talismen, etc.
- "Nazar Utarna" (rituals to cast away the influence of the evil eye), teeka (applying herbal paints on forehead, cheek etc.), and "Jhad Phuk".
- Massage of the anterior fontanelle.
- Using clothes and utensils begged from others for the newborn infant (a ritual often followed by a mother with a bad obstetric history and repeated infant deaths).

TPNC in India Needing Further Research

Some traditional practices still require further systematic study to discover their possible uses and dangers. Blind faith in such practices may interfere with the acceptance of modern systems of medicine as well as with proper understanding of traditional medicine.

- Use of a variety of preparations to promote lactation such as herbal medicines and preparations including ginger, fenugreek seeds, poppy seeds, and aniseed.
- The concept of "hot" and "cold" food for mothers.
- Avoiding exposure of pregnant women to eclipses.
- Use of certain herbal preparations for complaints (of the newborn infant) such as vomitting, diarrhoea, regurgitation of feeds, abdominal distension, and constipation.

Modern 'Traditional Practices'

The availability of modern medical facilities, the increasing education of mothers and affluence of the community, and the widespread dissemination of health education measures through health workers and the media (especially television), has led to a situation in which many traditional practices are changing or fading and a whole set of new practices making their presence felt. Some recent practices with potentially negative effects include:

- the widespread use of feeding bottles and ready-made expensive formula feeds;
- the use of costly baby soaps, oils, and powders (which drain the scant resources of middle-income women);
- the use of pacifiers;
- the use of thick diapers made of synthetic fibres which, particularly in hot and humid climates, increase problems like skin allergy and rashes;
- the use of synthetic fibre clothing;
- early separation of mothers and newborn infants;
- reduction in the time taken for handling, fondling, singing lullabies and other activities important for emotional bonding and stimulation;
- lack of support from elderly family women or neighbours because of the break-up of joint families and migration to cities;
- changing styles of living and socialising with the advent of the TV culture;
- unnecessary prescription of antibiotics and strong medicines for simple common problems of newborn infants; and
- undesirable use of multivitamins including Vitamin E, etc.

One definitely harmful trend is the increasing misuse of facilities for antenatal sex determination and selective female foeticide. There are some positive trends as well, especially in urban areas, including the increasing interest of fathers in newborn infant care, and the routine acceptance of vaccinations for newborn infants against various infectious diseases.

Conclusion

Evaluating TPNC is a complex task, especially in developing countries with widely diverse cultures and educational and socio-economic differences. Most TPNC appear to be based on common sense, logic and scientific justification; but many have undergone changes over time and some have become unacceptable. TPNC should be properly evaluated before they are encouraged or condemned: modern medical professionals should approach TPNC with an open mind, and evaluation should be ongoing and regionally specific because of the temporal and geographic variability.

Some widely prevalent TPNC should be selected immediately, their potential to reduce neonatal morbidity and mortality evaluated, and specific recommendations formulated, especially to develop simple messages that can be used by the media for community education and incorporated in training programmes for medical and paramedical personnel.

At the same time countries should seek to preserve their beneficial TPNC. Regional TPNC identified as scientifically rational and beneficial should be promoted in other regions of the same country, and perhaps other countries.

One point remains clear: considerable integrated research at national and regional level is required to classify existing TPNC as harmful, innocuous, beneficial, or of doubtful utility.

References

1. Report of the National Workshop on Traditional Practices of Neonatal Care in India, S.N.Vani ed., Available from the National Neonatology Forum.
2. Pitt D and Sterky G, "Culture and neonatal technology; values, views and neonatal practices," In: *Breathing and Warmth at Birth: Judging the Appropriateness of Technology*, Sterky G, Tafari N and Tunell R, eds, SAREC report, Stockholm, R2, (1985): 13–16.
3. Report of National Seminar on Traditional (including Tribal) Practices in Mothers and Child Care. National Institute of Public Co-operation and Child Development, New Delhi (1989).
4. Bhave S and Rao VN, "A study of prevalent cultural practices of mothers and child health," KEM Hospital, Pune (1980).
5. "Mother and child care. An evaluation of Lok Swasthya Parampara (First Draft)," Lok Swasthya Parampara samivardhan Samiti/CHETNA (1990).
6. Mokashi A, "Consumer Alert. Do we need gripe waters?" *Academy Today*, July (1990): 6–7.
7. Kulkarni M, Prabhu S and Chawla C, "Oil application in preterm newborn infants — A source of warmth and nutrition," *Indian Pediatrics* **23** (1986): 790–791.

8. Balkrishan S, "Lipoid pneumonia in infants and children in South India," *British Medical Journal* **4** (1973): 329–331.

9. Mahadevan S, Ananthakrishnan S and Srinivas S, "Lipoid pneumonia in South Indian infants," *Indian Pediatrics* **28** (1991): 1529–1530.

10. Mehta BP, "Study of beliefs and practices regarding perinatal care and measurement of neonatal birth weight," Thesis for MD (Pediatric), Department of Pediatrics, B.J. Medical College, Gujarat University, Ahmedabad (1988).

11. Athavle VB, *Bala Veda-Pediatrics and Ayurveda*, Published by VB Athavle, Sion, Bombay (1977): 101–106.

12. Ghosh S, "Strategies for lowering perinatal mortality," *Indian Pediatrics* **26** (1989): 1131–1132.

13. Bhargava SK, Singh KK and Saxena BN, "ICMR Task Force national collaborative study on identification of high risk families, mothers and outcome of their offsprings with particular reference to the problem of maternal nutrition, low birth weight, perinatal and infant morbidity and mortality in rural and urban slum communities. Summary, conclusion and recommendations," *Indian Pediatrics* **28** (1991): 1473–1480.

14. Natu M, "Review of traditional practices in mother and child care in Maharashtra," In: *Report of National Seminar on Traditional Practices in Mother and Child Care*, National Institute of Public Co-operation and Child Development, New Delhi (1989): 80–89.

15. Vani SN and Singh M, eds, Report and recommendations of National Neonatology Forum workshop on human resource development for neonatal care in India, Ahmedabad (1989): 9–10.

16. Rajadhan PA, "Customs connected with the birth and rearing of children," In: *South East Asian Birth Customs. Human Relations Area Files Press* Hart DV, Rajadhan PA and Coughumn RJ, eds, (1965): 121–204.

17. Ramji S, "The challenge of perinatal care in urban slums," Editorial, *Bulletin of National Neonatology Forum* **5**(2) (1991): 1–2.

18. Bhargava SK, Ramji S and Sachdev HPS, "Current status of neonatal care and alternate strategies of reduction of neonatal mortality in the decade of nineties," *Indian Pediatrics* **28** (1991): 1429–1436.

19. Bhakoo ON, Garg SK, Agarwal KC and Gupta AN, "Socio-epidemiological study of neonatal tetanus," *Indian Pediatrics* **13** (1976): 545–552.

20. Can G, "Neonatal traditional practice: A case report from Turkey," In: *Breathing and Warmth at Birth Judging the Appropriateness of Technology*, Sterky G, Tafari N and Tunell R, eds, Stockholm (1985): 16–18.

21. Mohapatra SS and Bang RK, "Customs and beliefs on neonatal care in a tribal community," *Indian Pediatrics* **19** (1982): 675–678.

22. Pandey H and Punetha S, "Traditional mother and child care practices of the Bhutia tribe of District Pithorgarh (UP) — A pilot research study," In: *Report of National Seminar on Traditional Practices in Mother and Child Care*, New Delhi, National Institute of Public Co-operation and child Development (1989): 192–212.

23. WHO, *Appropriate Technology for Thermal Control of Newborn Infants — An Update*, MCH unit, Division of Family Health, WHO Geneva (1986): 2–3.

24. Daga SR, "Warm chain is the key to newborn survival," *Chronick-NNF* **1**(2) (1991): 1–3.

25. Karan S, Rao M and Manorama, "A study of customs and beliefs relating to mothers and infants in rural India," *Current Topics of Pediatrics* 0507/04, XV International Congress Pediatrics, New Delhi (1977).

26. Gopaldas T, "Review of traditional practices in mother and child care in Gujarat," In: *Report of National Seminar on Traditional Practices in Mother and Child Care*, New Delhi, National Institute of Public Co-operation and child Development (1989): 42–68.

Commentary

TRADITIONAL BELIEFS AND PRACTICES IN NEWBORN CARE IN NEPAL

Munu Thapa
Reproductive Health and Gender Coordination,
Reproductive Health Project, GTZ

Care of the newborn, especially during the first 28 days of life, is vital in determining the survival and health of the child. There are a number of socio-cultural and traditional practices, local beliefs, and taboos which influence the quality of newborn care at home. Since 90% of deliveries take place at home,[1] these practices strongly influence the morbidity and number of deaths during the neonatal period. Health care workers, particularly midwives and neonatal paediatricians, need to be aware of traditional practices and beliefs in relation to neonatal care.

The following is a description of typical traditional practices used in Nepal, using data collected in two districts, Dhading and Nawalparasi — one hill, one Terai.[2,3]

Immediate Care of the Newborn: The Traditional Approach in Nepal

Resuscitation

Respiration is the first vital function a newborn has to establish at birth. In rural communities, families have limited knowledge of the correct process of resuscitation of the newborn. Most families think the newborn is dead if it fails to cry and breathe at birth. The following measures are sometimes used to make a newborn cry:

- Sprinkling water on the body of the newborn.
- Spilling water on the face of the newborn.
- Fanning the face of the newborn.
- Making a noise in the hope of wakening the newborn.
- Milking the umbilical cord.
- Massaging the soles of the newborn with oil.
- Holding the newborn upside down and patting its back. This special procedure is done by a trained birth attendant.

Few families know about cleaning the airway passage and providing first aid resuscitation procedures.

Hygiene and warmth

Delivery is considered a dirty process and it often takes place in a cowshed or an unused corner of the house, which is usually not cleaned or prepared for delivery. The surface used for delivery is either not covered or only scantily covered with straw, old bed sheets, old sacks, or a plastic sheet. The newborn is kept naked or covered by a thin piece of cloth on this surface until after the placenta is delivered at which time the cord is cut; thus the body temperature of the newborn is probably not maintained. This is mainly because birth attendants pay more attention to the delivery of the placenta, which is considered to be a very important procedure, than to the newborn. Few people realise that a newborn should be kept warm. Families do not usually have warm comfortable clothes ready for the new newborn. The tradition is to find clothes after the newborn is born. In the hills, the newborn is bathed in hot water after the cord is cut; in the Terai, in cold well water. The person attending the delivery usually washes her hands after completing the delivery procedure but not before.

Cord care

In the Terai, the majority of people use a clean razor blade to cut the cord, whereas in the hills many families still use a sickle or even a piece of wood. The majority apply mustard oil to the cord stump, but some families in the Terai use ash, and some families in the hills use turmeric and antiseptic powder. The cord is then tied with thread which is not necessarily clean. Coins or jewellery are placed under the cord to make it easy to cut. Tamang families in Dhading district leave the cord untied.

Prelacteal and early breastfeeding

In both the hills and Terai, people traditionally put honey, sugar or ghee into the mouth of a newborn. Families believe that the breasts start secreting milk only after the third day of delivery and attempts are not usually made to suckle the child immediately after birth. In the Terai, fresh undiluted goat's milk is given to the newborn with the help of a cotton swab or soft cloth for two to three days, whereas in the hills the newborn may be breastfed by other lactating mothers. Colostrum is usually discarded because families believe that the newborn will find it difficult to swallow because of its viscosity or because they think it is harmful. Breastfeeding is usually started on the third day in a sitting position. At night, mothers usually feed in a lateral position. This may sometimes be harmful, with reports of a babies being suffocated when the nose was covered by the breasts. The newborn is breastfed exclusively and on demand, unless the mother is ill or fails to secrete milk.

Later Care of the Newborn

Ghotti Chauthi

In the hills, the newborn is given a paste called "Gothi Chuthi", which is made of breastmilk, nuts and herbs, from the third week onwards. This is considered good for strengthening digestive processes, inducing sleep and providing additional protein.

Clothing

The newborn does not wear stitched clothes until after the naming ceremony, which usually takes place between the 6th and 11th day after birth. Until then the newborn is simply wrapped from head to toe in a soft cloth. The newborn infant's head is considered to be a special part requiring more heat, and is usually covered with a thick cap. A simple piece of cloth is used as a diaper and changed when needed. The wet cloths are dried without washing. Particularly in the hills, a soft piece of cloth called a "patuka" is tied around the newborn infant's abdomen. It is believed that this will prevent air from entering the abdomen and swelling of the umbilicus when crying. In the hills, families prepare special clothes for newborns called "Bhoto", which are made of two to three layers with simple string ties.

Sleeping

A mustard seed pillow is used in the hills. Families believe that it makes the infant's head round. The mother and newborn sleep in the same bed, and handling by others is minimal.

Massage

Mustard oil massage is considered very useful for preserving or providing heat and energy to the newborn. Oil is applied to the whole body two or three times a day in sunlight or firelight. Excess oil is softly patted or massaged into the fontanelle. Some herbs are also applied to the anterior fontanelle, which is thought to be very fragile. Oil is poured into the nostrils, eyes, ears, navel, anus and vagina. It is considered to be good for absorbing cold and for making the skin soft and shiny. The arms and legs are passively exercised during the massage. Hot compression is used on the extremities. Newborns are generally exposed to the sun, which is considered to be good for the development of the infant's bones.

Ambient temperature

The room with the newborn is kept warm by burning cow dung cake or firewood and closing the windows and doors. A kerosene lamp is often burnt throughout the night, mainly to provide heat and light. Families also believe that by keeping a fire near the newborn and a knife under his or her pillow, he or she will be protected from evil spirits. Some believe that prior to touching the newborn one should touch either water or fire in order to safeguard the newborn against illness.

Eye-liner

In the hills, kajal/gazal (a black eye-liner made by burning mustard oil) is applied to the eyes with a swab stick after the naming ceremony; in the Terai, both mustard oil and kerosene lampblack are used, applied with the fingers. This practice is thought to brighten, widen and clear the newborn infant's eyes.

Miscellaneous

The newborn infant's breasts are squeezed from five to six days after birth with the aim of preventing early enlargement of the breasts. A blue/black thread is tied around the wrists, ankles and groin of the newborn after the naming ceremony to protect him/her from spells. These threads are changed when they tighten, usually after a month, this provides a chance to assess weight gain. Some families believe that a newborn changes the colour of its skin seven times a day, which means that jaundice and cyanosis may go unnoticed. Refusal by the newborn to breastfeed is considered to be due to witchcraft. Excessive crying for a few days is considered normal. There is a tendency to think that a newborn is searching for its placenta, which was its company in the womb. These beliefs lead to delays in the family seeking health care services.

Conclusions

It is clear that traditional practices in newborn care can be both helpful and harmful. Health workers and educators need to understand the local culture, customs, practices, and beliefs about the newborn before trying to educate mothers on newborn care.

The benefits of some of the helpful practices should be appreciated, e.g. making the room warm, oil massage, exclusive demand feeding, use of razor blades for cord cutting, mother and newborn sleeping together, passive exercise, sunbaths, and assessing weight gain through ties. Some negative practices need to be discouraged, e.g. burning wood in closed rooms, discarding colostrum, delay in breastfeeding, not wrapping the newborn immediately after birth, immediate newborn bath, using oil in eyes/navel, not washing diapers, not washing hands, use of sickle and wood to cut the cord, using eye-liners made from kerosene, application of eye-liners with fingers, and squeezing of the infant's breasts. Health education also needs to focus on beliefs regarding skin colour change, crying behaviour, and refusal to breastfeed.

The use of TBAs and delivery kits are widely promoted in the country, and there is strong support for immediate breastfeeding and feeding the colostrum. Tradition and culture is deeply rooted in Nepal, however, especially in rural areas. Hence, changes in these practices and beliefs are slow. Even so, several studies, for example an educational session related to newborn care conducted for village women in the Thankre and Kusma villages in Dhading and Nawalparasi districts, have demonstrated that it is possible to introduce changes in practice and behaviour.[3]

Future ideas for action include:

- Auditing the implementation of guidelines on newborn care at the family and community level (included in the National Maternity guidelines of the MOH).
- Development of an IEC programme on appropriate newborn care with target communities, in the local language and based on local culture and tradition, with visual material, songs, and street dramas.
- Case studies and in-depth studies on newborn care to prove the scientific value of helpful traditional practices, and provide facts to help in changing harmful practices and beliefs.

References

1. *Nepal Family Health Survey 1990*, Family Health Division, Department of Heath Services, Ministry of Health, Kathmandu, Nepal.
2. Dali SM, Thapa M and Shrestha S, "Study on KAP of mothers-in-law regarding the intraconceptional care of their daughter's in law — Before and after educational service," IOM/WHO, Kathmandu, Nepal (1991).
3. Thapa M, "Action research on women's participation and leadership in maternal health and family planning," IOM/MOH/WHO/UNFPA, Kathmandu, Nepal (1994).

Section 3:

Cost-Effective Essential Newborn Care in Poor Communities: The Evidence-Base

Chapter 8

EFFECTIVE INTERVENTIONS IN PREGNANCY TO IMPROVE FOETAL GROWTH

Amali Lokugamage
Honorary Lecturer & Specialist Registrar in
Obstetrics and Gynaecology,
University College London Medical School

and

Charles H. Rodeck
Professor of Obstetrics and Gynaecology,
University College London Medical School

Introduction

Definition

A foetus that is small for gestational age may be constitutionally small, with no significant increase in risk of perinatal mortality or morbidity, or it may be growth-restricted due to failure to fulfill its growth potential — the result of genetic disease or environmental damage — or due to reduced placental perfusion and uteroplacental insufficiency.

The causation of foetal growth retardation (FGR) is poorly understood and often difficult to detect. Two patterns of FGR are generally described. *Symmetrical* growth retardation can be observed ultrasonically as both the head circumference and abdominal circumference measurements being below the fifth centile. An *asymmetrical* growth retardation pattern is depicted by a foetal abdominal circumference which is markedly below the centile on which the head circumference lies on a growth chart. When there is a curtailing of foetal growth, there is redistribution of foetal blood flow with more blood to the brain and heart and less to the peripheries and the liver and kidneys, a reduction of foetal movements, and a decrease in amniotic fluid.

There are many theories that speculate upon ways in which to improve foetal growth. However, most theories involve the use of expensive scientific technology which would make application very difficult in the developing world. It is interesting that in reviewing the clinical trials of measures to improve foetal growth, most complicated "advanced technology" interventions do not offer obvious solutions at all, and that basic improvements in the health and nutritional status of the mother still form the core of providing the best environment for foetal growth.

Assessment of Foetal Growth and Well Being

Several methods of foetal assessment are outlined below with reference to an evidence-based evaluation of their actual effectiveness in detection of foetal compromise.

Abdominal examination

Abdominal palpation[1] to postulate foetal size by experienced doctors and midwives has been disproved as a scientific method of estimating foetal size. 20% of such assessments just before birth are not within 450 g of actual birth weight and errors are worse at the extremes of the ranges where information is most needed.

Numerous studies have evaluated measuring symphyseal fundal height[2,3] and have shown it to have quite reasonable sensitivity and specificity in picking up small-for-gestational-age-foetuses, despite obvious difficulties such as intra- and inter-observer error in taking the measurements.

Abdominal girth measurement has not been scientifically evaluated.

Foetal movement counting

Two randomised control trials[4,5] collectively provide no evidence that routine formal foetal movement counting reduces the incidence of intrauterine foetal death in late pregnancy. However, there is a small possibility that an occasional woman might benefit from foetal movement counting to prevent foetal death, i.e. those in an at-risk group.

Non-stress cardiotocography

Interpreting foetal heart rate patterns, without induced contractions, in the antenatal setting was introduced in 1969. Its use is widespread, however evidence based analyses provide no support for the use of antepartum non-stress cardiotocography. In four trials[6-9] of non-stress testing that have been reported, perinatal deaths from causes other than malformations were more common in the groups whose test results clinicians had access to. Collectively, the increase in perinatal deaths among women tested was statistically higher (three-fold).

Antenatal cardiotocography is only truly an immediate assessment of foetal well being. With present knowledge it would seem sensible to reserve its use to situations in which acute foetal hypoxia may be present (e.g. sudden reduction of foetal movements or antepartum haemorrhage).

Contraction stress testing

The oxytocin challenge test or nipple stimulation stress test have not been found to be useful as they may potentially harm a compromised foetus, because uterine activity can be unpredictable.[10] Its use is contraindicated in pregnancies affected by antepartum bleeding, placenta praevia, history of preterm labour, or preterm rupture of membranes.

Biochemical tests

Biochemical tests such as oestriol[11] and human placental lactogen assays[12] are expensive and have a low predictive value for adverse outcome.

Unexplained elevation of maternal alpha-fetoprotein[13-15] levels may help to predict later intrauterine growth retardation but is not a very sensitive test. Elevated levels of AFP and *B*HCG, in the double test to screen for Down's syndrome and neural tube defects, indicate a pregnancy at greater risk of perinatal mortality. At present, there are no other substances, such as other hormones or enzymes, that have sufficient predictive properties that would be useful for clinical practice.

Ultrasound

Women in developing countries may not have access to routine ultrasonography for dating or foetal size and hence any possible attendant problems of over-scanning. Animal studies[16] have suggested that exposure to ultrasound may reduce birth weight, but non-randomised cohort studies and randomised trials[17,18] have failed to reach any conclusion about the effects of ultrasound on human birth weight.

Ultrasound techniques are available to confirm foetal size at a single point in time to clarify the clinical impression that the foetus is small for gestational age. It can also assess amniotic fluid volume, which is an indicator of placental function, via foetal urine output, grade placental appearance, and look at the movement and behaviour of the foetus.

Serial ultrasound measurements can reveal deviations from normal growth velocity and detect any asymmetry in foetal growth.

Doppler ultrasound

Doppler ultrasound techniques are helpful in looking at blood flow through the umbilical and uterine vessels. Abnormalities in foetal umbilical blood flow may occur due to placental insufficiency. Knowing that these abnormalities exist can prompt actions such as elective delivery. Uteroplacental Doppler ultrasound may be effective in decreasing perinatal mortality in high risk groups, but has not been proven to have any effect on pregnancy outcome when used as a screening test in low risk populations.[19,20,25]

At present trials are underway to investigate whether abnormalities in uterine artery blood flow can predict the risk of developing pre-eclampsia or intrauterine growth retardation. However, the cost of this technique would be prohibitive for use in many obstetric units in the developing world.

Foetal biophysical profile

This is a scoring system combining foetal movement, tone, reactivity, breathing, and amniotic fluid volume. Its intention is to reduce the frequency of false positive and false negative results compared to non-stress cardiotocography alone. In two controlled trials[21,22] comparing biophysical profile with non-stress (CTG) cardiotocography, the biophysical profile was more sensitive and specific than the non-stress test in predicting overall abnormal outcome. However, despite the slightly superior predictive value of the biophysical score it did not result in a statistically improved rate of perinatal deaths, foetal distress in labour, low Apgars, or low birth weight for gestational age.

Placental grading

One randomised trial[23] reporting placental "texture" grading performed at 30–32 weeks and 32–34 weeks gestation suggested that knowledge of placental appearance can result in clinical action to improve pregnancy outcome. Appropriate clinical action consisted of an increased use of other foetal assessment techniques or immediate delivery for foetal compromise. The findings of this trial resulted in less frequent meconium staining of amniotic fluid, fewer neonates with low Apgars at five minutes, and fewer deaths of normally formed foetuses during the perinatal period. Further studies are required to prove or refute the findings of this studies.

Cordocentesis

Cordocentesis can be used in tertiary referral centres to check foetal karyotype, blood gases and metabolites in small-for-gestational-age foetuses, but the risks of foetal death from the procedure has to be balanced against any potential benefit to the foetus.[24]

Treatments for Foetal Compromise

Once foetal compromise has been suspected or detected, the choice of clinical action lies between delivery or conservative management if there is prematurity. If management has to be conservative the following interventions have been examined: hospitalisation and bed rest, abdominal decompression, beta-mimetics, maternal oxygen therapy, hormone therapy, calcium blockers, plasma volume expansion, transcutaneous electrostimulation, and calf blood extract.[25] However, all of these methods, except for perhaps abdominal decompression, have not yet been proven to help treat a compromised foetus.

The latter treatments all need further rigorous and scientific trials to evaluate them properly. Elective delivery still seems to be the most effective clinical action. Monitoring foetal well being until delivery with Doppler ultrasound assessment of uteroplacental and foetal blood flow seems to be, at present, the most effective method of assessing whether immediate delivery is necessary or not.

Two out of three trials[26-28] examining abdominal decompression as a treatment when foetal compromise has been detected have shown a reduction in the incidence of low birth weight, low Apgar scores and perinatal mortality.

There are no trials[29] that give good evidence that hospitalisation and bed rest improves foetal growth even though this is a common practice among obstetricians.

Prevention of Intrauterine Growth Retardation

Pre-pregnancy advice

Cigarette smoking has been shown to clearly retard foetal growth, hence interventions that help women reduce cigarette smoking are beneficial.[30] Population strategies that aim to achieve a community wide reduction in smoking are best.

High levels of peri-conceptual alcohol consumption can lead to foetal growth retardation, mental retardation, and a dysmorphic syndrome.[25,31,32] No formal trials of interventions to reduce high levels of consumption in pregnancy have been reported and there is no consensus as to the degree of risk of low levels of regular alcohol consumption in the peri-conceptual period.

Pre-conceptual improvements in diet, although desirable for general health, have not been shown to prevent malformations or low birth weight except for supplementation with folic acid (4 mg/day) to reduce the risk of neural tube defects.[33,34] The peri-conceptual effects of extreme famine are not clear and evidence on the effects of physical activity, work, exercise and travel is still inconsistent.

In utero infections such as rubella or toxoplasmosis have been shown to produce intrauterine growth retardation.[35,36] Therefore, pre-pregnancy rubella vaccination and general health education advice to avoid toxoplasmosis, i.e. wearing gloves when touching soil or cat faeces, and avoiding consumption of raw or undercooked meat, are useful interventions.

Pregnancy advice

Diet and foetal growth

Severe dietary restriction during pregnancy[37-39] can cause a marked decrease in birth weight. In the studies that examine this issue, starvation had no effect on gestational age or rate of preterm birth, but may depress birth weight by 550 g.

Studies examining the effect on foetal growth in obese mothers whose diet were restricted, have been too small to demonstrate or exclude an effect on foetal growth.[25,40-42] The extent to which major suppression of foetal weight is associated with perinatal mortality and morbidity is unknown, therefore imposing dietary restrictions or major manipulation of dietary constituents upon them cannot be justified.

Attempts have been made to improve foetal growth by administering high protein nutritional supplementation,[43-45] but in fact trials of high protein nutritional supplementation provide no evidence of benefit to foetal growth

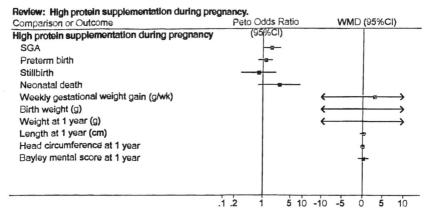

Figure 1 Trials of the effects of protein–energy supplementation during pregnancy.

and even suggest an increased incidence of small-for-gestational age births in higher protein intervention groups as compared to groups given supplements of similar calorific content but lesser protein concentration (see Figure 1).

Balanced energy and protein supplementation[44] results in only a small increase in average birth weight (~ 30 g) and a small decrease in the incidence of low birth weight. Although there is a small benefit shown with actual protein/energy supplementation in developed countries, it may prove to be of large benefit to mothers in developing countries.

A Gambian study[62] has shown that prenatal dietary supplementation with high energy foods can result in reduced rates of foetal growth retardation if this intervention is targeted at genuinely at-risk mothers. This was in turn linked to a reduction in the prevalence of stillbirth and neonatal mortality.

Prevention of pre-eclampsia

Pre-eclampsia is closely linked to intrauterine growth retardation. Evidence to suggest prophylactic dietary manipulation may help to prevent pre-eclampsia and hence perhaps growth retardation remains insufficient.[46,47]

Prophylactic fish oil in pregnancy has been studied and may provide a reduction in the incidence of proteinuric pre-eclampsia and preterm delivery, but there is not enough data to show a decrease in the incidence of any other measure of perinatal mortality or morbidity.[48-50]

A large randomised double-blinded trial[51] from Brazil attempted to settle the debate on whether there is any benefit in administering low dose aspirin to women at moderate risk of pre-eclampsia or intrauterine growth retardation. No significant differences were noted between the treatment group and the placebo group in the incidence of pre-eclampsia or foetal growth retardation.

Haematinic supplements

Routine supplementation may be of benefit if there is genuine evidence of iron deficiency and iron treatment is needed, or in countries where iron deficiency is a common problem, but at present there are no well conducted trials to verify this. In developed countries, no benefit has been detected by using iron or folate on any of the following outcomes: proteinuric hypertension, antepartum haemorrhage, maternal infection, preterm birth, low birth rate, stillbirth, or neonatal morbidity.[52-54]

Meta-analysis of studies investigating iron supplementation in well nourished communities show that this intervention may reduce the need for postpartum transfusions.[63]

Often, normal haematological dilutional adaptations to pregnancy are misread as evidence of iron deficiency that needs to be corrected. The supposition that a high level of haemoglobin in pregnancy puts a woman in a better position to withstand haemorrhage remains unsubstantiated.[25] A low haemoglobin of 10 or 10.5 g/dl in healthy women implies a large circulating blood volume, and it is plausible that healthy women with a low haemoglobin might better withstand a given loss.

It is unclear whether routine iron supplementation causes harm in well nourished communities. One previous reviewer has suggested[64] that iron supplementation may increase the prevalence of preterm birth and low birth weight. The foetal effects of administering iron are unclear despite theories which postulate that increasing maternal blood viscosity may impede uteroplacental blood flow and influence foetal growth.

Mineral supplementation

Many trials examining the role of calcium supplementation in pregnancy,[55,56] such as the Guatemalan study, have shown a marked reduction in the risk of women developing hypertension and proteinuric pre-eclampsia. But at present it is too premature to extrapolate to any other benefit such as improving foetal growth or reducing the incidence of perinatal death as the evidence is insufficient. Hence, larger trials are necessary to examine these issues.

Data from trials looking at magnesium supplementation[25,57,58] have suggested a reduced incidence of preterm birth and low birth weight, but the studies have been shown to be biased.

Malarial chemoprophylaxis

Improved foetal growth and higher maternal haemoglobin levels can be achieved by administering anti-malarials in malaria-endemic areas. The benefits of anti-malarial chemoprophylaxis are more prominent in primigravidae.[59,60]

Conclusion

We need better knowledge about the factors that control foetal growth. Presently, effective treatments to improve foetal growth are sparse. Preventative measures may possibly be improved if they are combined with the concepts proposed by the Barker studies.[61] Barker's group suggests that retarded foetal and infant growth are strongly related to adult death from obstructive lung disease and cardiovascular disease, and to risk factors for these diseases. They have also found that a large placenta is related to raised adult blood pressure in future life and that a large placenta may be due to sub-optimal maternal nutrition. Prevention and treatment of foetal growth retardation are part of a broad spectrum of interrelated variables that affect human health and have implications in improving the health of whole communities worldwide.

References

1. Loeffler FE, "Clinical foetal weight prediction," *Journal of Obstetrics and Gynaecology British Commonwealth* **74** (1967): 675–677.
2. Pearce JM and Campbell S, "A comparison of symphysis-fundal height and ultrasound as screening tests for light for gestational age infants," *British Journal of Obstetrics and Gynaecology* **94** (1987): 100–104.
3. Quaranta P, Currell R, Redman CWG and Robinson JS, "Prediction of small for dates infants by measurements of symphysial-fundal height," *British Journal of Obstetrics and Gynaecology* **88** (1981): 115–119.
4. Neldham S, "Foetal movements as an indicator of foetal wellbeing," *Danish Medical Bulletin* **30** (1983): 274–280.
5. Grant AM, Elbourne DR, Valentin L and Alexander S, "Routine formal foetal movement counting and risk of antepartum late death in normally formed singletons," *Lancet* **ii** (1989): 1345.
6. Brown VA, Sawers RS, Parsons RJ, Duncan SLB and Cooke D, "The value of antenatal cardiotocography in the management of high risk pregnancy: A randomized controlled trial," *British Journal of Obstetrics and Gynaecology* **89** (1982): 716–722.
7. Kidd LC, Patel NB and Smith R, "Non stress antenatal cardiotocography — a prospective randomised clinical trial," *British Journal of Obstetrics and Gynaecology* **92** (1985): 1156–1159.
8. Flynn AM, Kelly J, Mansfield H, Needham P, O'Conor M and Viegas O, "A randomized controlled trial of non stress antepartum cardiotocography," *British Journal of Obstetrics and Gynaecology* **89** (1982): 427–433.
9. Lumley J, Lester A, Anderson I, Renou P and Wood C, "A randomized trial of weekly cardiotocography in high risk obstetric patients," *British Journal of Obstetrics and Gynaecology* **90** (1983): 1018–1026.
10. Hill WC, Moenning RK, Katz M and Kitzmiller JL, "Characteristics of uterine activity during breast stimulation stress test," *Obstetrics and Gynecology* **64** (1984): 489–492.
11. Duenhoelter JH, Whalley PJ and MacDonald PC, "An analysis of the utility of plasma immunoreactive estrogen measurements in determining delivery time of

gravidas with a fetus considered at high risk," *American Journal of Obstetrics and Gynecology* **125** (1976): 889–898.

12. Spellacy WN, Buhi WC and Birk SA, "The effectiveness of human placental lactogen measurements as an adjunct in decreasing perinatal deaths. Results of a retrospective and a randomized controlled prospective study," *American Journal of Obstetrics and Gynecology* **15** (1975): 835–844.

13. Gordon YB, Lewis JD, Leighton M, Kitau MJ, Clarke PC and Chard T, "Maternal serum alpha-fetoprotein levels as an index of foetal risk," *American Journal of Obstetrics and Gynecology* **4** (1979): 422–424.

14. Wald NJ, Cuckle HS, Boreham J and Turnbull AC, "Maternal serum alpha-fetoprotein and birth weight," *British Journal of Obstetrics and Gynaecology* **87** (1980): 860–863.

15. Brock DJH, Barron L, Watt M, Scrimgeour JB and Keay AI, "Maternal alpha-fetoprotein and low birth weight: A prospective study throughout pregnancy," *British Journal of Obstetrics and Gynaecology* **89** (1982): 348–351.

16. Pizzarello DJ, Vivino A, Adden B, Wolsky A, Keegan AF and Becker M, "Effect of pulse ultrasound on growing tissues. 1. Developing mammalian and insect tissues," *Exp. Cell. Biol.* **46** (1978): 179–191.

17. Stark CR, Orleans M, Haverkamp AD and Murphy J, "Short and long term risks after exposure to diagnostic ultrasound *in utero*," *Obstetrics and Gynecology* **63** (1984): 194–200.

18. Smith CB, "Birth weight of fetuses exposed to diagnostic ultrasound," *Journal of Ultrasound Medicine* **3** (1984): 395–396.

19. Bewley S, Campbell S and Cooper D, "Uteroplacental Doppler flow wave forms in the second trimester. A complex circulation," *British Journal of Obstetrics and Gynaecology* **96** (1989): 1040–1046.

20. Bower S, Schochter K and Campbell S, "Doppler ultrasound screening as part of routine antenatal scanning: Prediction of pre-eclampsia and intrauterine growth retardation," *British Journal of Obstetrics and Gynaecology* **100** (1993): 989–994.

21. Manning FA, Lange IR, Morrison I, Harman CR and Chamberlain PF, "Foetal biophysical profile score and the non stress test: A comparative trial," *Obstetrics and Gynecology* **64** (1984): 326–331.

22. Platt LD, Walla CA, Paul RH, Trujillo ME, Loesser CV, Jacobs ND and Broussard PM, "A prospective trial of the fetal biophysical profile versus the non stress test in the management of high-risk pregnancies," *American Journal of Obstetrics and Gynecology* **153** (1985): 624–633.

23. Proud J and Grant A, "Third trimester placental grading by ultrasonography as a test of foetal well being," *British Medical Journal* **294** (1987): 1641–1644.

24. Nicolaides KH, Economides DL, Thorpe-Beeston JG and Snijders RJM, "Cordocentesis in the investigation of the small-for gestational age foetuses," In: *Progress in Obstetrics & Gynaecology*. Vol 11, Churchill Livingstone (1994): 75–95.

25. Enkin M, Keirse MJNC, Renfrew M and Neilson J, *A Guide to Effective Care in Pregnancy and Childbirth*. 2nd Ed, Oxford University Press (1995).

26. Blecher JA and Heyns OS, "Abdominal decompression in the treatment of toxaemia of pregnancy," *Lancet* **2** (1967): 621–625.

27. MacRae DJ, Mohamedally SM and Willmot MP, "Clinical and endocrinological aspects of dysmaturity and the use of intermittent abdominal decompression in pregnancy," *Journal of Obstetrics and.Gynaecology British Commonwealth* **78** (1971): 636–641.

28. Varma TR and Curzen P, "The effects of abdominal decompression on pregnancy complicated by the small for dates foetus," *J. Obstet. Gynaecol. Br. Commonwlth* **80** (1973): 1086–1094.

29. Laurin J and Persson P-H, "The effect of bed rest in hospital on fetal outcome in pregnancies complicated by intrauterine growth retardation," *Acta Obstetricia et Gynecologica Scandinavica* **66** (1987): 407–411.

30. MacArthur C, Newton JR and Knox EG, "Effect of anti-smoking health education on foetal size. A randomised controlled trial," *British Journal of Obstetrics and Gynaecology* **94** (1987): 295–300.

31. Abel EL, Fetal Alcohol Syndrome and Fetal Alcohol Effects, CRC Press, Boca Raton.

32. Blessed WB, Hannigan JH, Welch RA and Sohol RJ, "The prenatal effects of alcohol," In: *Progress in Obstetrics & Gynaecology* Vol. 11 Churchill Livingstore (1994): 141–159.

33. Medical Research Council Vitamin Study Research Group, "Prevention of neural tube defects: Results of the Medical Research Council Vitamin Study Research Group," *Lancet* **338** (1991): 131–137.

34. Rush D, "Nutrition in preparation of pregnancy," In: *Pre Pregnancy Care*, Chamberlain GVP and Lumley J, eds, Chichester: John Wiley (1996): 113–139.

35. Miller CL, Miller E, Sequera PJL, Cradock-Watson JE, Longson M and Wiseberg EC, "Effect of selective vaccination on rubella susceptibility and infection in pregnancy," *British Medical Journal* **291** (1985): 1398–1401.

36. Desmonts G and Couvieur J, "Congenital toxoplasmosis: A prospective study of 378 pregnancies," *New England Journal of Medicine* **290** (1974): 1110–1116.

37. Antonov AN, "Children born during the siege of Leningrad in 1942," *Journal of Pediatrics* **30** (1947): 250–259.

38. Dean RFA, "The size of baby at birth and the yield of breast milk," In: *Studies of Under-Nutrition. Wuppertal 1946–9*, Medical Research Council Special Report Series, No 275. London: Her Majesty's Stationary Office (1951): 346–378.

39. Stein Z, Susser M, Saenger G and Marolla F, "Famine and human development: The Dutch Hunger Winter of 1944/45," New York: Oxford University Press (1975).

40. Campbell DM and MacGillivery I, "The effect of a low calorie diet or a thiazide diuretic on the incidence of pre eclampsia and on birth weight," *British Journal of Obstetric and Gynaecology* **82** (1975): 572–577.

41. Campbell DM, "Dietary restriction in obesity and its effect on neonatal outcome," In: *Nutrition in Pregnancy. Proceedings of the Tenth Study Group of the Royal College of Obstetricians and Gynaecologists* (1983): 243–250.

42. Barsa Gregory P and Rush D, "Iatrogenic calorie restriction in pregnancy and birth weight," *American Journal of Perinatology* **4** (1987): 365–371.

43. Osofsley HJ, "Relationship between prenatal medical and nutritional measures, pregnancy outcome and early infant development in an urban poverty setting. I : The role of nutritional intake," *American Journal of Obstetrics and Gynaecology* **123** (1975): 682–690.

44. Rush D, Stein Z and Susser M, "A randomized controlled trial of prenatal nutritional supplementation in New York City," *Pediatrics* **65** (1980): 683–697.

45. Adams SO, Barr GD and Huenemann RL, "Effects of nutritional supplementation in pregnancy. I: Outcome of pregnancy," *J. Am. Diet. Assoc.* **72** (1978): 144–147.

46. Dyerberg J and Bang HO, "Pre eclampsia and prostaglandins," *Lancet* **1** (1985): p. 1267.

47. Romero R, Lockwood C, Oyarzum E and Hobbins JC. Toxaemia, "New concepts in old disease," *Seminars in Perinatology* **12** (1988): 302–323.

48. Olsen SF, Sorensen JD and Secher NJ, "Randomized controlled trial of the effect of fish oil supplementation on pregnancy duration," *Lancet* **339** (1992): 1003–1007.

49. Onwude JL, Lilford RJ, Hjartardottir H, Staines A and Tuffnell D, "A randomised double blind placebo controlled trial of fish oil in high risk pregnancy," *British Journal of Obstetrics and Gynaecology* **102** (1995): 95–100.

50. Onwude JL, Hjartardottir H, Tuffnell D, Thornton J and Lilford RJ, "Fish oil in high risk pregnancy, a randomized double blind controlled trial," *Proceedings of the 26th British Congress of Obstetrics and Gynaecology*, Manchester UK (1992): p. 430.

51. ECPPA, "Randomised trial of low dose aspirin for prevention of maternal and foetal complication in high risk pregnant women," *British Journal of Obstetrics and Gynaecology* **103** (1996): 39–47.

52. Paintin DB, Thomson AM and Hytten FE, "Iron and haemoglobin level in pregnancy," *Journal of Obstetrics and Gynaecology British Commonwealth* **73** (1966): 181–196.

53. Taylor DJ, Mallen C, McDougall N and Lind T, "Effect of iron supplementation on serum ferretin levels during and after pregnancy," *British Journal of Obstetrics and Gynaecology* **89** (1982): 1011–1017.

54. Wills L, Hill G, Bingham K, Miall M and Wrigley J, "Haemoglobin levels in pregnancy. The effects of the rationing scheme and routine administration of iron," *British Journal of Nutrition* **1** (1947): 126–138.

55. Chaudhuri SK, "Calcium deficiency and toxaemia of pregnancy," *Journal of Obstetrics and Gynaecology India.* **19** (1969): p. 31.

56. Belizan JM and Villar J, "The relationship between calcium intake and edema, proteinuria and hypertension-gestiosis: A hypothesis," *American Journal of Clinical Nutrition* **33** (1980): 2202–2210.

57. Spating L and Spating G, "Magnesium supplements in pregnancy. A double blind trial," *British Journal of Obstetrics and Gynaecology* **95** (1988): 120–125.

58. Conradt A, Weindinger H and Algayer H, "The role of magnesium on foetal hypertrophy, pregnancy-induced hypertension and pre-eclampsia," *Magnesium Bulletin* **6** (1984): 68–76.

59. Taha TE, Gray R and Mohamedari A, "Malaria and low birth weight in Central Sudan," *American Journal of Epidemiology* **138** (1993): 318–325.

60. Garner P and Brabin B, "A review of randomized controlled trials of routine antimalarial drug prophylaxis during pregnancy in endemic malarious areas," *Bulletin of the World Health Organization* **72** (1994): 89–99.

61. "Foetal and infant origins of adult disease," The Medical Research Council Enviromental Epidemiology Unit, Barker DJP, ed., *British Medical Journal* (1992).

62. Ceesay SM, Prentice AM, Cole TJ, Foord F, Weaver LT, Poskitt EME and Whitehead RG, "Effects on birth weight and perinatal mortality of maternal dietary supplements in rural Gambia: Five year randomised controlled trial," *British Medical Journal* **315** (1997): 757–824.
63. Mahomed K, "Routine iron supplementation during pregnancy," *The Cochrane Library. The Cochrane Collaboration*; Issue 2, Oxford: Update software (1997).
64. Koller O, "The clinical significance of haemodilution during pregnancy," *Obstetrical and Gynecological Survey* **37** (1983): 649–652.

Chapter 9

HYPOTHERMIA: EPIDEMIOLOGY AND PREVENTION

Ragnar Tunell
Emeritus Professor of Pediatrics, Stockholm, Sweden

Definition

Hypothermia is an abnormally low body temperature. The normal body temperature range of a newborn infant is 36.5–37.5°C (97.7–99.5°F) when measured rectally or in the axilla. Mild hypothermia is a body temperature of 36.0–36.4°C (96.8–97.5°F), moderate hypothermia 32.0–35.9°C (89.6–96.6°F), and severe hypothermia less than 32°C (< 89.6°F).[1]

Causes of Neonatal Hypothermia

Before birth, the infant lies in the mother's womb surrounded by amniotic fluid at a temperature at 38°C. The foetus does not regulate its own body temperature. Heat produced by the foetus is transferred via the placenta to the mother and the foetus has a body temperature about 1°C higher than the mother. If the mother has fever, the foetus also has fever.

At birth, the newborn infant is exposed to a colder environment and the skin and body temperature decrease, mostly because of evaporative heat loss from the wet skin. This heat loss is normal and helps to stimulate spontaneous breathing at birth. It is essential though that heat loss is limited to a 1–1.5°C decrease in body temperature. The surface area of the skin is about two to three times the surface area of an adult per kilogram body weight. During the first few days after birth the infant has difficulty maintaining its body temperature when exposed to a cold environment.[2] Immediately after birth, the infant does not increase its heat production when exposed to cold and is therefore dependent on the environmental temperature. Avoiding naked exposure to room air, being wet, or contact with cold surfaces, such as metal weighing scales, are the basic principles of neonatal thermal care.[3,4] A newborn infant that is wet cannot cope with an environmental temperature less then 32°C.[5] If the infant is dried immediately and dressed, or placed in skin-to-skin contact with its mother, it can cope with an environmental temperature of 25°C.

Low birth weight is an important risk factor for hypothermia. Thermal insulation of the body depends on subcutaneous fat. Preterm and low birth weight (LBW) infants have little fat so the skin temperature will be similar to the deep body temperature and heat loss from the skin will increase. In neonatal units in developing countries, hypothermia is a frequent finding at admission of sick, LBW infants. In one study in India, the neonatal mortality in infants with a birth weight below 2 kg was 130/1,000 live born, between 2–2.5 kg was 52/1,000, and above 2.5 kg was 20/1,000.[6] Hypothermia may have been an important contributor to this mortality.

Measurement of Temperature

In order to recognise hypothermia, use thermometers which can read temperatures below 35°C. Special low reading thermometers are available from many UNICEF offices, including Copenhagen. Every neonatal unit ought to have a low reading thermometer, but many units in the developing world lack any type of thermometer.

Epidemiology of Hypothermia

The prevalence and patterns of hypothermia in developing countries has not been rigorously studied. Most infants are born at home and their temperatures are not measured.

Sclerema

One serious manifestation of hypothermia in the newborn is sclerema, a hard oedema under the skin of the back and legs. A study in six regions of China in 1988–89 used sclerema as a marker for hypothermia.[7] 14,809 infants were repeatedly examined at home by a local doctor during the first 28 days after birth. For each case of sclerema three control infants were examined for comparison. Less then 50% of deliveries were in hospital. The overall prevalence of sclerema was 6.7 per 1,000 with regional variations from 15.7 to 2.5 per 1,000. The region with the highest incidence of home deliveries (88%) and the lowest income per capita had the highest prevalence of sclerema. There was a strong relationship between birth weight and the prevalence of sclerema: the odds ratio was 57 (95% confidence limits 17–191) comparing infants weighing below 2.5 kg with infants weighing more than 2.5 kg at birth. A significantly higher incidence of sclerema was found also among infants not dried and covered properly at birth, and in those living in houses with a low room temperature (5–10°C) and homes where the specially heated bed, "Kang", was not used.

Hypothermia on admission to hospital

In 1989 in Xian, China, a study of 700 infants admitted to a neonatal clinic[8] showed an average body temperature of 34.9°C with a lower range value of 24°C. 68% of infants had an admission temperature below 36°C. In other studies from Turkey,[9] Ethiopia[10] and Thailand,[11] most LBW, sick infants (70–90%) were hypothermic on arrival at the neonatal unit.

Hypothermia after the first two hours

Christensson *et al.* in Zambia[12] found that 50% of infants had a body temperature below 36°C at discharge from the hospital 14 hours after birth. The hypothermic infants at discharge had also experienced a temperature decline of more than 2°C after delivery because they were not properly dried. The room air temperature was 26°C. A similar result, also in infants not adequately dried after birth, was reported from Nigeria[4] where the air temperature was 27°C.

In Kathmandu (1988–89), Johansson *et al.*[13] found that 85% of 495 infants had a rectal temperature below 36°C two hours after birth. At 24 hours, 49% were still hypothermic (rectal temperature below 36°C) and 3% had a body temperature below 34°C. The room air temperature was 17–19°C. In 111 LBW infants 21% had severe hypothermia (rectal temperature below 34°C) two hours after birth. In infants with a birth weight above 2.5 kg 3% were severely hypothermic at two hours. Infants were rarely properly dried after birth.

Clinical Effects of Hypothermia

Mortality

Early neonatal mortality is associated with the degree of hypothermia. In China,[8] mortality increased sharply when the infants' body temperature fell below 32°C. A linear increase in mortality in infants with body temperature below 36°C was found in Ethiopia.[10] In three controlled clinical trials performed from 1958 to 1964 a decrease in mortality of 21–67% was found in preterm normothermic infants compared with hypothermic infants.[14–16]

Morbidity

An important early sign in infants with hypothermia is poor sucking, which may set up a vicious cycle particularly in LBW infants. A randomised controlled trial has shown that preterm and LBW infants do not grow properly if they are hypothermic.[17] (See Figure 1.)

There is also a close association between infection and hypothermia although it is difficult to know which comes first. Sclerema is often associated with septicaemia.[8] One common reason for death in severely hypothermic infants is pulmonary and/or intracranial haemorrhage[18,19] because of coagulation disturbances and left heart failure. Oliguria is also a common finding in infants with severe hypothermia.[20]

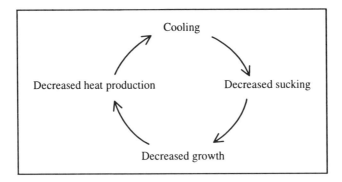

Figure 1 The vicious circle in hypothermic LBW infants with low insulation and increased risk of hypothermia.

Avoiding Hypothermia at Home and in Primary Care Health Facilities

Ambient temperature

The room temperature is of central importance and cannot be over-emphasised. A high skin temperature, especially in LBW infants, means heat loss from the skin to the ambient air is increased. The exposure of a naked infant to 25°C room temperature has the same thermal effect as exposing of an adult nude person to 0°C.[21]

In a cool room it does not matter which method is used to provide warmth to the newborn infant: it will not function properly. Solar energy has been shown to be a good method to achieve an acceptable ambient temperature.[22] This is true also for expensive modern air-heated incubators. When the main door of the incubator is opened the temperature inside the incubator will fall rapidly, especially in a cool room (see Table 1).

Care of the healthy newborn infant at birth

Many studies have shown that drying the infant, putting him in skin-to-skin contact with the mother, and covering him with a blanket will result in a

Table 1 The effect of two different room temperatures (15 and 25°C) on total non-evaporative heat loss measured on a thermal mannekin.[23]

Mode of care	Room temperature (15°C)	Room temperature (25°C)
	Total non-evaporative heat loss (W/m²)	
Dressed and cot-nursed without heated bed	58*	43*
Dressed and cot-nursed with heated bed at 36°C, or in skin-to-skin contact	37	25
Dressed and tightly swaddled with bands	85*	–
Air heated incubator with air temperature at 35.8°C	21	13
Air-heated incubator with main door open	82*	26
Radiant heater of 400 watt at 80 cm distance	165*	25

*Heat loss exceeding maximal heat production of $\cong 40$ W/m². Basal level of heat production $\cong 20$ W/m².

normal temperature after birth: these methods also rewarm infants cooled after birth.[24,25] After delivery, the skin temperature of the mothers' chest will be close to 36–37°C and thus the infant and the mother will soon reach the same skin and body temperatures. The advantage of this procedure is that it is completely safe, gives the infant the chance to start breastfeeding, and promotes mother–infant bonding.[26]

There is no reason to bathe an infant after birth. Just drying it with a clean towel will remove blood and meconium. In many Asian countries, there is a tradition to use oil on the skin. Evaporative heat loss is certainly decreased but the skin might absorb the oil, and little is known about the toxicity of these substances. The tragic experience from the use of hexachlorophene baths has to be remembered. This substance was absorbed by the skin and caused toxic effects.[27,28] The use of the so-called silver swaddler will decrease heat loss by reducing evaporation.[29,30] The same effect can also be achieved with plastic material.[31,32] These methods improve thermal stability, and can be used during transportation, but are not suitable for prolonged stationary care.

The dressing of the normal infant

In a draught-free room at 25°C room temperature an infant dressed in locally available clothes and covered with a blanket in the cot will be in completely neutral thermal conditions for the first critical month after birth. For a newborn infant weighing less than 1.5 kg, a room temperature of about 29°C (with covering of the head) is necessary to ensure comparable conditions, during the first week.[21]

Swaddling is a method used for more than 1000 years. Most probably the method of wrapping the infant in a blanket, and putting bands around, was used to protect the infant from being eaten by wild animals.[33] During the last 100 years this method has not been used in Western Europe and North America, but it is still widely practised in East Europe, Asia and parts of Africa. The reason for its prolonged use is probably that it decreases crying.[33] The swaddled infant is, however, separated from its environment, under-stimulated, and the skin-to-skin contact method cannot be used. Also, heat loss is increased when bands compress the blanket and thereby reduce the enclosed layer of insulating air (see Table 1).

Breastfeeding

Promotion of exclusive breastfeeding is a high priority. Early, within 30 minutes after birth, the healthy infant should be put to the mother's breast. Implementing the ten steps to improve breastfeeding through the Baby Friendly Hospital initiative advocated by WHO/UNICEF is of great importance.

Table 2 The ten steps to successful breastfeeding, as recommended by WHO/ UNICEF.[34]

---

1. Have a written breastfeeding policy that is routinely communicated to all health care staff.

2. Train all health care staff in skills necessary to implement this policy.

3. Inform all pregnant women about the benefits and management of breastfeeding.

4. Help mothers initiate breastfeeding within half an hour of birth.

5. Show mothers how to breastfeed.

6. Give the newborn infant no food or drink other than breastmilk, unless *medically* indicated.

7. Practice rooming-in 24 hours a day.

8. Encourage breastfeeding on demand.

9. Give no artificial teats or pacifiers.

10. Foster the establishment of breastfeeding support groups and refer mothers to them on discharge from the hospital or clinic.

When breastfeeding well the infant increases in weight, and growth will increase the use of energy and improve thermal stability. The widespread habit of giving newborn infants fluids such as sugar water, honey, or butter as the first feed may introduce harmful infections, and potentially counteracts successful breastfeeding. On the other hand, colostrum (the very first thick yellowish milk) is often discarded. This is a harmful habit because colostrum contains more proteins and antibodies than mature milk.

Separation of mother and infant is not acceptable unless the infant is sick, and even then mothers should have open access to their sick infant. Close contact between mother and infant (e.g. skin-to-skin) has the advantage not only of providing warmth but also food and establishing mother–infant bonding.[26]

Care of the sick and preterm infant

Resuscitation

In about 5–10% of newborn infants spontaneous breathing does not start within the first minute after birth and the infant needs resuscitation. During resuscitation oxygen consumption and heat production is low and increased heat loss occurs.

To avoid severe hypothermia in this situation the use of radiant heat from a non-focussing radiant heater is recommended. In a draught-free room with a room temperature of 25°C, a radiant heater with about 400–600 Watts at a distance of 80 cm from the bed with the infant, results in an effective warm environment (see Table 1). Also, in this situation it is important to dry the infant because cutaneous stimulation will also help to induce spontaneous breathing.

Extra warmth

In many instances extra warmth must be supplied, e.g. to a LBW infant or an infant after resuscitation who is hypothermic. These infants have cold hands and feet — a sign of early thermal stress. Feeling the temperature of their hands and feet by touch has been shown to be a useful strategy in primary health care.[35] Also, in this situation the safest and most effective method is to use the mother as an extra heat source and let the newborn infant stay in skin-to-skin contact with her.[36–38] No infant has been burnt by its mother, yet almost all other tools for providing warmth carry a risk of burns or overheating. Hot water bottles, hot stones, and other locally available heating devices must be used with great caution to avoid burns to the infant. Such tools must be placed so that a blanket is kept between the heating device and the infant, and the temperature of the heating device has to be kept below 39°C.

However, mothers cannot be a heat source 24 hours per day. They have to eat and sleep. This became obvious in Bogota, Colombia, when mothers were sent home with very small preterm infants using the "kangaroo mother" method.[39,40] The results were not very good: poor growth, and cases of cold injury and death were reported. There is a place for a heated bed for the infant. This can be achieved using a radiant heater placed over the bed, with ordinary electrical lamps placed below the bed, or with a more sophisticated thermo-controlled heated mattress kept at 36–37°C.[41]

Transporting Sick or Preterm Infants from Homes or Health Facilities to Neonatal Care Units

In many developing countries, infants must be carried without any special equipment. Here, the use of the skin-to-skin method is possible and effective. The infant is placed in a thin skirt in contact with the mother or father or whoever is transporting it. The head is covered by several layers of cloth[42] and the body by the clothes of the mother or transporting person. The advantage, apart from the thermal protection, is that the transporting adult can feel the infant's condition: its tone, breathing and movements.

In a health centre or small hospital it is advantageous to prepare for this situation by making thick blankets available. There is increased thermal protection if special insulating material[30] or plastic material[31] is used. Building a simple transport incubator can be done by making a box of polystyrene or a simple non-electrically heated transport incubator.[42,43]

Conclusion

1. Hypothermia is a common problem in developing countries, mainly affecting preterm and LBW infants even when the room temperature is high. It is associated with impaired feeding and growth, increased risk of invasive infections, and if severe, pulmonary or intracranial haemorrhage. There is a close relation between mortality and the degree of hypothermia: mortality is high in severe hypothermia (below 32°C).
2. Lack of knowledge rather than a lack of equipment is the problem. Poor handling — mainly improper drying of the newborn infant — is the main cause for hypothermia. To prevent hypothermia at birth: dry the infant, put

it in skin-to-skin contact with the mother, and cover it with a blanket in a room temperature above 25°C.

3. The simple use of the mother as a heat source in skin-to-skin contact with the infant is the easiest method to be practised after birth when treating preterm and LBW infants, and during transportation.

4. The use of additional heat can solve the problem of round-the-clock care, but great caution has to be taken to avoid overheating and burns.

5. Promotion of breastfeeding is of crucial importance to avoid hypothermia. Promoting skin-to-skin contact also encourages exclusive breastfeeding.

6. Monitoring the peripheral temperature of infants by feeling the temperature of the hands and feet is a simple and effective method for early recognition of thermal stress.

References

1. WHO, "Thermal Protection of the Newborn. A practical guide," In: *Maternal and Newborn Health and Safe Motherhood Programme*, Division of Reproductive Health, World Health Organization, Geneva (1997): p. 2.

2. Brück K, "Temperature regulation in the newborn infant," *Biologia Neonatorum* **3** (1961): 65–119.

3. Dahm LS and James LS, "Newborn temperature and calculated heatloss in the delivery room," *Pediatrics* **49** (1972): 504–513.

4. Omene JA, Diejomaoh FM, Faal M, Diakparomre MA and Obiaya M, "Heat loss in Nigerian newborn infants in the delivery room," *International Journal of Gynecology & Obstetrics* **16** (1979): 300–302.

5. Hey EN and Katz G, "The optimum thermal environment for naked infants," *Archives of Disease in Childhood* **45** (1970): 328–334.

6. WHO report of the director general, "Child health and development," WHO EB 89/26 (1991): 1–30.

7. Ji XC, Zhu CY and Pang RY, "Epidemiological study on hypothermia in newborns," *Chinese Medical Journal* **106** (1993): 428–432

8. Ruhei T, Jie M, Xiaocheng K and Jianping Z, "Analysis of temperature records of 700 newborn infants at admission," (unpublished data).

9. Sarman I, Can G and Tunell R, "Rewarming preterm infants on a heated water-filled mattress," *Archives of Disease in Childhood* **64** (1989): 687–692.

10. Tafari N, "Hypothermia in the tropics: Epidemiologic aspects," In: *Breathing and Warmth at Birth. Judging the Appropriateness of Technology.* Sterky G, Tunell R and Tafari N, eds., SAREC Report R 2 (1985): 53–58.

11. Pura Flor I, "Hypothermia and birth: A case report from Manila," In: *Breathing and Warmth at Birth. Judging the Appropriateness of Technology.* Sterky G, Tunell R and Tafari N, eds., SAREC Report R 2 (1985): 58–61.

12. Christensson K, Rahnsjö-Arvidson AB, Kakoma C, Lungo F *et al.* "Midwifery care routines and prevention of heat loss in the newborn. A study in Zambia," *Journal of Tropical Pediatrics* **34** (1988): 208–212.

13. Johansson RB, Spencer SA, Rolfe P and Malla DS, "Effect of post-delivery care on neonatal body temperature," *Acta Paediatrica* **81** (1992): 859–863.

14. Silverman WA, Fertig JW and Berger AP, "The influence of the thermal environment upon the survaval of newly born premature infants," *Pediatrics* **22** (1958): 876–886.

15. Beutow KC and Klein SW, "Effect of maintenance of "normal" skin temperature on survival of infants of low birth weight," *Pediatrics* **34** (1964): 163–170.

16. Day RL, Caliguri L, Kamenski C *et al.* "Body temperature and survival of premature infants," *Pediatrics* **34** (1964): 171–181.

17. Glass L, Silverman WA and Sinclair JC, "Relationship in thermal environment and caloric intake to growth and resting metabolism in the late neonatal period," *Biologia Neonatorum* **14** (1969): 324–340.

18. Rowe S and Avery ME, "Massive pulmonary haemorrhage in the newborn infant," *Journal of Pediatrics* **69** (1966): 12–20.

19. Mann TP and Elliott RIK, "Neonatal cold injury due to accidental exposure to cold," *Lancet* **1** (1957): 229–234.

20. Tafari N and Olsson EE, "Neonatal cold injury in the tropics," *Ethiopian Medical Journal* **11** (1973): 57–63.

21. Hey EN and O'Connell B, "Oxygen consumption and heat balance in the cot-nursed infant," *Archives of Disease in Childhood* **45** (1970): 335–343.

22. Daga SR, Sequera D, Goel S, Desai B and Gajendragadkar A, "Adequacy of solar energy to keep infants warm," *Indian Pediatrics* **33** (1996): 102–104.

23. Sarman I, Bolin D, Holmér I and Tunell R, "Assessment of thermal conditions in neonatal care: Use of a manikin of premature size," *American Journal of Perinatology* **9** (1992): 239–246.

24. Färdig JA, "A comparison of skin-to-skin contact and radiant heaters in promoting neonatal thermoregulation," *Journal of Nurse Midwifery* **25** (1980): 19–28.

25. Christensson K, Siles C, Moreno L, Belaustequi A *et al.* "Temperature, metabolic adaptation and crying in healthy full term newborns cared for skin-to-skin contact or in a cot," *Acta Paediatrica* **81** (1992): 488–493.

26. Klaus M and Kennell JH, "Human maternal and paternal behavior," In: *Maternal-Infant Bonding*, Mosby Comp (1976): 38–98.

27. Curley A, Hawk RE, Kimbrough RD, Nathanson G and Finberg L, "Dermal absorbtion of heaxachlorophene in infants," *Lancet* **2** (1971): 296–297.

28. Kimbrough RD and Gaines TB, "Hexachlorophene effects on the rat brain," *Archives of Environmental Health* **23** (1971): 114–116.

29. Baum JD and Scopes JW, "The silver swaddler: Device for preventing hypothermia in the newborn," *Lancet* **1** (1968): 672–673.

30. Girling DJ and Scopes JW, "Value of the silver swaddler in preventing evaporative heatloss," *Lancet* **4** (1970): 46–47.

31. Besch NJ, Perlstein PH, Edwards NK, Keenan WJ and Sutherland JM, "The transparent infant bag. A shield against heat loss," *New England Journal of Medicine* **284** (1971):121–124.

32. Holland BM, Bates AR, Gray OP and Wardrop CC, "New insulating material in maintenance of body temperature," *Archives of Disease in Childhood* **60** (1985): 47–50.

33. Lipton EL, Steischneider A and Richmond JB, "Swaddling, a child care practice: Historical,cultural, and experimental observations," *Pediatrics* Suppl. Part II (1965): 521–567.

34. Protecting, Promoting and Supporting Breast-feeding: The Special Role of Maternity Services. A Joint WHO/UNICEF Statement. WHO, Geneva.

35. Singh M, Malhotra AK and Deorari AK, "Assessment of newborn infant's temperature by human touch: A potentially useful primary care strategy," *Indian Pediatrics* **29** (1992): 449–452.

36. Sloan NL, Camacho LW, Rojas EP, Stern C and Ayora I, "Kangaroo mother method: Randomized controlled trial of an alternative method of care for stabilsed LBW infants," *Lancet* **344** (1994): 782–785.

37. Colonna F, Uxa F, da Graca AM, de Vonerweld U, "The "Kangaroo-mother method": Evaluation of an alternative model for the care of low birth weight newborns in developing countries," *International Journal of Gynecology & Obstetrics* **31** (1990): 335–339.

38. Bergman NJ and Jürisoo LA, "The "Kangaroo-method" for treating low birth weight infants in a developing country," *Tropical Doctor* **24** (1994): 57–60.

39. Whitelaw A and Sleath K, "Myth of the marsupial mother: Home care of very low birth weight infants in Bogota, Colombia," *Lancet* **1** (1985):1206–1208.
40. Whitelaw A and Liestöl K, "Mortality and growth of low birth weight infants on the kangaroo mother program in Bogota, Colombia," *Pediatrics* (1994): 931–932.
41. Sarman I and Tunell R, "Providing warmth to preterm infants by a heated, waterfilled mattress," *Archives of Disease in Childhood* **64** (1989): 29–33.
42. Templeman MC and Bell EF, "Head insulation for premature infants in servocontrolled incubators and radiant warmers," *American Journal of Diseases in Childhood* **140** (1986): 940–942.
43. Constantidinides A, Colletti PM and Snyder RA, "A nonelectrical incubator for developing countries," *Medical and Biological Engeneering* **11** (1973): 65–68.

Chapter 10

NEW METHODS FOR MONITORING NEONATAL HYPOTHERMIA AND COLD STRESS

Anthony Costello
Reader in International Child Health and Consultant Paediatrician, Centre for International Child Health, Institute of Child Health, London, UK

Introduction

As Professor Tunell has shown, neonatal hypothermia is a common problem in many developing countries.[1-3] It is associated with an increased risk of mortality,[4] and also with an increased risk of morbidity such as hypoglycaemia, apnoea and acidosis.

Thermal control of the newborn is currently being incorporated into the World Health Organization (WHO) Safer Motherhood Programme[5] and is an important element of the Baby Friendly Hospital initiative led by UNICEF.

Previous studies of neonatal temperature control and the epidemiology of hypothermia in developing countries have relied upon discrete measurements using mercury thermometers taken from single sites at wide time intervals. The act of measurement may disturb the behavioural and thermal status of the infant, and single measurements make no estimate of the duration of hypothermia experienced by infants. In addition, many hospitals lack low reading mercury thermometers; in the field, thermometers are fragile and not easily understood by TBAs or mothers.

Two new methods which may overcome some of these problems are continuous ambulatory multiple site temperature monitoring and liquid crystal thermometry.

Continuous Ambulatory Temperature Monitoring

Method

This method is potentially useful as a research and audit method in the routine postnatal environment of a developing country maternity hospital, and may shed light on weak links in early thermal care, i.e. when the "warm chain" breaks down. It may be of use to any agency or institution concerned with the evaluation of early infant care in developing country settings, for example, under the Baby Friendly Hospital initiative.

The method uses microthermistor skin probes for the forehead and axilla, and a black ball probe placed next to the infant for ambient temperature. Continuous rectal temperature monitoring is less successful than axillary monitoring as a measure of core temperature, and previous studies have shown axillary temperatures to be reliable estimates of core temperature in neonates.[6] We have confirmed these findings by showing no significant difference between rectal and axillary temperature values on the datalogger if the rectal probe is inserted at least 5 cm. At 3 cm or less the rectal temperature value was up to 0.5°C lower than the axillary value. All probes are connected to a compact battery-powered Squirrel Memory Logger giving a temperature reading to 0.2°C at 5-min intervals for 24 hours. The equipment and computer software costs about US$1,400 but cheaper equipment is being developed.

Use in newborns in Nepal

The method was used in a study in the main government maternity hospital in Kathmandu, Nepal, to describe the pattern of post-delivery hypothermia and cold stress among the normal neonatal population.[7] The aim of the study was to provide practical advice to improve thermal care in a resource-limited maternity hospital. The maternity hospital has 15,000 deliveries annually (constituting 40% of all Kathmandu Valley deliveries), but severe resource limitations (annual budget £350,000), and a cold winter climate. Continuous ambulatory temperature monitoring was carried out on a series of 35 healthy term newborns not requiring special care, enrolled for study within 90 minutes of birth. There were three important findings from this study:

Ambient temperature

24-hour mean ambient temperatures were generally lower than the WHO-recommended level of 25°C (median 22.3°C, range 15.1–27.5°C), especially in the winter months, showing that attempts to keep the environment warm were unsatisfactory. This was not altogether surprising given the lack of resources for heating and insulating the hospital, but highlights the need for vigilance and efficiency in monitoring and maintaining a reasonable ambient temperature on postnatal wards.

Hypothermia

Over the winter months most infants were moderately hypothermic by WHO criteria (32–36°C)[5] for much of the first eight hours of life. Postnatal hypothermia was prolonged with axillary core temperatures only reaching 36°C after a mean of 6.4 hours (range 0–21.1; s.d. 4.6). However, all of the newborns studied had recovered to 36°C before 24 hours had elapsed. This represents an improvement since Johanson *et al.*'s observational study[3] performed at the same hospital five years previously when 49% of babies were found to be still moderately hypothermic at 24 hours of age in the cold season. Since then, training of staff had emphasised early drying and wrapping, and early breastfeeding, as essential elements of the "warm chain". Our study suggests the intervention was reasonably effective and sustained if the achievement of a core temperature of 36°C by 24 hours is taken as the desired endpoint.

Cold stress

Cold stress was defined using cut-off values of core-skin (axilla-forehead) temperature difference greater than 3°C and 4°C. There was persistent and increasing cold stress over the first 24 hours with core-skin (axilla-forehead) temperature difference exceeding 3°C for more than half of the first 24 hours. When the 24-hour record for individual infants was studied a characteristic pattern was seen (see Figure 1). For this infant there was a period of hypothermia immediately after birth lasting several hours. Whilst under the labour room radiant heater cold stress was kept to a minimum with a core-skin gap of just over 1°C. As the newborn was taken to the cold postnatal wards cold stress increased, as demonstrated by the rapid development of a core-skin gap of over 5°C. Cold stress persisted throughout the whole of the remaining 24 hour period.

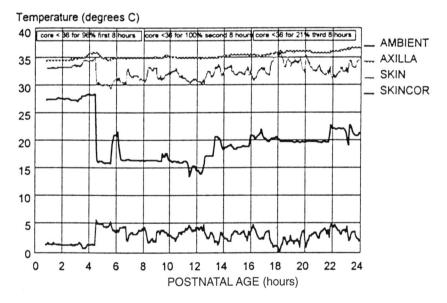

Figure 1 A representative 24-hour temperature record from a LBW term infant showing axillary (core), forehead (skin), and ambient temperatures, and the core-skin temperature difference.

Table 1 Severity and duration of hypothermia and cold stress experienced by newborn infants in the first 24 hours.

	Birth–8 hours	*9–16 hours*	*17–24 hours*
Hypothermia (Core temperature) n = 35			
% time < 36°C [mean (10th–90th centile)]	72 (4–100)	31 (0–96)	15 (0–56)
% time < 34°C	13 (0–49)	4 (0–3)	3 (0–0)
% time < 32°C	2 (0–30)	0.1 (0–0)	0.1 (0–0)
Cold stress (Core-skin temperature difference) n = 20			
% time > 3°C [mean (10th–90th centile)]	46 (14–72)	50 (10–87)	60 (32–88)
% time > 4°C	14 (0–35)	14 (1–50)	18 (1–49)

Table 1 presents data on the duration of different levels of severity of hypothermia (low axillary temperature) and cold stress (axillary-forehead temperature difference) for each of the first three eight-hour periods after birth. The mean percentage of time spent at a core temperature less than 36°C fell from 72% during the first eight hours to 31% and 15% in the second and third eight-hour periods. In contrast, axillary-forehead temperature differences tended to widen over the 24 hour period. In 20 infants for whom complete data sets were available the temperature gap exceeded 3°C for 46%, 50% and 60% of the time in the first three eight-hour periods after birth. The same infants spent 14–18% of the time with a core-skin difference of greater than 4°C.

Identifying weak links in the "warm chain"

Continuous ambulatory recording can identify weak links in the "warm chain" for newborns. The severity and duration of thermal problems was greater than expected in the Kathmandu hospital even though some of the WHO recommendations for improving the "warm chain" for newborns had been implemented previously. This technique, not previously reported from a developing country setting, may be of use to those concerned with the evaluation of early infant care by institutions with limited resources. 24-hour records graphically illustrate when the "warm chain" breaks down. In the example shown (Figure 1) early drying and wrapping in conjunction with temporary placement beneath an overhead radiant heater did indeed minimise early temperature loss. But as the infant was transferred to the postnatal ward a marked increase in the core-skin temperature gap occurred with an associated drop in core temperature. This represented an avoidable additional cold stress on the infant and prolonged the time taken for the core temperature to recover to 36°C.

Cold stress

Mechanisms

Our data on core-skin temperature differences suggest that many infants are subjected to unnecessary cold stress. Other possible explanations for core-skin differences include local vasoconstriction on the forehead when exposed to cold air, or a contraction in circulating blood volume perhaps as a result of early cord clamping.

One advantage of selecting the forehead as a site for skin temperature measurement is that vasomotor nerves exert only a slight effect on the forehead and there is practically no vasoconstriction in response to cold stress.[8] Local vasoconstriction therefore seems to be an unlikely explanation. The contribution of changes in circulating blood volume cannot be ruled out, especially as the usual practice in the hospital is to clamp the cord early. Certainly, inspection of all individual 24-hour records does not show a consistent pattern of a late fall in skin temperature, which might be expected if circulatory changes are the primary cause. In many cases, the core-skin temperature difference closely tracks the ambient temperature suggesting that this is likely to be more important than circulatory factors.

Does cold stress matter?

Non-shivering thermogenesis is triggered when the skin temperature falls to 35–36°C even when core temperature remains normal.[9] There is also evidence that infants exposed to a slightly sub-thermoneutral environment compared to those nursed within the thermoneutral zone have a higher mortality rate,[4,10] slower growth on a fixed calorie intake,[11] and a lower consumption of colostrum.[12] Ingestion of colostrum is in turn associated with a considerable increase in metabolic rate which contributes to the maintenance of body temperature. Conversely, cold stress may have some positive effects, acting as a ventilatory stimulus and as an inducer of mechanisms favouring cold resistance.[13] Further research is needed to evaluate the significance of high levels of cold stress among newborn infants in a developing country setting like Nepal, and its effects on metabolic adaptation, morbidity and mortality.

Singh *et al.*[14] in India noted that nearly 20% of term infants had a core-skin difference greater than 2°C at ambient temperatures of 26–28°C. They demonstrated the sensitivity of skin temperature assessment by experienced observers using touch alone to detect both early cold stress and hypothermia. Our findings suggest cold stress is much more common at lower ambient temperatures, and staff training in "touch assessment" may be important in identifying vulnerable infants.

Liquid Crystal Thermometry

For temperature measurement in developing countries, mercury-in-glass thermometers are generally used. Rectal temperature measurement carries a small risk of bowel perforation[15] and cross infection.[16] Several studies have shown a close correlation between rectal and axillary temperatures using this method,[7,17] and axillary temperature measurements are recommended by the American Academy of Pediatrics. More recently, the World Health Organization recommended the use of low reading thermometers in newborn care to detect hypothermia below 35°C.[5]

Unfortunately, mercury-in-glass thermometers, especially the low reading variety, are fragile and difficult to obtain in many parts of the developing world. LCT is potentially a simple, low-cost, and valid method for identifying core hypothermia in newborns. It is ideal for isolated rural communities where LCT strips could be added to delivery kits.

The LCT technique

In a liquid crystal, selective light scattering occurs at a specific wavelength. The wavelength of maximum scattering changes inversely with temperature. Thus, an appropriately calibrated strip of liquid crystals appears to "light up" in different places according to its temperature. An experimental 'colour contact thermometer' utilising this principle has been manufactured by TALC.[*] This reinforced plastic strip allows the visual recognition of temperatures in 1°C gradations between 30°C and 41°C. Three separate bands, i.e. cold (35°C and below), normal (36–37°C), and hot (38°C and above) are clearly distinguished. With a foam backing it is robust and easily cleaned before re-use.

LCT for neonatal hypothermia?

A previous study of 498 under-three year olds in Africa showed that LCT reads lower than rectal mercury thermometers by around 1.7°C.[18] The authors concluded that although LCTs underestimated fever in children the method was useful for detecting hypothermia (sensitivity 100%, specificity 92%) in that population.

---

[*]Teaching Aids at Low Cost, PO Box 49, St. Albans, Herts, AL1 5TX, UK.
Fax: 44-172-784 6852

Recently, an evaluation of the use of LCT for detecting neonatal hypothermia in the same Nepali maternity hospital described above was reported.[19] Temperature recordings from mercury, ambulatory, and LCT strips were compared in 76 newborns. LCT strips were placed between the infant's central chest area (in skin contact) and the mattress. A mercury-in-glass thermometer was placed in the axilla. Temperature readings were taken contemporaneously after allowing ten minutes for equilibration.

The sensitivity (83%, 95% CI: 70–92), specificity (96% 95% CI: 82–100) and likelihood ratio[23] for the detection of neonatal hypothermia were calculated for the LCT method in comparison with the gold standard. The likelihood ratio for a test result compares the likelihood of that result in patients with disease (hypothermia) to the likelihood of that result in patients without disease. Using estimates of the pre-test probability of neonatal hypothermia based on the measured prevalence using mercury thermometry in this population of first-day newborns, the likelihood ratio was applied to a nomogram for Bayes theorem to estimate the post-test probability of detecting hypothermia.[20,21] This gives a measure of the usefulness of the test for health workers.

Our study has shown that LCT is a valid method for identifying core hypothermia in newborns. From a clinical standpoint, the use of LCT to monitor newborns reliably identifies from 70–97% of hypothermic newborns depending upon the pre-test probability. This suggests that LCT could be a useful tool for use by paediatricians, midwives and other health workers in the developing world.

Can LCT be introduced on a large scale in developing countries?

The production cost of an LCT is comparable to that of a mercury thermometer. At present LCTs are made for TALC as a prototype, at a production cost of less than one pound sterling, and are not commercially available. The LCT strip has two important advantages compared to a mercury thermometer: it is not fragile, and the colour coding is easily understood by illiterate health workers or mothers who may have difficulty with a graded scale.

One caveat is that, as discussed earlier, the relative advantage of LCTs compared with temperature assessment by touch alone has not yet been assessed. Singh and colleagues in Delhi showed that paediatricians using touch alone could identify hypothermia in newborns with a high level of accuracy, which correlated with the experience of the observer.[14] It would be interesting to evaluate the accuracy of the "touch assessment" by midwives, nurses, and mothers, compared with using LCT strips. Pilot studies are also needed to evaluate the use of LCTs by traditional birth attendants, and whether addition of LCTs to delivery kits should be considered in Safer Motherhood programmes.

References

1. Ji XC, Zhu CY and Pang RY, "Epidemiological study on hypothermia in newborns," *Chinese Medical Journal* **106** (1993): 428–432.
2. Karan S, Rao MN, Urmila S and Rajaji S, "The incidence, clinical profile, morbidity and mortality of hypothermia in the newborn," *Indian Pediatrics* **12** (1975): 1205–1210.
3. Johanson RB, Spencer SA, Rolfe P, Jones P and Malla DS, "Effect of post-delivery care on neonatal body temperature," *Acta Paediatrica* **81** (1992): 859–863.
4. Tafari N, "Hypothermia in the tropics: Epidemiologic aspects," In: *Breathing and Warmth at Birth. Judging the Appropriateness of Technology* Sterky G, Tunell R and Tafari N, eds., Stockholm: SAREC report R2 (1985): 45–50.
5. WHO, "Thermal control of the newborn: A practical guide," In: *Maternal Health and Safe Motherhood Programme*, Division of Family Health, World Health Organization, Geneva.
6. Schiffman RF, "Temperature monitoring in the neonate. A comparison of axillary and rectal temperatures," *Nursing Research* **31** (1982): p. 274.
7. Ellis M, Manandhar N, Shakya U, Manandhar DS, Fawdry A and Costello AM de L, "Postnatal hypothermia and cold stress among newborn infants in

Nepal monitored by continuous ambulatory recording," *Archives of Disease in Childhood* **75**(1) (1996): F42–45.

8. Fox RH, "Cutaneous vasomotor control in the human head, neck and upper chest," *Journal of Physiology* **161** (1962): p. 298.

9. Bruck K, "Temperature regulation in the newborn infant," *Biology of the Neonate* **3** (1961): 65–119.

10. Silverman WA, Fertig JW and Berger AP, "The influence of thermal environment upon the survival of newly born premature infants," *Pediatrics* **22** (1958): 876–885.

11. Glass L, Silverman WA and Sinclair JC, "Effect of the thermal environment on cold resistance and growth of small infants after the first week of life," *Pediatrics* **41** (1968): 1034–1046.

12. Le-Dividich J and Noblet J, "Colostrum intake and thermoregulation in the neonatal pig in relation to environmental temperature," *Biology of the Neonate* **40** (1981): 167–174.

13. Sinclair JC, "Management of the thermal environment," In: *Effective Care of the Newborn Infant*, Sinclair JC and Bracken MB, ed., Oxford University Press (1992): 40–56.

14. Singh M, Rao G, Malhotra AK and Deorari AK, "Assessment of newborn baby's temperature by human touch: A potentially useful primary care strategy," *Indian Pediatrics* **29** (1992): 449–452.

15. Frank JD and Brown S, "Thermometers and rectal perforations in the neonates," *Archives of Disease in Childhood* **53** (1978): 284–285.

16. Im SW, "Rectal thermometer mediated cross-infection with Salmonella Wandsworth in a paediatric ward," *Journal of Hospital Infection* **2** (1981): 171–174.

17. Mayfield SR, Bhatia J, Nakamura KT, Rios GR and Bell EF, "Temperature measurement in term and preterm infants," *Journal of Pediatrics* **104** (1984): 271–275.

18. Valadez JJ, Elmore-Meegan M and Morley D, "Comparing liquid crystal thermometer readings and mercury thermometer readings of infants and children in a traditional African setting: Implications for community-based health," *Tropical and Geographical Medicine* **47**(3) (1995): 130–133.

19. Manandhar N, Ellis M, Manandhar DS, Morley D and Costello AM de L, "Liquid crystal thermometry for the detection of neonatal hypothermia in Nepal," *Journal of Tropical Pediatrics* **44** (1998): 15–17.

20. Fagan TJ, "Nomogram for Bayes theorem," *New England Journal of Medicine* **293** (1975): p. 257.

21. Jaeschke R, Guyatt G and Sackett D, "Users' guides to the medical literature. III. How to use an article about a diagnostic test," *Journal of the American Medical Association* **271**(9) (1994): 703–707.

Chapter 11

BIRTH ASPHYXIA IN DEVELOPING COUNTRIES: EPIDEMIOLOGY, SEQUELAE AND PREVENTION

Matthew Ellis
Research Fellow, Institute of Child Health, London

Introduction

Birth asphyxia refers to the impairment of the normal exchange of respiratory gases during the birth process and the ensuing adverse effects on the foetus. It is an important cause of stillbirth and early neonatal death in developing countries and contributes to the burden of neurodevelopmental disability. Clinical access to the foetus is limited during the birth process. In practical terms, the identification and quantification of birth asphyxia is problematic. For the birth attendant this makes it difficult to target interventions, such as caesarian sections, to high risk mothers. At a population level it complicates our attempts to quantify the scale of the problem posed by birth asphyxia.

This chapter reviews the epidemiology of birth asphyxia and its sequelae in developing countries as follows:

- Discussion of the case definition of birth asphyxia, crucial for understanding the epidemiology. Industrialised country data is briefly summarised to provide a comparative baseline.

- A review of published studies of birth asphyxia in developing countries (including personal research experience of a prospective follow-up study in Kathmandu, Nepal). Global estimates are made for death and disability resulting from birth asphyxia. Specific interventions (e.g. methods of foetal monitoring) and broader maternity care strategies (e.g. TBA programmes) to reduce asphyxia are critically reviewed.
- A review of possible preventive strategies and their potential impact on death and disability due to birth asphyxia; and priorities for research and development.

Approaches to the Study of Birth Asphyxia

Case definition

Birth asphyxia has been formally investigated for at least 135 years. Over this time the concept of what we mean by "birth asphyxia" has undergone much re-definition.The different perspectives of the labour room, the paediatric ward and the public health office have led investigators to a variety of definitions of birth asphyxia, with varying relevance for developing country settings.

Foetal distress

The concept of foetal distress developed from the 19th century obstetric experience with intermittent auscultation of the foetal heart.[1] Due to their relative oxygen requirements hypoxia theoretically adversely affects the foetal heart before causing hypoxic-ischaemic damage to the neonatal brain. This may be manifest in abnormalities of the foetal heart rhythm or rate (normally between 120 and 160 beats per minute). These may be detected by intermittent auscultation, recommended by one authority for one full minute every fifteen minutes in the first stage of labour and after each contraction in the second stage of labour,[2] or by continuous electronic fetal monitoring (EFM).

Hypoxia is not the only cause of an abnormal heart rate. Foetal tachycardia may also result from maternal fever and maternal anxiety whilst foetal bradycardia may be found in the postmature or hypothermic foetus. Rhythm abnormalities are common during labour and are often difficult to interpret. EFM has delineated four categories of abnormal foetal heart rate patterns:

- Loss of, or diminished, beat-to-beat variability may be observed with numerous conditions including foetal hypoxia.
- Early decelerations which coincide with contractions are a normal vagal response to cranial compression.
- Variable decelerations are common, affecting up to half of all foetuses, and are due to varying degrees of cord compression.
- Late decelerations appear to be causally related to foetal hypoxia due to uteroplacental insufficiency. But it is not clear what duration of cardiac compromise is necessary before foetal cerebral damage occurs.

Nineteenth century obstetricians also observed that many asphyxiated newborns passed meconium prior to delivery. More recent studies have demonstrated that meconium passage *in utero* is common and found in 10–15% of apparently normal pregnancies.[3] In the postmature infant, it is a normal result of increasing vagal tone occurring in up to 50% of all postdate pregnancies. However, when heavy meconium staining is found early in labour there is an association with poor condition at birth and early neonatal death.[4] But the vast majority of infants born with either or both of these signs of foetal distress display no outward signs of cerebral injury. Clearly, the presence of foetal distress is not *sufficient* to predict an adverse neonatal outcome.

More recently, techniques for the sampling of foetal blood in selected cases have been developed.[5] This represents an important advance since it allows direct estimation of foetal blood acidosis, a secondary effect of the switch from aerobic to anaerobic metabolism. Given the requirement for expensive blood gas measuring equipment it is unlikely that this technique will achieve wide coverage in developing countries in the foreseeable future. Intermittent auscultation remains the mainstay of foetal monitoring in the majority of developing country hospitals. Staff constraints often do not permit the ideal scheme described above to be followed. There is usually no attempt to monitor the foetal condition of infants born outside the hospital in rural settings.

Condition at birth

In 1953, Virginia Apgar, an American anaesthetist, described her popular scoring system for the evaluation of the newborn infant.[6] This permitted a quantitative expression of the early postnatal condition of infants and was designed to be a guide to assess the need for resuscitation of newborns.

An infant suffering from birth asphyxia is usually in poor condition at birth and therefore has a low Apgar score. Over time the universality and convenience of the Apgar score led many investigators to adopt it as a marker for birth asphyxia. This remains the case in many developing country studies. Varying definitions of birth asphyxia based on Apgar scores are found in the literature. The International Classification of Diseases (10th revision) classifies mild/moderate birth asphyxia with reference to Apgar score at one minute of four to seven whilst severe birth asphyxia is reserved for infants with an Apgar at one minute of three or less.[7] The National Neonatology Forum of India suggest that "gasping and ineffective breathing or lack of breathing at one minute", which, it is argued, corresponds to an Apgar at one minute of three or less "should be designated as birth asphyxia".[8]

Unfortunately, Apgar scores correlate poorly with outcome, which limits their usefulness in epidemiological studies.[9] This is because there are many causes other than birth asphyxia for a low Apgar score. Healthy premature infants have low Apgar scores due to their immature nervous system. Nasopharyngeal suction, maternal drugs, and anaesthesia may also temporarily depress the Apgar score. There is also considerable inter-observer disagreement in the allocation of Apgar scores.[10]

In the Collaborative Perinatal Project of the National Institute of Neurological and Communicative Disorders and Stroke (NCPP) conducted in the USA in the 1950s, a specially trained independent observer recorded the Apgar score in over 50,000 newborn infants up to 20 minutes after birth. Subsequent follow-up demonstrated the poor specificity of the early Apgar score. However, the extended Apgar score recorded 20 minutes after birth had much better specificity for the prediction of both early death and disability.[11] It is apparent that continuing depression of the infant after the first minutes of life is more significant than the early responses immediately after birth.

Apgar scores are almost always recorded in developing county hospitals at one minute and five minutes after birth. The extended Apgar score up to 20 minutes is rarely available.

Hypoxic-ischaemic encephalopathy

Brown and colleagues studied 760 neonates thought to have suffered birth asphyxia by contemporary criteria (with evidence of foetal distress or poor condition shortly after birth).[12] They found that only 11% of these infants displayed abnormal neurological behaviour in the neonatal period of whom two-thirds either died or developed neurodevelopmental disability. None of the neurologically normal neonates in this study subsequently appeared on the district handicap register. It was apparent that the neurological condition of infants over the first few days of life was a far more specific predictor of subsequent outcome than signs of foetal distress or low Apgar scores.

Two years later, Sarnat and Sarnat published a combined clinical and EEG study of 21 term infants who displayed evidence of foetal distress.[13] They described a syndrome of neurological and electroencephalogram (EEG) features that they labelled *neonatal encephalopathy following foetal distress.* As described in their original study, the syndrome was divided into three stages, with severely affected infants typically progressing from grade one to grade three. This scheme was later modified by Fenichel, who grouped the clinical features of what he termed *hypoxic-ischaemic encephalopathy* (HIE) into three different patterns (mild, moderate, and severe).[14] The asphyxiated infant was not considered to progress through the grades but rather to exhibit the characteristic features and time course (of either deterioration or resolution) consistent with a particular grade.

Whilst the Sarnat system continues to be used by investigators in specialised centres with neonatal EEG expertise, the Fenichel approach, or minor modifications thereof, has been widely adopted in clinical studies.[15-19] The clinical features including modifications from various studies are reproduced in Table 1.

As with all neurological clinical examination there remains a subjective element in the assessment procedure. The most difficult is the operational

Table 1 Syndromic diagnosis of neonatal encephalopathy (after Fenichel[9]).

	Grade 1 (mild)	Grade 2 (moderate)	Grade 3 (severe)
Conscious level	**irritable/ hyper-alert**	**lethargic**	**comatose**
Tone	**either**[a] mildly abnormal (hypo/hyper)	**moderately abnormal** (hypotonic or dissociated)	**severely abnormal** (hypotonia)
Suck	**or**[b] abnormal	**poor**	**absent**
Primitive reflexes	exaggerated	**depressed**	**absent**
Seizures	**absent**	present	present
Brain stem reflexes	**normal**	**normal**	**impaired**
Respiration	tachypnoeic	occasional apnoeas	**severe apnoea**

NB: The features in bold must be as described to meet the minimum requirements for each grade. Features not in bold may be present, but are not required to make the syndrome assignation.

[a,b]: either abnormal tone or abnormal suck should accompany altered conscious level to assign grade one.

definition of mildly affected infants. Irritability alone is difficult to define objectively. We have found reduced inter-observer variability if irritability is combined with *either* poor suck *or* abnormal tone for the minimal requirements for grade one. Five non-specialist assessors using this scheme on 27 neurologically abnormal newborns in Kathmandu achieved an overall kappa value for inter-observer agreement on grading NE of 0.87 (which according to standard interpretations is "almost perfect"). When the individual grade kappa values were calculated, only that for grade one fell below 0.8 (0.79) indicating that the operational definition of mild encephalopathy remains less secure than the more severe grades.

Neonatal encephalopathy

More recently, the definition of HIE has been criticised.[20] Most investigators have included some marker of foetal distress and/or low Apgar score in their case definition of HIE. There are two problems with this approach. In the absence of a practical method of directly measuring foetal asphyxia during the birth process these secondary markers have problems of interpretation, as described above.[21] Secondly, high quality information on the condition of the foetus during labour is often lacking in the context of developing countries.

In 1992, a task force set up by the World Federation of Neurology Group for the Prevention of Cerebral Palsy and Related Disorders concluded that researchers should employ a wider definition of neurobehavioural abnormality in the newborn infant — *neonatal encephalopathy of early onset* (NE).[22] NE has been described as a *disturbance of neurological function in the earliest days of life in the term infant manifested by difficulty initiating and maintaining respiration, depression of tone and reflexes, subnormal level of consciousness and often by seizures.*[20]

Some investigators have chosen a much broader definition of NE.[23] This makes the concept less useful. By including, for example, isolated neonatal seizures it widens the aetiological spectrum of the syndrome. It also makes epidemiological comparison with earlier work on HIE less useful. In clinical practice in a developing country setting NE has the advantage of being a clinical case definition requiring neither detailed investigation nor obstetric information. It does, however, require a reasonably thorough active surveillance system if mild cases are to be detected.

Differential diagnosis of NE

The task force recognised that birth asphyxia is not the only cause of NE and recommended that "clinical information be recorded as to possible antecedents of the encephalopathy". Causes of neonatal encephalopathy recognised to-date include:

- perinatal hypoxic-ischaemia
- hypoglycaemia

- infection
- severe hyperbilirubinaemia
- cerebral trauma
- intracranial haemorrhage
- idiopathic cerebral infarction
- inherited metabolic disorders
- congenital neuromuscular disease
- congenital dysmorphic syndromes

The causes of NE are likely to differ according to the population studied and the exact definition of encephalopathy employed. There are few reported studies. A recent Australian study found evidence of adverse intrapartum events in only 13 of 89 cases (15%) in a large population based study of NE in full-term singleton infants.[23] This series includes 15 congenital malformation syndromes. Such industrialised country studies should not be taken as a predictor of the distribution of NE by cause in developing countries.

Non-clinical methods

There is a growing literature on biochemical[24-26] and imaging aspects of birth asphyxia.[27] Such investigations are undoubtedly useful for evidence of acute disturbance in encephalopathic neonates. However, they lack the sensitivity to replace clinical diagnosis. Some investigators have used measures of cord blood acidosis assayed shortly after birth as an indirect measure of birth asphyxia. Low proposed an umbilical artery buffer base concentration of < 34 mmol/L as a definition for birth asphyxia.[18] However, this correlates poorly both with clinically defined NE and with long-term neurodevelopmental outcome. One research group speculate that the presence of acidosis is a good sign indicating healthy adaptation to intrapartum anoxic stress.[25]

Fresh stillbirth

In a minority of fresh stillbirths (SB) there is evidence of other pathology, notably infection, trauma, and congenital dysmorphic syndromes. However, most fresh stillbirths result from birth asphyxia.[28-30] Wigglesworth has proposed the following scheme for the pathophysiological classification of perinatal deaths (including both stillbirths [SB] and neonatal deaths [NND]):[31]

1. Normally formed macerated (SB)
2. Congenital malformations (SB or NND)
3. Conditions associated with immaturity (NND)
4. Asphyxial conditions developing in labour (fresh SB/NND)
5. Specific conditions other than the above

He argues convincingly that perinatal mortality is so closely related to birth weight that without birth weight-banding perinatal mortality statistics are virtually meaningless.

Clearly, fresh stillbirths should also be taken into account in developing country studies of birth asphyxia. Many developing country paediatric units prioritise care for term infants. In some settings, extremely premature infants do not receive active care and are recorded as fresh stillbirths. Ideally, preterm fresh stillbirths should be excluded to ensure comparability with NE data from the term liveborn population. Unfortunately, there is no simple way of assessing the gestation of stillborn infants and we must rely on a birth weight cut-off. Low birth weight is common amongst developing country term infants[32] and intrauterine growth retardation is associated with an increased risk of stillbirth.[33] Therefore, in the Kathmandu birth asphyxia study we included all fresh stillbirths with a birth weight of 2,000 g or above.

Retrospective interview

Estimating the incidence of NE and fresh stillbirths may be practical for developing country hospital settings. Community based studies of sufficient size to measure the incidence of birth asphyxia must adopt an entirely different methodology. The crucial observation in this context is the fact that the neonatal neurological syndrome associated with morbidity and mortality is not subtle. Therefore, to gauge the incidence of neonatal encephalopathy it is possible to retrospectively interview parents and birth attendants. This has recently been attempted in northern India.[34] Kumar employed a broad definition of birth asphyxia, including as cases those infants with delayed or absent cry and infants appearing pale after birth. Future studies should seek firmer evidence of moderate/severe encephalopathy signs such as an inability to suck, floppiness, and fits.

Birth asphyxia in preterm infants

It should be noted that the HIE/NE syndrome describes early neurological abnormality in the *term* and *post-term* infant. The immature central nervous system of the premature infant renders the clinical neurological definition of HIE more problematic for this group. There is diminished tone and a lower level of arousal in the healthy premature infant, making it difficult to apply the criteria developed for the term infant. Furthermore, there does not appear to be a striking acute clinical neurological syndrome associated with birth asphyxia in this group. In the absence of operational definitions of HIE in premature infants this group will remain outside the scope of syndromically defined birth asphyxia studies for the present. It should be noted that the neurological pathology seen in premature infants (typically periventricular leucomalacia) develops over the first days and weeks of life and is different from that encountered in term infants. There is good evidence that much of this pathology results from postnatal hypoxic-ischaemia.[35]

Therefore, it seems unlikely that premature infants make a significant contribution to morbidity resulting from *birth* asphyxia. In industrialised countries, preterm infants make an increasingly important contribution to overall cerebral palsy rates.[36] In the absence of neonatal intensive care they remain a much less important contributor to overall cerebral palsy rates in developing countries.

Birth asphyxia and cerebral palsy

There are many causes of cerebral palsy (CP). How much cerebral palsy is caused by birth asphyxia? There are two main approaches to answering this question. Prospective cohort studies seek to identify all NE occurring at birth in a defined population. Obstetric records are assessed retrospectively for evidence of intrapartum asphyxia. Subsequent follow-up is designed to identify all cases of CP amongst the NE population. This is then compared with expected rates of CP in the total population from which the NE cases were identified. The alternative approach is to identify all disabled children and attempt to assign causation retrospectively. Investigators conducting either type of study should be aware of the problematic causal chain involving birth asphyxia, NE, and CP. A recent summary of these issues uses flow diagrams to illustrate the logical possibilities (Figure 1).[37] This clarifies two key problems with this field of research. Firstly, we do not yet understand the antenatal events which may predispose to or directly cause neonatal encephalopathy. Secondly, as stated above, we have no way of directly measuring birth asphyxia.

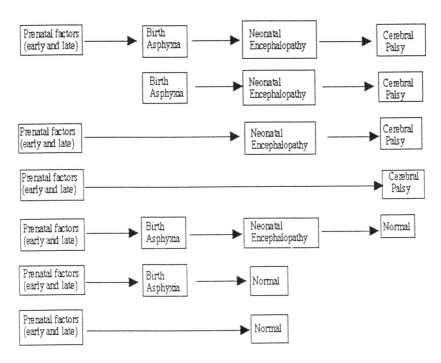

Figure 1 Summary of causal factors resulting in neonatal encephalopathy and cerebral palsy (after Stanley).

It is clear in industrialised countries that birth asphyxia is the main mechanism of injury in only 10–25% of CP cases (after the exclusion of postnatally caused CP).[38,39] In other words, CP often results from antenatal disease processes. If a disability is to be ascribed to birth asphyxia each of the following four criteria should be met:[11]

- evidence of adverse intrapartum events (foetal distress and poor condition at birth);
- evidence of neonatal encephalopathy (clinically defined);
- disability of a nature consistent with presumed hypoxic ischaemic pathology; and
- adequate neurological assessment to exclude other conditions.

It is almost impossible to retrospectively gather intrapartum data for disabled children surveyed in the developing world. Using a simple set of screening questions it is usually possible, however, to retrospectively identify moderate/severe neonatal encephalopathy.

Industrialised Country Studies

Prevalence data

The most recent studies suggest the prevalence of moderate/severe HIE lies around 1–2/1,000 livebirths.[40,41] This rises to nearly 4/1,000 in the Perth study where the investigators adopt a broad definition of NE.[23]

Outcome studies

Many groups have reported cohort studies of HIE. Some of these studies were designed to assess the predictive power of early investigative techniques and were not population based. A meta-analysis of the largest equivalent studies covers a total of 459 cases of HIE born in North America or Europe between 1974 and 1984.[42] Mild cases of HIE suffer no short-term mortality nor long-term morbidity; moderate cases have a low risk of death (5%) and a moderate risk of severe disability (20%); and severe cases a high risk of death (78%) and a moderate risk of severe disability (24%).

The wider context in industrialised countries

It is important to consider birth asphyxia-related mortality and morbidity in the wider contexts of both perinatal mortality and childhood disability.

Perinatal mortality

1993 national data from the UK includes a combined estimate for perinatal death due to intrapartum asphyxia/trauma of 1.1/1,000 total births — approximately 10% of overall perinatal mortality.[43]

Childhood disability

The best estimates suggest CP rates are around 2.0–2.5 per thousand of the population (at birth) in industrialised countries excluding those due to post-neonatal causes.[37] Prevalence studies in later childhood show some decline to 1.5–2.0 per thousand due to increased death rates in this disabled population. Many studies have attempted to assess the contribution made by birth asphyxia to cerebral palsy. As discussed above, establishing causal factors for CP is problematic. However, several studies have estimated the proportion of CP resulting directly from birth asphyxia at between 10% and 25%. Applying this to the CP rates above it seems likely that the prevalence of serious disability due to birth asphyxia is considerably less than one per thousand amongst industrialised country school-age populations.

The historical context

There have been striking trends in the short historical record since regional handicap registers have permitted epidemiologically rigorous studies. Stillbirth rates have fallen steadily and CP rates have remained steady.[37] The implication is that improving maternal health and perinatal services in industrialised countries have had a huge impact on perinatal mortality but relatively little impact on long-term disability.

Birth Asphyxia in Developing Countries

Investigators in developing countries have major problems with data collection. Many deliveries occur outside institutional settings and a significant proportion are unattended by any trained person. In India, for example, it is estimated that at least 80% of deliveries take place at home often attended by untrained birth attendants.[34] Many births are not registered at the time of delivery. Stillbirths and neonatal deaths are usually never registered with the authorities. These factors make population based studies difficult.

There are two significant trends which are gradually changing this picture. Many developing countries (especially in Asia and South America) are urbanising fast. With urbanisation come "modern" aspirations which include the desire for an institutional delivery. In the growing metropolitan area of Nepal's capital, Kathmandu (urban growth rate 9% annually), over 50% of deliveries now occur in hospital, including the vast majority of first deliveries.[44] This means the population delivering in the larger government hospitals is now more representative of the wider population.

The second encouraging trend is for community oriented studies which attempt to assess morbidity and mortality for rural populations. New methodological techniques, such as verbal autopsy, are undergoing field validation.[45] However, the non-specific signs and symptoms of neonatal disease make this type of study especially challenging.

Descriptive studies

Descriptive studies of birth asphyxia in developing countries have generally used methods of ascertainment based on Apgar scores or the pathophysiological classification of perinatal mortality. More recently, there have been three important studies looking specifically at encephalopathy rates in the neonatal period.

Perinatal mortality studies

The contribution of birth asphyxia to perinatal mortality in developing countries is a useful and important way of describing the prevalence of birth asphyxia. A literature search identified all developing country studies in which the contribution of birth asphyxia to either perinatal mortality, stillbirth, or early neonatal death rates was noted in the abstract. Table 2 presents data from 20 studies published in the last 15 years mainly from South Asia and Sub-Saharan Africa.[34,46–55] Six studies looked at defined populations, and the remainder were hospital based.

A variety of methods were employed. Several used pathophysiological criteria as advocated by Wigglesworth. The proportion of perinatal mortality attributed to birth asphyxia ranges from 24–61%. Where sufficient data was available a cause-specific perinatal mortality rate for birth asphyxia has been calculated. This lies between 10–20/1,000 total births with the exception of Rajasthan and rural Nepal, where the overall perinatal mortality was exceptionally high.

These estimates give a useful indication of the scale of the perinatal mortality associated with birth asphyxia in the total population. However, they do not distinguish between term and preterm infants. There are important differences between these two groups both in terms of the pathophysiology of hypoxic-ischaemia and the likely effect of particular interventions. In the perception of many developing country clinicians the prevention of birth asphyxia amongst term infants remains the top priority. Therefore, it would be useful to develop a separate methodology for estimating perinatal mortality due to birth asphyxia amongst term infants. We have attempted to do this in Kathmandu. We included all fresh stillbirths of 2,000 g or more and all term HIE cases dying in the first week. The denominator was the estimated number of all term livebirths and all stillbirths of 2,000 g or more. We conclude that there were 11.7 perinatal deaths per thousand total term births. This is 24% of the total perinatal mortality.[56]

Apgar studies

A recent review of birth records at the main hospitals in Central, East and Southern Africa based on a five-minute Apgar score of less than seven found an incidence of birth asphyxia of 21.3% of all births.[57] A prospective study of low Apgar scores (< / = 3 at 1 minute) in India over the 1980s

Table 2 Review of perinatal mortality studies published over the last 15 years which have assessed the relative importance of birth asphyxia in developing countries.

Place	Year of Publication	Study Population Hospital Community (denominator = total deliveries)	Estimated PNMR (per 1,000 total births)	Estimated SBR (per 1,000 total births)	Method of cause of death attribution (clinical where not specified)	Proportion of PNMR attributed to birth asphyxia	Proportion of neonatal deaths attributed to birth asphyxia	Birth asphyxia cause specific PNMR (per 1,000 total births)
Northern India (rural)	1995	C (2,243)	62	31	Interview		41%	
Nepal (multicentre, a, b — urban, c — periurban, d — rural)	1995	H[a] (2,783)	23	15	Wigglesworth	35%		8
		H[b] (10,436)	48	28		44%		21
		C[c] (470)	42	23		48%		20
		C[d] (1,278)	96	34		45%		43
Jamaica	1993	C (10,482)	41			61% (term infants only)		
Bangalore, India	1992	H (5,000)	43		Wigglesworth	24% (term infants only)		
S. Africa	1992	C (1,795)	38	18	Outcome of previous child		29%	11
Trivandrum, S. India	1991	H (13,964)	43	24		31%		13
Bangladesh	1990	C	75	37		26%		20
Zimbabwe	1989	C	31		Wigglesworth	35%		11
Thailand	1987	H (52,433)	9	4				
India (ten urban regional centres combined)	1986	H (ten studies)	57–106		Wigglesworth	26–41%		
Maharashtra, India (rural)	1984	C (3,173)		28.4		36%		
Nairobi, Kenya	1983	H (5,293)	36		Post mortem (71% sample)	38%		14
Rajasthan, India (rural)	1983	C (4,443)	106	63		59%		62

found an overall incidence of 7.6%.[58] In Kathmandu, we recorded 734 infants with birth asphyxia by this definition — an overall incidence of 5.1% of all livebirths.[59] However, over the same period prospective case finding identified 96 cases of NE, 91 of which were attributed to birth asphyxia; of these 84 had a one-minute Apgar less than or equal to three. In our study the WHO Apgar definition ($< / = 3$ at 1 minute) overestimates the degree of significant birth asphyxia (using NE as our gold standard) *eightfold*. This confirms similar findings in industrialised country hospital settings.[59]

Neonatal encephalopathy

Causes of NE in developing countries

In our hospital based study of NE in Kathmandu we followed Fenichel's syndromic approach to the definition of three grades of encephalopathy. All encephalopathic neonates presenting within 24 hours of birth were included. We excluded infants with major dysmorphic syndromes and hypoglycaemia if the neurological signs resolved once normoglycaemia was demonstrated.

We used cranial ultrasound imaging to exclude major intracranial haemorrhage and pre-existing porencephalic cysts due to prenatal idiopathic cerebral infarction. Ultrasound is rapidly becoming available in most developing country urban centres. In practice, lesser degrees of intracranial haemorrhage (especially of the subarachnoid space) commonly accompany HIE and therefore the distinction between trauma and hypoxic-ischaemia is blurred.[30,60] All encephalopathic infants were screened for infection. Lumbar puncture and examination of cerebrospinal fluid was included in those with moderate or severe encephalopathy to exclude meningitis. All cases developing clinical jaundice underwent serum bilirubin estimation. The remaining causes of NE are rare in the absence of preferential endogamous marriage patterns and may be identified retrospectively at follow-up.

Over a 12-month period we identified 96 cases of NE in term infants which met these entry criteria. Five cases grew pathogenic organisms on blood culture taken within the first 24 hours of life, which we assumed to be due to infection. The progression of neurological signs in this group was atypical. Of the remaining 91 cases 84 (92%) had one-minute Apgar scores of three or less and all had both one- and five-minute Apgar scores of less than seven. Fifty-three (58%) had some evidence of foetal distress despite the fact that monitoring of the foetal heart rate was much less than that described as best practice. Of the other 38 cases six had instrumental or operative delivery and one was a multiple birth. We conclude that the majority of neonatal encephalopathy of early onset which met our entry criteria in this setting was caused by hypoxic-ischaemic insult.

Incidence of NE in developing countries

There are three studies reporting encephalopathy rates in neonatal populations in developing countries. These are summarised in Table 3.

The Kuwait[16] and Kathmandu[61] studies were conducted in government hospitals with high numbers of non-selected deliveries (18,000 and 15,000 per annum respectively). Both studies used a similar syndromic approach to the prospective recruitment of cases. The Nigerian study[15] was performed in a tertiary referral teaching hospital delivering 2,000 infants per annum. This study used a slightly different syndromic approach for the retrospective case definition of cases of HIE. It reported significantly higher rates than the other two studies. It seems likely that this reflects the more selected population or methodological differences in case definition, but it remains possible there was a genuinely higher incidence of birth asphyxia amongst this African population.

In comparison to industrialised countries this data suggests that NE is more common in developing countries, tends to be more severe, and carries a higher early mortality. Early neonatal mortality from birth asphyxia defined in the most accurate manner available to us appears to be between one and five per thousand live births. This suggests the majority of foetuses experiencing severe birth asphyxia in developing countries die during the delivery process.

Table 3 Comparison of developing country HIE rates and associated early neonatal mortality rates.

	Nepal	*Kuwait*	*Nigeria*
Year of study	1995	1989	1987–1989
Study population	14,771	4,591	6,261
Setting	main hospital	main hospital	referral hospital
Study design	prospective single centre	prospective single centre	retrospective single centre
Grade 2/3 NE/total NE (%)	65/96 (68%)	22/43 (51%)	76/166 (46%)
NE Rate (/1,000 LB) (/1,000 TLB)	6.7	9.4	26.5
Grade 1 NE rate (/1,000 LB) (/1,000 TLB)	2.2	4.6	14.4
Grade 2/3 NE rate (/1,000 LB) (/1,000 TLB)	4.5	4.8	12.1
Early case fatality (%)	33	12	18.7
Early neonatal cause-specific mortality rate NE (/1,000 LB) (/1,000 TLB)	2.2	1.1	4.9

Case-control studies

Before interventions can be designed to reduce the incidence, we need to understand the relative contribution of antenatal and perinatal factors in the causation of birth asphyxia in developing countries. Birth asphyxia appears to be multifactorial with both antenatal and intrapartum factors coming into play.[23,62,63] There is good clinical evidence that significant antenatal hypoxic-ischaemic damage occurs in up to 30% of cases of apparent birth asphyxia in industrialised countries.[35] Even in the absence of actual antenatal damage it appears likely that some infants are more vulnerable to perinatal hypoxic-ischaemic insult than others. Thus, a moderately difficult labour with associated hypoxia may cause lasting hypoxic-ischaemic damage in a vulnerable infant whilst leaving a more robust foetus undamaged. To what extent such vulnerability may be due to maternal factors affecting the intrauterine environment and developing foetus, or to genetic factors operating only in the foetus, remains speculative.

From a public health perspective the relative contribution of antenatal and intrapartum factors to the incidence of birth asphyxia in developing countries is a central question. To reduce birth asphyxia should scarce resources be targeted more at antenatal care or better delivery care? Women of reproductive age are clearly different from their industrial country counterparts. They are more likely to be illiterate, have poor nutrition, to be burdened with a heavy workload into late pregnancy, and to be exposed to a higher risk of ascending vaginal infections. They are also less likely to receive antenatal care or be attended by a trained person during delivery. Even with a hospital delivery, foetal monitoring and early intervention may be far less intensive than in industrialised countries. How much do these various factors contribute to the excess of birth asphyxia seen in developing countries? There have been few attempts to address this issue.

The Kuwait study

The Kuwait study, from a country far from representative of developing countries, is the only case-control study of clinically defined neonatal encephalopathy. Approximately 75% of the cases and controls in this study were from either professional or semi-professional families. Also, virtually all mothers had received antenatal care. No data was collected on indicators of maternal nutritional or micronutrient status, but we can assume that nutritional status in Kuwait is far better than most of Africa and South Asia. The socio-economic status of the family was not significantly associated with HIE. Consanguinity was significantly more common in HIE cases. It should be noted that there was no long-term follow-up of cases and, therefore, some recessive genetically determined conditions masquerading as birth asphyxia may have been missed. Of the obstetric factors primiparity and hypertension were both significantly more common in HIE cases than controls. The study also found that HIE cases were more likely to have meconium stained liquor and to have undergone longer labour than controls. The latter may simply reflect the excess of primigravid deliveries in this group. Surprisingly, there was no excess of low birth weight infants or breech deliveries amongst the HIE group. In conclusion, the Kuwait study identified only hypertension as a risk factor amenable to intervention.

The Mumbai study

A controlled study of risk factors associated with low Apgar scores was conducted amongst 1,811 admissions to a special care baby unit between 1984 and 1986 in Mumbai, India.[63] Five hundred and forty-one cases, infants with an Apgar of seven or less at one minute, were compared with 1,270 controls who were also receiving special care. This study found primigravidity, pre-eclampsic toxaemia, and breech presentation to be significantly associated with birth asphyxia. Unfortunately, even accepting the pragmatic definition of birth asphyxia and the choice of abnormal infants as controls, there remains the problem that the vast majority of both cases and controls were of preterm gestation.

Nutritional and other risk factors

A priority is to assess the importance of risk factors amenable to public health interventions. Whilst low birth weight has been repeatedly shown to be an important risk factor for birth asphyxia in developed countries, this has not been confirmed in developing countries. Furthermore, there has been little progress in improving low birth weight rates by public health interventions. We know that maternal nutrition and workload, especially in late pregnancy, are important contributory factors for low birth weight, but these aspects of maternal experience are notoriously difficult to change by a targeted intervention. They relate to wider socio-economic forces which lie beyond the scope of affordable public health interventions. No study has assessed the contribution of micronutrient deficiency, an area which is proving to be extremely promising in attempts to lower infant mortality. Other potentially important factors are maternal anaemia and hypothyroidism, both of which are common, amenable to affordable public health interventions, and are biologically plausible predisposing factors for birth asphyxia.

Outcome studies

Early outcome and management

Early mortality in HIE cases in developing countries is higher than that seen in industrialised countries. Comparing the early case fatality proportions shown in Table 2 these vary from 5–17% in industrialised country studies to 12–33% in the three developing country hospital studies to date. This may reflect increased severity of the hypoxic-ischaemic insult and perhaps the increased vulnerability of this population to hypoxic-ischaemia. 46–68% of HIE in the developing country hospital studies was moderate or severe (grades two to three) compared to 37–47% in industrialised country studies.

Is the relatively less intensive neonatal care available in developing countries a factor? Ventilation of severe HIE cases, which by definition show evidence of compromised ventilatory drive, does undoubtedly prolong life. Ventilation of infants with severe HIE is rarely performed in developing countries. However, death rates for severe HIE remain high (over 50%) in both settings and this seems unlikely to be an important factor. No "magic bullet" interventions for the treatment of HIE are yet available even in the most advanced centres. It seems that careful attention to fluid status, serum glucose levels and the prevention of secondary sepsis all positively affect outcome. Whilst these are affordable low-technology interventions appropriate to developing country hospitals it is likely that their management remains sub-optimal in many understaffed departments.

The only study to look at early mortality of syndromically defined birth asphyxia amongst a home delivering population found an overall case fatality of 74%.[34] This suggests that the absence of appropriate early neonatal care is associated with a very high risk of early mortality.

Long-term outcome: How much disability is due to asphyxia?

No study has yet reported the longer term outcome of HIE in a developing country setting. This is due to the problems of poor communication and population mobility common in these countries. Although no convincing evidence of neurodevelopmental abnormality following mild HIE has been demonstrated in industrialised countries it is possible that studies to date may have been too small to detect a weak effect. In developing countries, where early neonatal death rates are high, mild HIE may carry an increased risk of death or later disability over and above that of the normal population. Possible reasons include earlier discharge to deprived domestic settings where any increased vulnerability to infection or to feeding difficulties may tip the balance in the neonatal period.

Given the high prevalence of moderate and severe encephalopathy in developing countries one might expect a proportionately larger contribution to the overall disability prevalence than in industrialised countries. But if NE carries a disproportionately higher mortality risk in developing countries the disability prevalence may remain unchanged. The interim results from Kathmandu suggest disabled survivors are no more likely in a deprived urban setting than in published studies from industrialised countries. No study has estimated the overall contribution of NE to disability rates found in developing countries. These are all public health issues of the highest importance.

In developing countries, disability surveys, such as the ten-question screening approach, suggest 60–70/1,000 of the school-age population have some disability.[64] This survey method was backed up by clinical assessment amongst a representative population of 2,500 children in Dhaka, Bangladesh.[65] This identified 10–20/1,000 of two- to nine-year olds as having serious disability. 3–4/1,000 were found to have serious physical disability, a category which includes not only cerebral palsy but acquired lower motor neurone disorders such as polio. A huge population based study of 1,579,316 children under 14 years of age in China used a similar methodology to screen (using a 41-questionnaire tool) and then clinically assess the identified cases.[66] This group found a slightly higher overall disability rate of 26.6/1,000.

However, when broken down by sub-category the prevalence of purely physical disability was 2/1,000, which rose to 3–4/1,000 when the mixed disability category was also included. These estimates are surprisingly similar to the CP prevalence of 2–3/1,000 found in many studies in developed countries.

Intervention studies

When discussing childbirth in developing countries there are two perspectives to consider:

- service delivery — 'who' attends labour 'where'?
- service content — 'what' does the attendant do during the labour and delivery process?

Service delivery

Place of delivery

Institutional delivery rates are rising in urban centres of the developing world. In Kathmandu, which is rapidly urbanising, institutional delivery has gone from virtually zero in 1950 to over 50% in 1995. Nevertheless, in rural areas there remains a very low institutional delivery rate; for Nepal as a whole it is estimated that more than 90% deliver at home, mainly due to poor access to obstetric services in remote rural areas. A comparison of the perinatal mortality data in Table 2 strongly suggests that the likelihood of perinatal death (including the component due to birth asphyxia) is higher in rural areas where obstetric services are less well developed.

Late pregnancy hostels are proving an effective approach to this problem in parts of Africa.[67] These are places neighbouring an obstetric unit where higher risk mothers are encouraged to come and spend the last week or so of their pregnancy. There is growing evidence that this measure reduces perinatal mortality. It is becoming increasingly popular in parts of Africa where low population density makes service provision problematic. It inevitably makes high demands on the user population who must be convinced of its value if uptake is to be satisfactory.

Another approach is the provision of low-cost *midwife-run birthing centres* accessible to the target population. These allow for the prompt recognition of intrapartum complications and speed referral to more sophisticated obstetric units. Siting birthing centres in periurban areas can relieve the pressure on central specialist units which may translate into improved quality of care for a selected high risk population.

Even when health services are geographically accessible utilisation rates may differ widely from programme to programme. Perceptions of service quality and cost considerations are clearly relevant to user choice.

Training for birth attendants

There is an inverse relationship between the assistance of a trained birth attendant and perinatal mortality according to the WHO sub-regional statistics.[68] In the cluster of highest PMR sub-regions (West, Middle and East Africa and South-Central Asia) less than half of all deliveries are assisted by a trained attendant. Many TBA programmes suffer from poor referral pathways to centres where foetal monitoring, instrumental or surgical obstetric intervention, and appropriate neonatal care is available. TBAs lacking such backup are less likely to affect significantly the incidence of birth asphyxia. However, early resuscitation may modify the effects of intrapartum asphyxia in some cases. In 1989, one group of Indian investigators recommended that TBAs conducting more than 30 deliveries a year should be given a bag, mask, and disposable mucus suction traps; while those handling less cases should be given the disposable mucus suction traps and training in mouth-to-mouth resuscitation.[69]

A recent study from northern India in a population with a perinatal mortality rate of 55/1,000 births claimed a 20% reduction in perinatal mortality for the sub-group attended by more highly trained TBAs compared to those less well trained.[69] The training emphasised the recognition of signs of asphyxia, the importance of clearing the airway and providing mouth-to-mouth resuscitation in severe cases. If this finding is confirmed by other studies it would be important validation of TBA programmes from the neonatal perspective. It would serve to strengthen the case for resuscitation training and equipment for TBAs — a measure yet to generate widespread support. There are also exciting developments in the use of low-cost mouth-to-mask technology for resuscitation with air which is now undergoing a multicentre trial.[71] However, an individual TBA deals with comparatively few births per year and will see very few asphyxiated babies. Supervision and training may not therefore be cost-effective.

Formal risk scoring during pregnancy

The identification and referral of high risk patients during pregnancy is an attractive concept. It underlies much of the rationale for antenatal check-ups. Evaluation of formal risk-scoring systems has shown surprisingly equivocal results, partly for methodological reasons. The introduction of a scoring system formalises obstetric management and usually brings with it a host of co-interventions which makes it difficult to identify the effect of risk scoring in isolation. Improvements in outcome usually result from a whole package of change of which formal risk assessment is only one part. This suggests the initiation of a system of risk assessment can be an effective strategy for introducing a new package of service delivery.

Different scoring systems have different objectives. Of interest in the context of birth asphyxia are those designed to predict either perinatal mortality or low Apgar scores. In an excellent review of the published literature only two of 15 studies had a positive predictive value for perinatal death greater than 10%.[72] All had high negative predictive values greater than 90%. In other words, the risk assessment was good at identifying those at low risk of perinatal death, but incorrectly assigned to the high risk group large numbers of women with a normal infant outcome. Since the proportion of the total delivering population considered at risk was high (10–50%) this has major service implications. Six studies are reported which have specifically predicted infants with low Apgar scores. The best of these achieved a positive predictive value of 41%, with 27% of the population considered to be at risk.[73] The setting was a remote rural community where the incidence of low Apgar scores was high (13%).

All screening tests will perform differently according to the frequency of the target condition and the characteristics of the target population. Many risk assessment schemes include information on prior pregnancies which makes them less useful in primigravid women, as nulliparity is an independent risk factor for birth asphyxia.

In conclusion, risk assessment is commonly used in developing countries where resources are limited. Particular systems need to be evaluated on the target population bearing in mind the operational constraints of the programme.

Service content: The management of delivery

Foetal monitoring

Several studies in industrialised countries have reported the disappointing impact of foetal monitoring on presumed outcomes of birth asphyxia. In the influential Dublin Study of foetal monitoring, continuous electronic foetal monitoring (EFM) was found to have no advantage over intermittent auscultation when the outcome of cerebral palsy was considered.[74] A recent review concludes that foetal monitoring generates a huge proportion of false positives that receive unnecessary and, in some cases, harmful interventions in order to prevent a handful of adverse outcomes.[75]

Application of this study finding to developing country situations can be misleading. The study methodology of the Dublin trial compared the best possible foetal auscultation practice with CTG in a setting of individual one-to-one care where birth asphyxia was relatively rare. In practice, both the technique and frequency of foetal auscultation is often far from optimal in maternity hospitals in developing country. Studies comparing different techniques should be conducted in the real developing world settings of busy, understaffed maternity units where birth asphyxia is common.

An important recent randomised trial of intrapartum foetal monitoring in Zimbabwe has done just that.[76] The investigators compared the detection rate of abnormal foetal heart rates in 1,255 labours randomly assigned to:

- EFM;
- hand-held Doppler ultrasound monitor;

- scheduled auscultation for the last ten minutes of every half-hour by research midwives; and
- routine ausculation by the duty midwife.

Compared with routine monitoring the relative risk (and 95% confidence intervals) of detecting abnormal foetal heart rate was EFM 6.1 (4.2–8.8), Doppler 3.6 (2.4–5.3), and scheduled auscultation 1.7 (1.1–2.7) respectively. HIE rates were lowest in the first two groups and highest in the last two groups, but the power of the study was insufficient to assess the significance of this difference. Ironically, perinatal deaths were equally common in the EFM group as the routine auscultation group. The investigators ascribe this to delays in intervention either due to failure to follow protocols or to lack of available operating facilities.

From this study it appears that the detection rate of foetal heart rate monitoring is dependent on both the motivation of staff and the technique of foetal monitoring used. It remains to be seen if in developing country hospital settings this can be translated into lower birth asphyxia rates.

Partograms

The concept of the active management of labour requires close monitoring of the progress of labour and a commitment to intervene when the labour process is found to be deviating from normal. The WHO, as part of the Safe Motherhood initiative, has developed a partograph to facilitate the monitoring of labour. The central feature is a cervicograph which plots cervical dilatation against time. An "alert line" (recommending referral to a central hospital) is crossed when the rate of cervical dilatation falls below 1 cm/hour. An "action line" (recommending active intervention) lies parallel to and four hours beyond the alert line. An important multicentre historically controlled trial of this partograph was performed in South-East Asia involving over 35,000 women in 1990.[77] No new interventions were introduced in any of the eight participating hospitals as part of this study but the same formalised protocol for partography and the subsequent management of labour was introduced to all centres. The proportions of prolonged labour, labours requiring augmentation, and emergency caesarian sections all fell significantly following the intervention. In this study, intrapartum stillbirth refers to stillbirths with evidence of life at the time of hospital presentation. These fell from 93 of 516 total stillbirths in 18,254 total deliveries before the intervention to 55 of 413 total stillbirths in 17,230 total deliveries after the intervention. There was a significant reduction in the risk of stillbirth (risk ratio 0.85, 95% C.I. 0.75–0.96) which was much more marked for intrapartum stillbirth (risk ratio 0.63, 95% C.I. 0.45–0.87). Survivors of birth asphyxia were assessed crudely only by Apgar scores and admission rates to neonatal special care, which showed no significant changes. This study provides important evidence that partography, provided it is accompanied by agreed intervention protocols which are adhered to, can reduce stillbirth rates where these are currently high (around 28/1,000 in this case).

Strategies for Prevention of Perinatal Death due to Birth Asphyxia

What proportion of birth asphyxia-related perinatal deaths can be prevented? Historically, we know that perinatal mortality rates have fallen to around 10/1,000 in industrialised countries. About 10% are due to birth asphyxia in term infants, i.e. 1/1,000. By analogy, in developing countries over the long term, the vast majority of birth asphyxia-related perinatal deaths will prove preventable. In the best available study described above, where district health centres and hospital facilities were well integrated, correctable perinatal care deficiencies were still implicated in 50% of the 10/1,000 asphyxial perinatal deaths. Where services are less well developed asphyxial perinatal death rates are higher and the proportion preventable by perinatal obstetric care is likely to be higher.

Female education

Evidence from South India suggests that female education and literacy, even without improved economic conditions, significantly improves perinatal health. But educational programmes take a generation to have an appreciable impact. What should be the focus of more specific programmes to prevent birth asphyxia in the shorter term? Should resources be directed to antenatal or perinatal care? Most successful obstetric interventions comprise a package of care which make this division rather artificial. Antenatal care programmes are important to identify and advise high risk women. Little is currently known about the effect, if any, of specific micronutrient supplements during the antenatal period on neonatal mortality and morbidity. This is an area of increasing interest.

Trained birth attendants

Which perinatal interventions can reduce asphyxial perinatal death rates cost effectively? The emphasis differs in rural and urban areas. Access to a trained person able to assess and assist women during pregnancy and labour is an essential precondition for any perinatal service. This has not yet been achieved for over 50% of the population of South Asia and Africa. TBA programmes will remain the mainstay of primary obstetric care in rural areas until health services can train and employ literate young women as nurse/ midwives in sufficient numbers. However, even programmes promoting good training of TBAs are unlikely to have much impact in the absence of an effective support and referral system. The secondary centre must be able to intervene effectively by way of emergency operative delivery.

Better referral to secondary care

There has been little action research into the links between primary and secondary levels. Referral problems are clearly important. Ideally, secondary services should be available close to people's locale, or referral time should be short, or the target population must be brought to the secondary services. Scattered villages with relatively good roads and telephone services (on the Gangetic plain of India, for example) may find ambulance referral of intrapartum problems satisfactory. For more remote and inaccessible areas, such as parts of Nepal or Ethiopia, prepartum referral of women considered at risk to low-cost birthing centres with good links to specialist centres will probably prove more effective. It seems likely that until secondary obstetric services are accessible to the rural poor there will be little improvement in birth asphyxia-related mortality.

In urban areas, the problem is to make obstetric care affordable to the most impoverished strata of society. The hidden social costs of maternal mortality are so high as to make free maternity services cost effective to governments in the long term. Structural adjustment programmes should exempt mothers and young infants from health care charges. Where, as in India, private sector maternity services are flourishing, adequate incentives must be maintained to foster both the quality and commitment of government health staff.

Efficient identification and targeting of the sub-population at risk is essential if antepartum referral is to be effective. Monitoring of both foetal condition and the progress of labour needs to be performed regularly and competently. In this regard, innovations such as hand-held doppler and partography are likely to prove cost effective. However, monitoring will only prove effective if agreed management protocols are followed. There is evidence from both the NCPP and Dublin studies that the injudicious use of oxytocin augmentation during labour is associated with birth asphyxia. Local management guidelines should explicitly restrict its use to appropriate situations accompanied by careful monitoring. The WHO S.E. Asia trial has shown that this can be done in specialist centres. The next challenge is to prove that these management innovations can be made to work at secondary birthing centres.

Resuscitation

Secondary prevention of birth asphyxia by prompt resuscitation is helpful in limiting the further exacerbation of cerebral injury. The impact of TBA resuscitation has been found to be promising in the only study to date. More research needs to be done in evaluating the sustainable impact and cost-effectiveness of this strategy before firm conclusions can be drawn.

Various potential candidates for the treatment of cerebral hypoxic-ischaemia have been proposed. These need further evaluation in sophisticated settings, where their impact on subcellular metabolic processes and asphyxia related cerebral pathology can be studied directly. Pilot studies in specialist units should be followed by field trials in developing countries where the problem is common.

Birth Asphyxia and Disability

The discussion above has been limited to mortality. How much disability results from birth asphyxia? The available evidence, which is extremely scanty, suggests disability arising from birth asphyxia is significantly less than previously estimated. The best available evidence suggests that NE is more severe and is associated with a disproportionately higher risk of early mortality than in industrialised settings. Survival is probably even less likely after home delivery. The net result is probably similar numbers of disabled survivors of birth asphyxia as are found in the industrialised countries, i.e. 0.2–0.4/1,000. Regarding CP in developing countries what little evidence there is suggests rates are broadly equivalent to those of the industrialised world. Historically, the CP rate in the industrialised world has remained disappointingly unchanged despite improving obstetric care and falling stillbirth rates over the last 40 years. By extension, it seems likely that this will also prove to be the case in the developing world.

What More do We Need to Know?

This review has highlighted numerous gaps in our knowledge of perinatal health issues in developing countries. The following types of study may yield information of direct relevance to the prevention and treatment of birth asphyxia in developing countries:

Descriptive data from developing countries

Descriptive studies will be valuable, especially for perinatal mortality data for remote rural populations, more refined antepartum risk assessment developed and tested on appropriate populations, to measure NE rates in all types of population and long-term outcome studies of NE, and to conduct CP and disability population based surveys.

Case-control studies

These can explore the association of birth asphyxia with preventable antenatal exposures (e.g. maternal anaemia, hypothyroidism, and micronutrient deficiencies).

Intervention trials

Priorities for intervention trials include an evaluation of foetal monitoring systems in the prevention of birth asphyxia (large trials where birth asphyxia is common will also have the power to detect a significant reduction in perinatal death); trials of partography and management protocols at secondary centres such as birthing units; and more studies on the effectiveness of resuscitation training for TBAs/midwives (with and without appropriate low-technology bag and masks).

Action research

We need different ways of linking primary, secondary, and tertiary levels of obstetric care using referral rates and referral delays as the key measures. We need evaluation of quality assessment tools for maternity services, and methods to introduce agreed protocol-driven intervention strategies. We also need to assess the overall cost-effectiveness of programmes per perinatal death averted.

A Real World Research and Development Strategy

Many programmes worldwide seek to improve perinatal health under the auspices of the WHO Safe Motherhood policy. Any programme needs to collect basic monitoring data which should include the numbers of stillbirths classified by Wigglesworth's method. The fresh stillbirth rate in infants of 2,000 g or more is probably the single most useful and practical indicator to use as a proxy for birth asphyxia rates. Interventions designed to reduce birth asphyxia should be assessed with reference to this outcome indicator.

Once the fresh stillbirth rate falls below 5/1,000, NE rates should also be included in the monitoring programme.

Ideally, programmes should aim to monitor all deliveries occurring in their district. Therefore, early identification and inclusion of home birth attendants by the programme is vital. Many areas lack a culturally recognised traditional birth attendant. Birth attendant training programmes are probably a vital first step in such areas. Early emphasis should be placed on building durable links between these primary workers and the district centre. The quality of the service available at the centre (including staff–patient communication) and total patient charges will be important determinants of user uptake. Antepartum risk assessment, referral practices, and resuscitation training are priority areas for TBAs in relation to birth asphyxia. In the district centre, the effective management of labour is the priority. This requires appropriate foetal monitoring, some form of partography, and agreed protocols governing interventions. Early neonatal care at district level should emphasise prompt bag and mask resuscitation, thermal care, and appropriate early feeding.

Acknowledgments

The Kathmandu birth asphyxia study involved a large team of doctors, nurses, and research assistants without whom the input for this work would not have been possible. My research fellowship was generously funded by the Wellcome Trust. The Maternal and Infant Research Activities programme (MIRA) in Kathmandu also receives funding from the British Government Department for International Development.

References

1. Grant A, "Monitoring the foetus during labour," In: *Effective Care in Pregnancy and Childbirth*, Chalmers I, Enkin M and Keirse MJNC, eds, Oxford: Oxford University Press (1989): 345–365.
2. O'Driscoll K, Meagher D and Boylan P, *Active Management of Labour*, 3rd ed., London: Mosby (1993).

3. Wiswell TE and Bent RC, "Meconium staining and the meconium aspiration syndrome," *Pediatric Clinics of North America* **40** (1993): 955–981.

4. Meis PJ, Hall M and Marshall JR, "Meconium passage: A new classification for risk assessment during labour," *American Journal of Obstetrics and Gynecology* **131** (1978): 509–513.

5. Mires GJ and Patel NB, "Advances in the diagnosis and management of foetal distress in labour," In: *Recent Advances in Obstetrics and Gynaecology*, Bonnar J, ed., Edinburgh: Churchill Livingstone (1994).

6. Apgar V, "A proposal for a new method of evaluation of the newborn infant," *Anaesthesia and Analgesia* **32** (1953): p. 260.

7. World Health Organization, *International Classification of Diseases and Related Health Problems*, tenth revision (1992).

8. Singh M, "Diagnosis and management of perinatal asphyxia," *Indian Pediatrics* **31** (1994): 1169–1174.

9. Nelson KB and Ellenberg JK, "Apgar scores as predictors of chronic neurological disability," *Pediatrics* **68** (1981): 36–44.

10. Marlow N, "Do we need an Apgar score?" *Archives of Disease in Childhood* **67** (1992): 765–769.

11. Freeman JM and Nelson KB, "Intrapartum asphyxia and cerebral palsy," *Pediatrics* **82** (1988): 240–249.

12. Brown JK, Purvis RJ, Forfar JO and Cockburn F, "Neurological aspects of perinatal asphyxia," *Developmental Medicine and Childhood Neurology* **16** (1974): 567–580.

13. Sarnat HB and Sarnat MS, "Neonatal encephalopathy following foetal distress," *Archives of Neurology* **33** (1976): 696–705.

14. Fenichel JM, "Hypoxic-ischaemic encephalopathy in the newborn," *Archives of Neurology* **40** (1983): 261–266.

15. Airede AI, "Birth asphyxia and hypoxic-ischaemic encephalopathy: Incidence and severity," *Annals of Tropical Paediatrics* **11** (1991): 331–335.

16. Al-Alfy A, Carroll JE, Devarajan LV and Moussa Maa, "Term infant asphyxia in Kuwait," *Annals of Tropical Paediatrics* **10** (1990): 355–361.

17. Archer LNJ, Levene MI and Evans DH, "Cerebral artery Doppler ultrasonography for prediction of outcome after perinatal asphyxia," *Lancet* **1** (1986): 67–69.

18. Low JA, Galbraith RS, Muir DW, Killen HL, Pater EA and EJ. K, "The relationship between perinatal hypoxia and newborn encephalopathy," *American Journal of Obstetrics and Gynecology* **152** (1985): 256–260.

19. Levene ML, Sands C, Grindulis H and Moore JR, "Comparison of two methods of predicting outcome in perinatal Asphyxia," *Lancet* **1** (1986): 67–69.
20. Nelson KB and Leviton A, "How much of neonatal encephalopathy is due to birth asphyxia?" *American Journal of Diseases in Childhood* **145** (1991): 1325–1331.
21. Blair E, "A research definition for birth asphyxia?" *Developmental Medicine and Childhood Neurology* **35** (1993): 449–455.
22. Editorial, "Birth asphyxia: A statement," *Developmental Medicine and Child Neurology* **35** (1993): 1022–1024.
23. Adamson SJ, Alessandri LM, Badawi N, Burton PR, Pemberton PJ and Stanley F, "Predictors of neonatal encephalopathy in full term infants," *British Medical Journal* **311** (1995): 598–602.
24. Naeye RL and Localio AR, "Determining the time before birth when ischemia and hypoxemia initiated cerebral palsy," *Obstetrics and Gynecology* **86** (1995): 713–719.
25. Dennis J, Johnson A, Mutch L, Yudkin P and Johnson P, "Acid-base status at birth and neurodevelopmental outcome at 4.5 years," *American Journal of Obstetrics and Gynecology* **161** (1989): 213–220.
26. Fernandez F, Verdu A, Quero J and Perez-Higueras A, "Serum CPK-BB Isoenzyme in the assessment of brain damage in asphyctic term infants," *Acta Paediatr Scand* **76** (1987): 914–918.
27. Flodmark O, "Imaging of the neonatal brain," In: *Foetal and Neonatal Neurology and Neurosurgery*, Levene MI, Lilford RJ, Bennett MJ and Punt J, eds., 2nd ed., Edinburgh: Churchill Livingstone (1995).
28. Low JA, Robertson DM and Simpson LL, "Temporal relationships of neuropathological conditions caused by perinatal asphyxia," *American Journal of Obstetrics and Gynecology* **160** (1989): 608–614.
29. Hovatta O, Lipasti A, Rapola J and Karjalainen O, "Causes of stillbirth: A clinico-pathological study of 243 patients," *British Journal of Obstetrics and Gynaecology* **90** (1983): 691–696.
30. Lucas SB, Mati JKG, Aggarwal VP and Sanghvi H, "Pathology in perinatal mortality in Nairobi, Kenya," *Bulletin de la Société de Pathologie Exotique* **76** (1983): 579–583.
31. Wigglesworth JS, "Monitoring perinatal mortality — A pathophysiological approach," *Lancet* **2** (1980): 684–686.

32. Rajbhandari S, Manandhar DS and Costello AM de L, "Anthropometry of term newborn infants in Nepal," *Journal of the Nepal Medical Association* (1996) (in press).
33. Hellier JL and Goldstein H, "The use of birthweight and gestation to assess perinatal mortality risk," *Journal of Epidemiology and Community Health* **33** (1979): 183–185.
34. Kumar R, "Birth asphyxia in a rural community of North India," *Journal of Tropical Pediatrics* **41** (1995): 5–7.
35. Volpe JJ, *Neurology of the Newborn*, 3rd ed., Boston: WB Saunders (1995).
36. Pharoah POD, Cooke T, Rosenbloom L and Cooke RWI, "Trends in the birth prevalence of cerebral palsy," *Archives of Disease in Childhood* **62** (1987): 379–382.
37. Stanley FJ and Blair E, "Cerebral palsy," In: *The Epidemiology of Childhood Disorders*, IB P, ed., New York: Oxford University Press (1994): 473–497.
38. Paneth N and Kiely J, "The Frequency of Cerebral Palsy: A review of population studies in industrialised nations since 1950," In: *The Epidemiology of the Cerebral Palsies*, Stanley FJ and Alberman E, eds.,Oxford: Blackwell Scientific (1984): 46–56.
39. Yudkin PL, Johnson A, Clover LM and Murphy KW, "Assessing the contribution of birth asphyxia to cerebral palsy in term singletons," *Paediatric and Perinatal Epidemiology* **9** (1995): 156–170.
40. Hull J and Dodd KL, "Falling incidence of hypoxic-ischaemic encephalopathy in term infants," *British Journal of Obstetrics and Gynaecology* **99** (1992): 386–391.
41. Thornberg E, Thiringer K, Odeback A and Milsom I, "Birth asphyxia: Incidence, clinical course and outcome in a Swedish population," *Acta Paediatrica* **84** (1995): 927–932.
42. Peliowski A and Finer NN, "Birth asphyxia in the term infant," In: *Effective Care of the Newborn Infant*, Sinclair JC and Bracken MB, eds., Oxford: Oxford University Press (1992): 249–279.
43. *Confidential Enquiry into Stillbirth and Deaths in Infancy*, Third Annual Report: Department of Health (1996).
44. Bolam AJ, Manandhar DS, Shrestha P, Manandhar B, Ellis M and Costello AM de L, "Maternity care utilisation in the Kathmandu Valley: A community based study," *Journal of the Nepal Medical Association* **35** (1997): 122–129.

45. Bang AT and Bang RA, "Diagnosis of causes of childhood deaths in developing countries by verbal autopsy — Suggested criteria," *WHO Bulletin* **70**(4) (1992): 499–507.

46. de Muylder X, "Perinatal mortality audit in a Zimbabwean district," *Paediatric and Perinatal Epidemiology* **3** (1989): 284–293.

47. Bai NS, Mathews E, Nair PM, Sabarinathan K and Harikumar C, "Perinatal mortality rate in a South Indian population," *Journal of the Indian Medical Association* **89** (1991): 97–98.

48. Fauveau V, Wojtyniak B, Mostafa G, Sarder AM and Chakraborty J, "Perinatal mortality in Matlab, Bangladesh: A community-based study," *International Journal of Epidemiology* **19** (1990): 606–612.

49. Geetha T, Chenoy R, Stevens D and Johanson RB, "A multicentre study of perinatal mortality in Nepal," *Paediatric and Perinatal Epidemiology* **9** (1995): 74–89.

50. Raghuveer G, "Perinatal deaths: Relevance of Wigglesworth's classification," *Paediatric and Perinatal Epidemiology* **6** (1992): 45–50.

51. Keeling JW, "Perinatal mortality of mothers and children: The Jamaica studies," In: *Nestle Nutrition Workshop Series*, Baum D, ed., New York: Raven Press (1993): 25–33.

52. Singh M, "Hospital based data on perinatal and neonatal mortality in India: Special review article," *Indian Pediatrics* **23** (1986): 579–584.

53. Shah U, Pratinidhi AK and Bhatlawande PV, "Perinatal mortality in rural India: A strategy for reduction through primary care. 2. Neonatal Mortality," *Journal of Epidemiology and Community Health* **38** (1984):138–142.

54. Mati JK, Aggarwal VP, Lucas S, Sanghvi HC and Corkhill R, "The Nairobi Birth Survey IV. Early perinatal mortality rate," *Journal of Obstetrics and Gynaecology in East and Central Africa* **2** (1983): 129–133.

55. Buchmann EJ, Crofton Briggs IG and McIntyre JA, "Previous birth outcome of antenatal attenders in northern Kwazulu — Perinatal and infant mortality rates," *South African Medical Journal* **81** (1992): 419–421.

56. Ellis M, Manandhar N, Wyatt J, Manandhar DS, Bolam AJ and Costello AM de L, "Stillbirths and neonatal encephalopathy, Kathmandu, Nepal: An estimate of the contribution of birth asphyxia to perinatal mortality in a low income urban population," *Paediatric and Perinatal Epidemiology*. In Press.

57. Kinoti SN, "Asphyxia of the newborn in East, Central and Southern Africa," *East African Medical Journal* **70** (1993): 422–433.

58. Kumari S, Sharma M, Yadav M, Saraf A, Kabra M and Mehra R, "Trends in neonatal outcome with low Apgar scores," *Indian Journal of Pediatrics* **60** (1993): 415–422.

59. Ellis M, Manandhar N, Manandhar DS and Costello AM de L, "An Apgar score of three or less at one minute is not diagnostic of birth asphyxia but is a useful screening test for neonatal encephalopathy," *Indian Pediatrics* **35** (1998): 415–421.

60. Fenichel G, Webster D and Wong W, "Intracranial haemorrhage in the term newborn," *Archives of Neurology* **41** (1984): 30–34.

61. Ellis M, Manandhar N, Manadhar DS, Wyatt JS and Costello AM de L, "Incidence and severity of neonatal encephalopathy in Nepal, a least developed country," (abstract) *Paediatric and Perinatal Epidemiology* **10** (1996): p. A17.

62. Macdonald HM, Mulligan JC, Allen AC and Taylor PM, "Neonatal asphyxia. 1. Relationship of obstetric and neonatal complications to neonatal mortality in 38,405 consecutive deliveries," *Journal of Pediatrics* **96** (1980): 898–907.

63. Daga AS, Daga SR and Patole SK, "Risk assessment in birth asphyxia," *Journal of Tropical Pediatrics* **36** (1990): 34–39.

64. Khan N and Durkin M, "Framework: Prevalence," In: *Disabled Children and Developing Countries*, Zinkin P and McConachie H, eds., Oxford: Mackeith Press (1995).

65. Zaman SS, Khan NZ, Islam S, Banu S, Dixit S, Shrout P *et al.*, "Validity of the 'ten questions' for screening serious childhood disability: Results from urbam Bangladesh," *International Journal of Epidemiology* **19** (1990): 613–620.

66. Li R, "A study of the current situation regarding disabled children in China and its countermeasures," *Chinese Journal of Population Studies* **3** (1991): 17–26.

67. Chandramohan D, Cutts F and Millard P, "The effect of stay in a maternity home on perinatal mortality in rural Zimbabwe," *Journal of Tropical Medicine and Hygiene* **98** (1995): 261–267.

68. World Health Organization, "Perinatal mortality: A listing of available information," (1996).

69. Raina N and Kumar V, "Management of birth asphyxia by traditional birth attendants," *World Health Forum* **20** (1989): 243–246.

70. Kumar R, "Effect of training on the reuscitation practices of traditional birth attendants," *Transactions of the Royal Society of Tropical Medicine and Hygiene* **88** (1994): 159–160.

71. Ramji S, Ahuja S, Thirupurum S, Rootwelt T, Rooth G and Saugstad OD, "Resuscitation of asphyxic newborn infants with room air or 100% oxygen," *Pediatric Research* **34** (1993): 809–812.

72. Alexander S and Keirse MJNC, "Formal risk scoring during pregnancy," In: *Effective Care in Pregnancy and Childbirth*, Chalmers I, Enkin M and Keirse MJNC, eds., Oxford: Oxford University Press (1989): 345–365.

73. Smith M, Stratton WC and Roi L, "Labour risk assessment in a rural community hospital," *American Journal of Obstetrics and Gynecology* **151** (1985): 569–574.

74. Macdonald D, Grant A, Sheridn-Pereira M, Boylan P and Chalmers I, "The Dublin randomised controlled trial of intrapartum foetal heart rate monitoring," *American Journal of Obstetrics and Gynecology* **152** (1985): 524–539.

75. Nelson KB, Dambrosia JM, Ting TY and Grether JK, "Uncertain value of electronic foetal monitoring in predicting cerebral palsy," *New England Journal of Medicine* **334** (1996): 613–618.

76. Mahomed K, Nyoni R, Mulambo T, Kasule J and Jacobus E, "Randomised controlled trial of intrapartum foetal heart rate monitoring," *British Medical Journal* **308** (1994): 497–500.

77. Kwast BE, Lennox CE and Farley TMM, "World Health Organization partograph in management of labour," *Lancet* **343** (1994): 1399–1404.

Chapter 12

EFFECTIVE RESUSCITATION

Siddarth Ramji

Professor of Neonatal Medicine,
Maulana Azad Medical School, Delhi, India

According to World Health Organization estimates there are an estimated seven million perinatal deaths each year and about four million neonates who suffer from moderate to severe asphyxia at birth. About 800,000 of these die and probably an equal number are left with residual developmental sequelae such as cerebral palsy, mental retardation, language delays, hearing and visual disorders, and learning disabilities.[1] A significant proportion of handicap consequent to asphyxia in the perinatal period are preventable by improved perinatal care. An important component contributing to this improvement is ensuring effective resuscitation of the asphyxiated newborn at birth. A large proportion of the world's asphyxiated neonates are delivered in the developing nations by poorly or untrained personnel lacking in knowledge, skills and equipment needed for effective neonatal resuscitation.

The issues that need to be addressed are the appropriateness of equipment for resuscitation, training guidelines and the cost-effectiveness of interventions. The standard equipment used for resuscitation, i.e. self-inflating bag and mask, laryngoscopes, endotracheal tubes and supplemental oxygen are expensive, difficult to maintain and not easily available in most places where births take place in the developing world. Most birth attendants at the primary level are difficult to reach for training. This chapter will review alternative interventions that have been tried and tested for neonatal resuscitation, which can be effectively adapted for use in disadvantaged communities.

Resuscitation Equipment: Alternative Technologies

Mouth-to-mouth breathing was the technique used as an alternative to bag and mask ventilation in situations where either the bag/mask was not available or the skills for its use were non-existent. The technique is difficult to standardise for training guidelines and has a risk of infection, so more viable, cost-effective and scientifically acceptable techniques have been sought as a substitute for bag and mask ventilation.

Mouth-to-tube to Mask Resuscitation

Experimental studies

Milner first described the use of the modified face mask connected to a mouth piece for neonatal resuscitation.[2] It was tested by 150 volunteers, of whom 82 had no previous resuscitation experience. It was observed that the volunteers ventilated at rates appropriate for the newborn (between 35–42 breaths per minute), and achieved a mean peak inspiratory pressure of about 20 cm of water and a mean ventilatory pressure of 15 cm of water. There were no significant differences in rates and pressures achieved between the groups of volunteers. Having demonstrated the efficacy of the device, especially in the hands of personnel with no previous resuscitation experience, and its low production cost (approx. US$5), it was suggested as a device for domiciliary neonatal resuscitation.

A more refined prototype of this device, manufactured by the Laerdal Company, Norway, underwent laboratory tests.[3] The Laerdal mouth-to-tube-to-mask device had a bacterial filter and a 20 cm non-compressible tube for resuscitation. The volunteers for this study included doctors, nurses, midwives and the lay public (parents or visiting relatives). The efficacy in terms of pressure and ventilatory rates were comparable in the four groups of volunteers. The study clearly underscored the fact that unskilled personnel with minimal training could be trained to effectively ventilate asphyxiated neonates.

Clinical trials

The data comparing mouth-to-mask ventilation and bag and mask ventilation from Dar-es-Salaam (Tanzania) and Bombay (India) in the resuscitation of asphyxiated newborns suggest that the two methods are equally effective.[4] It was observed that the mean insufflation pressures and respiratory rates achieved were similar with the two devices. The proportion of newborns with five-minute Apgar scores > 3, the number with first gasp or cry within five minutes and the number with pulse oximetry values > 75% at five minutes were comparable in the two groups. These benefits were also observed in the preterm subset of the study population who had an average gestation of about 34–35 weeks. Personnel could carry on ventilation with the mouth-to-mask device without tiring for five to ten minutes, which would be an important break-point to decide how resuscitation would continue thereafter. The results of the present study need to be validated in a community setting in the hands of TBAs and nurse midwives. However, several questions need to be answered before it can be recommended for large-scale use — issues related to training approaches, equipment maintenance, and the evaluation of the long-term outcome of these infants.

Room Air vs 100% Oxygen in Neonatal Resuscitation

Standard clinical protocols for neonatal cardiopulmonary resuscitation have all recommended the use of 100% oxygen as supplementation.[5] Recent evidence suggests that oxygen radicals are produced in excess in the posthypoxic reoxygenation period with the potential to increase tissue damage.[6] The hypoxanthine that accumulates during hypoxia, in the presence of high oxygen concentrations generates free oxygen radicals through the activation of the xanthine oxidase system. It has been suggested that the use of 100% supplemental oxygen may be detrimental in the resuscitation of asphyxiated newborns.[7] These observations led to investigations comparing room air and 100% oxygen in neonatal resuscitation.

Experimental studies

Rootwelt *et al*. compared 21% and 100% oxygen in asphyxiated newborn piglets.[8] The animals were made hypoxic till the systolic blood pressure fell to 20 mm Hg or the heart rate fell below 80 beats per minute. The animals were randomised to be reoxygenated with either 21% or 100% oxygen. The base deficits at the end of hypoxemia were comparable in the two groups (29 ± 5 and 27 ± 4 mmol/L in 21% and 100% groups respectively). During reoxygenation there were no significant differences between the two groups with regard to blood pressure, heart rates, base deficit or plasma hypoxanthine. Blinded pathologic examination of the cerebral cortex, cerebellum, and hippocampus after four days showed no significant differences with regard to brain damage.

Studies in asphyxiated newborn piglets resuscitated with 21% or 100% oxygen have demonstrated no differences between the two groups with regard to cerebral blood flow, oxygen uptake and somatosensory evoked potentials in the posthypoxic period.[9] Measurements of oxypurines in plasma in porcine models during the posthypoxic period, an indicator of hypoxia, were similar in the groups resuscitated with 21% or 100% oxygen.[10] More recently, Feet and co-workers found that hypoxanthine from microdialysis in the brain cortex of piglets during resuscitation reaches a higher peak in those resuscitated with 100% oxygen compared to room air, indicating a metabolic impairment in the brain cortex of animals receiving 100% oxygen.[11]

Clinical trials

Ramji *et al*.[12] in a clinical trial compared the efficacy of room air and 100% oxygen in 84 asphyxiated neonates with birth weights greater than 999 g. The serial heart rates during the first ten minutes after birth, the median time to first breath and cry, and the arterial pO_2, pH and base deficit at ten and 30 minutes were comparable between the two groups. The median Apgar score at five minutes was significantly better in the room air group compared to the 100% oxygen group (eight vs seven). The two groups were also comparable with regards to death and short-term neurologic sequelae up to 28 days of life.

A recent multicentre clinical trial[13] enrolling over 600 asphyxiated newborn infants (birth weights > 999 g), showed that the room air and 100% oxygen resuscitated groups had comparable heart rates, pH and base deficits in the post-resuscitation period. The mortality and neonatal neurologic sequelae were also similar in the two groups, but Apgar scores were significantly higher in the room air group during the first ten minutes after birth. It has also been observed that the time to reach 75% oxygen saturation (measured by pulse oximeter) after birth was significantly longer in asphyxiated newborns resuscitated with 100% oxygen compared to room air.[13,14]

Most of the clinical trials have a predominant population of term newborn infants and the extrapolation of the trial results to preterm asphyxiated infants remains unclear. Lundstrom *et al.* have recently shown that two hours after resuscitation with 80% oxygen, there was reduced cerebral blood flow in preterm infants(< 32 weeks) compared to 21% oxygen.[15] This may suggest a possible deleterious effect of 100% supplemental oxygen in asphyxiated newborns across all gestational groups.

The body of information that has accumulated in recent years from experimental and clinical studies indicate that ambient air is efficient in resuscitating most asphyxiated newborn infants. Some studies even suggest a possible deleterious effect of oxygen. The efficacy of room air in asphyxiated preterm neonates still needs to be tested. However, the large majority of perinatally related asphyxial deaths and the long-term neurological sequelae observed amongst the survivors are amongst term infants; the group in which ambient air's efficacy in resuscitation has been demonstrated.

The implications for the developing world, where supplemental oxygen is rarely available for any delivery, are obvious. These observations could have important implications with regards to training of health and para-health personnel in neonatal resuscitation at the primary level.

Impact of Neonatal Resuscitation Training in the Community

The need for neonatal resuscitation training for health care providers in the community, who attend close to 80% of the births in the developing countries, needs no further emphasis. Making available appropriate technology for resuscitation and training community level health care providers, especially the traditional birth attendants (TBAs), is visualised as the major step in grappling with the effects of birth asphyxia.

TBAs depend on crying, breathing and activity of the baby to judge the need for resuscitation. This combination of symptoms has been found to correlate well with blood pH and Apgar score.[16] TBAs conventionally use a variety of methods (e.g. instillation of onion juice in nostril, milking the cord, warming the placenta, mouth-to-mouth ventilation) as resuscitative interventions for an asphyxiated newborn. However, there is evidence that they can be trained in the use of more modern resuscitative methods with a beneficial impact on survival. It has been shown that the asphyxia case fatality rate declined from 7.1% to 0.45% in a Chinese province after the grass root level health functionaries were trained in modern methods of neonatal resuscitation.[17]

More recently, the impact of training TBAs in neonatal resuscitation was prospectively evaluated over a two to three year period in a community development block in North India.[18,19] As part of a continuing training programme at the Primary Health Centre, the TBAs were trained in neonatal resuscitation using conventional techniques which included physical stimulation, postural drainage and clearance of the mouth with a finger wrapped in gauze, mouth-to-mouth breathing, and chest compressions. An additional group (advanced group) were trained in the use of bag and mask ventilation. The advanced trained group had cleared the airway in 65% and ventilated 75% of the asphyxiated newborns compared to the conventionally trained TBAs who cleared the airways in 45% and used mouth-to-mouth breathing in 63% of cases. Traditional methods were used less frequently by the advanced trained group. The perinatal mortality was significantly lower in babies delivered by the advanced trained TBAs (49.4/1,000 births) compared to those delivered by the conventionally trained TBAs (61.0/1,000 births).

It is evident that with training, TBAs can change their practices in favour of modern resuscitation procedures with a beneficial effect in favour of improved perinatal survival. However, TBAs are not likely to encounter many asphyxiated newborns each year. There is therefore a need to maintain the resuscitation skills by periodic retraining. Mannequins with inflatable lungs are ideal but expensive, training tools. Alternative training models such as dolls or balls with painted heads need to be considered. Milner and colleagues[3] have demonstrated that a 12–15 cm diameter ball with a painted face can be an effective substitute for a mannequin. Using an attached water manometer with a tube dipped 30 cm under water could improve its effectiveness as a training tool, especially at the community level.

Resuscitation Guidelines

There is a need to simplify neonatal resuscitation guidelines so that they can be practiced effectively even at the peripheral health care units and in the community. Outlined below are some practical resuscitation guidelines that may be adapted for use at all levels of health care, particularly considering the constraints in the developing world.

1. Oropharyngeal suction

There is insufficient evidence to show that all neonates require airway clearance at birth. There is however evidence to show that over-enthusiastic oropharyngeal suction can delay the onset of spontaneous respiration. It may be prudent to restrict airway clearance to infants whose upper airway is contaminated with blood or meconium. In the case of institutional deliveries, the need to clear the oropharynx at delivery of the head in all births occurring through meconium-stained liquor, needs to be strongly advocated in order to reduce the risk of meconium aspiration.

2. When to resuscitate?

The poor utility of Apgar score as an indicator of resuscitation needs is now well recognised. The respiration of the newborn (cry and breathing) and heart rates are the main assessment tools for this decision. If the heart of the baby is > 80/min, delaying intervention up to a minute may be acceptable even if there are no breathing efforts.[20] In a hospital setting while both respiration and heart rates are useful, at the community level, cry and then breathing are the critical tools for decision making and not heart rates.

Therefore, TBA training programmes should exclude training in cardiac compression, so that they do not complicate the training and dilute the ventilation skills being provided.

3. Assisted ventilation and use of oxygen

A neonate with a heart rate > 80/min but making insufficient respiratory effort at one minute should be provided assisted ventilation with room air. In hospital deliveries a heart rate < 80/min under one minute should also be considered an indication for assisted ventilation. All medical personnel should be trained in the use of bag and mask ventilation. In situations where bag and mask ventilation is not available or cannot be used, personnel should be trained in the use of alternate methods such as mouth-to-mask ventilation.

It is important to emphasise that in oxygenating the asphyxiated newborn the attendant uses sufficient inflation pressure. The available evidence base probably does not justify the use of 100% oxygen routinely in all asphyxiated neonates (op. cit). Oxygen supplementation (when available) may be considered in neonates who, after about two minutes of assisted ventilation, remain cyanosed or have heart rates less than 80 per minute.

4. Use of drugs

There is presently insufficient evidence to justify the use of glucose and calcium during initial neonatal resuscitation. The use of sodium bicarbonate has been most controversial. Evidence available suggests that the risks of rapid infusion of bicarbonate in hypoxemia outweigh its benefit. The potential hazards include decreased myocardial contractility, decreased cerebral blood flow, intraventricular haemorrhage, intracellular calcium influx and possible cell death.[21] In over 10,000 hospital births, with almost 5% neonates needing assisted ventilation at birth, sodium bicarbonate was used in less than 3% of the asphyxiated neonates, with no difference in outcome between those who did and did not receive bicarbonate.[22] Since blood gas analytical facilities are generally not available at birth, bicarbonate therapy may be recommended for empirical use in neonates with poor respiratory efforts or perfusion after about ten minutes of birth, although these infants are more likely to benefit from volume expansion and inotrope therapy rather than alkali therapy.

5. When to stop resuscitation?

There is sufficient evidence to suggest that all resuscitative efforts may be discontinued if a neonate fails to establish spontaneous breathing 30 minutes after birth.[23]

While these guidelines are not comprehensive, they emphasise the current changing trends in neonatal resuscitation practices that may be incorporated in future guidelines and protocols.

References

1. Costello AM de L and Manandhar DS, "Perinatal asphyxia in less developed countries," *Archives of Disease in Childhood* **71** (1994): F1–3.
2. Milner AD, Upton C, Green J and Stokes GM, "A device for domiciliary neonatal resuscitation," *Lancet* **335** (1990): 273–274.
3. Milner AD, Stokes GM, Tunel R, McKeugh M and Martin H, "Laboratory assessment of Laerdal mouth-tube-mask prototype resuscitation device," *Medical and Biological Engineering and Computing* **30** (1992): 117–119.
4. Massawe A, Kilewo C, Irani S, Verma RJ, Chakrampam AB, Ribbe T *et al.* "Assessment of mouth-to-mask ventilation in resuscitation of asphyxic newborn babies. A pilot study," *Tropical Medicine and International Health* **1** (1996): 865–873.
5. American Heart Association, "Guidelines for cardiopulmonary resuscitation and emergency cardiac care," *Journal of the American Medical Association* **268** (1992): 2276–2281.
6. Saugstad OD, "Role of xanthine oxidase and its inhibitor in hypoxia: Reoxygenation injury," *Pediatrics* **98** (1996): 103–107.
7. Saugstad OD, "Oxygen toxicity in the neonatal period," *Acta Pediatrica Scandinavia* **79** (1990): 881–892.
8. Rootwelt T, Loberg EM, Moen A, Oyasaeter S and Saugstad OD, "Hypoxemia and reoxygenation with 21% or 100% oxygen in newborn pigs: Changes in blood pressure, base deficit, and hypoxanthine and brain morphology," *Pediatric Research* **32** (1992): 107–113.

9. Rootwelt T, Odden JP, Hall C, Ganes T and Saugstad OD, "Cerebral blood flow and evoked potentials during reoxygenation with 21% or 100% O_2 in newborn pigs," *Journal of Applied Physiology* **75** (1993): 2054–2060.

10. Poulsen JP, Oyasaeter S and Saugstad OD, "Hypoxanthine, xanthine and uric acid in newborn pigs during hypoxemia followed by resuscitation with room air or 100% oxygen," *Critical Care Medicine* **21** (1993): 1058–1065.

11. Feet BA, Yu X-Q, Oyasaeter S and Saugstad OD, "Effects of hypoxia and resuscitation with 21% and 100% O_2 in newborn piglets: Extracellular hypoxanthine (Hx) in brain cortex and femoral muscle," *Critical Care Medicine* **25** (1997): 1384–1391.

12. Ramji S, Ahuja S, Thirupuram S, Rootwelt T, Rooth G and Saugstad OD, "Resuscitation of asphyxic newborn infants with room air or 100% oxygen," *Pediatric Research* **34** (1993): 809–812.

13. Saugstad OD, Rootwelt T, Aolen O, "Resuscitation of Asphyxiated Newborn Infants with Room Air or Oxygen: An international controlled trial: The Resair 2 study," *Pediatrics* **102** (1998): E1.

14. Rao R, "Pulse oximetry evaluation of oxygenation during resuscitation of asphyxiated newborns with 21% or 100% oxygen," Thesis for Doctor of Medicine (Pediatrics), University of Delhi, Delhi, India (1995).

15. Lundstrom K, Pryds O and Greisen G, "Oxygen at birth and prolonged cerebral vasoconstriction in preterm infants," *Archives of Disease in Childhood* **73** (1995): F81–86.

16. Ghosh D, "Evaluation of traditional criteria for assessment of birth asphyxia," Thesis for Doctor of Medicine, Postgraduate Institute of Medical Education and Research, Chandigarh, India (1989).

17. Zhu X, "Neonatal resuscitation," *World Health Forum* **14** (1993): 289–290.

18. Kumar R, "Training traditional birth attendants for resuscitation of newborns," *Tropical Doctor* **25** (1995): 29–30.

19. Kumar R, "Effect of training on the resuscitation practices of traditional birth attendants," *Transactions of the Royal Society of Tropical Medicine and Hygiene* **88** (1994): 159–160.

20. Milner AD, "Resuscitation of the newborn," *Archives of Disease in Childhood* **66** (1991): 66–99.

21. Burchfield DJ, "Medication use in neonatal resuscitation: Epinephrine and sodium bicarbonate," *Neonatal Pharmacology Quarterly* **2** (1993): 25–30.

22. Ramji S. *Personal communication.*

23. Nadkarni V, "Pediatric resuscitation: An advisory statement from the Pediatric Working Group of the International Liaison Committee on Resuscitation," *Circulation* **95** (1997): 2185–2195.

Commentary

EFFECTIVE RESUSCITATION: RESEARCH FROM BOMBAY ON THE USE OF A MOUTH-TO-MASK METHOD

Simin Irani

Professor of Paediatrics, Bombay

A recent WHO report invited research and development of "appropriate procedures and devices required for resuscitation of the newborn infant at the community and health centre level". Today, the use of bag and mask for ventilation is an established procedure. In most developing countries, however, facilities for neonatal resuscitation are limited to maternity units in hospitals, where less than 10% of deliveries take place. Instruction of village health workers in techniques of mouth-to-mouth resuscitation was rejected, because such techniques are difficult and often culturally unacceptable, and may spread infection, including HIV. The question of replacing the unhygienic mouth-to-mouth resuscitation with a mouth-to-mask method was first discussed in 1985 and different devices have been tested on mannequins. Incorporation of a bacteriological filter created high airway resistance so Laerdal Medical company constructed a prototype with low airway resistance (less than 1 cm H_2O at an air flow of 300 ml/s).

The Bombay Study

In Bombay, we joined a multicentre study to examine the utility of this simple, inexpensive Laerdal prototype which potentially can be used with little training by TBAs, reduces the risk of cross-infection, and can withstand repeated sterilisation by boiling water. A safety blow-off valve was not included because of cost, the increased difficulty of sterilisation, and the risk of deterioration with age. The aim of our study was to compare the effectiveness of the new method of mouth-to-mask ventilation with the established bag and mask ventilation.

Resuscitation procedures

Up to 5% of the newborn infants in our hospital need resuscitation at birth. In this study ventilation was started if the infant has not started spontaneous breathing within 30 seconds of birth. Newborn infants with a birth weight below 1,000 g and those with obvious life-threatening malformations were excluded. Suctioning was performed with the help of a laryngoscope before ventilation was started in infants with meconium-stained amniotic fluid. All other newborn infants had suctioning of their mouth and nose before ventilation commenced. The ventilation continued until regular spontaneous breathing occurred. If the heart rate at five minutes was below 100 beats per minute the baby was incubated and ventilated. Then, if necessary, bag and mask ventilation was used.

Mouth-to-mask ventilation was performed with a soft, circular silicon rubber face mask (Laerdal medical No. 0) for newborn infants with a birth weight above 1,200 g. For smaller newborn infants face mask number 00 was used. This mask was connected to a one-way valve and to a mouth piece.

The bag and mask used was the Laerdal Neonatal Resuscitation Bag with a volume of 250 ml and a 'pop-off' valve opening at approximately 30 cm of water. If necessary, the 'pop-off' valve was occluded.

The insufflation pressure was adjusted to produce visible chest expansion. Pure oxygen was not used during the initial ventilation period; 100% oxygen was used if the baby required intubation and ventilation.

Outcome indicators

Efficacy was assessed by comparing the Apgar scores at one, five and ten minutes, time to first gasp, time to first cry, oxygen saturation levels measured by pulse oximeter at five minutes, and the time to achieve a heart rate level exceeding 130 beats per minute. The end point also included the clinical condition of the newborn infants at discharge.

External cardiac message was not given to any of the infants in this study.

Training

The investigation was started after a training period of approximately one month at each centre. During the period, the personnel practised using the ventilation device on a dummy baby consisting of a ball of 10 cm diameter, while the paper-recorder and water manometer were connected. Pressure was regulated to 30 cm of water to accustom the trainee to that pressure level.

Results

There was no significant difference between mouth-to-mask and bag and mask groups with maternal and intrapartum factors, or with anthropometric data from term and preterm newborn infants.

Insufflation pressures and respiratory frequencies

The mean peak insufflation pressure in the bag and mask group was significantly higher than in the mouth-to-mask group ($p = 0.001$), but the respiratory frequency was the same in both groups.

Clinical effects of resuscitation

Some outcome parameters are seen in Table 1. Neonatal convulsions and neonatal deaths occurred frequently in both term and preterm newborn infants.

Table 1 The clinical effects of resuscitation using mouth-to-mask compared with bag and mask in the Bombay study.

	Mouth-to-mask	Bag and mask
Term Infants (*n*)	20	16
Apgar score 4 at one minute	0	2
Apgar score 4 at five minutes	16	14
Apgar score 4 at ten minutes	19	16
First gasp in five minutes	17	15
First cry in five minutes	14	14
Heart rate > 130 at five minutes	16	16
Survival without convulsions	16	12
Preterm infants (*n*)	10	8
Apgar score 4 at one minute	0	0
Apgar score 4 at five minutes	7	8
Apgar score 4 at ten minutes	8	8
First gasp in five minutes	7	8
First cry in five minutes	2	8
Heart rate > 130 at five minutes	5	8
Survival without convulsions	4	3

Most of the convulsions and deaths occurred in infants who had moderate asphyxia, with an Apgar score of more than three at five minutes.

Discussion

We have shown that in term infants in Bombay the response to resuscitation was not significantly different with the two methods. Physiological measurements of lung expansion and pulmonary gas exchange during spontaneous breathing and neonatal resuscitation have shown that in both spontaneously breathing and assisted ventilated infants the mean peak inspiratory pressure is high (30–70 cm of water). The insufflation pressures in our study were in agreement with these figures.

Of our outcome parameters, time to heart rate above 130/min and a pulse oximeter value above 75% at five to six minutes are objective criteria reflecting effectiveness of assisted ventilation.The other parameters — Apgar score less than four at five and ten minutes, first gasp and cry within five minutes — only partly reflect the efficacy of ventilation because they are also determined by the duration and severity of prenatal asphyxia. Within five minutes after birth at least 75% of the infants had an Apgar score greater than four which is in good agreement with previous studies using bag and mask ventilation. Studies have shown that even five minutes of mouth-to-mask ventilation is tiring when 40–50 breaths per minute are used. During the first breaths, prolonged insufflation has been shown to promote establishment of the functional residual capacity of the resuscitated baby.

The present results were obtained after a training period when the water manometer was used. After training with a water manometer, performance improves so that the pressures generated are close to 30 cm of water.

Mouth-to-mask ventilation is effective, provided there is proper training and a normal respiratory frequency is used. If ventilation fails with room air then oxygen should be administered if available. Careful monitoring of the heart rate and oxygenation is then required, but it must be remembered that the alternative to the mouth-to-mask method of ventilation in many situations is no assisted ventilation at all.

Chapter 13

EFFECTIVE INTERVENTIONS TO REDUCE NEONATAL MORTALITY AND MORBIDITY FROM PERINATAL INFECTION

Zulfiqar Ahmed Bhutta
Professor of Child Health and Director of Neonatal Services,
The Aga Khan University Medical Center, Karachi, Pakistan

Any programme of intervention that is geared towards the prevention and eradication of neonatal infections in developing countries, requires a close understanding of their epidemiology, spectrum and predisposing risk factors. This review will focus on the available epidemiological evidence and known risk factors for important neonatal infections in developing countries. Although the impact of perinatally acquired HIV-1 infection is mainly in the post-neonatal period, given the devastating effect of this infection in the developing world the pathogenesis and predisposing factors for HIV-1 infection will also be considered.

Epidemiology

Despite advances in antimicrobial therapy, neonatal infections still account for considerable morbidity and mortality globally. Almost 23% of all deaths among children under five occur in the first week of life and almost 33%

within the neonatal period.[1] In 1993, of an estimated 3.7 million neonatal deaths, 15% were due to neonatal tetanus and a further 8% were directly attributable to neonatal sepsis or meningitis.[1] In a longitudinal study of lethal and potentially lethal episodes in a birth cohort in rural Guatemala, 92% of the episodes were identified as infectious diseases, with half the episodes occurring in the neonatal period.[2] In a similar longitudinal follow-up of a birth cohort in Pakistan, almost 40% of all first week deaths were found to be related to infectious disorders[3] (Figure 1). Although hepatitis B, cytomegalovirus and toxoplasmosis are also important,[4] the bulk of serious perinatal infections are bacterial. The recent emergence of perinatal HIV infection, however, has changed the entire spectrum of morbidity from infectious diseases in the developing world. In sub-Saharan Africa, perinatally acquired HIV infections now account for a substantial and increasing burden of childhood illnesses.[5] In addition, an important global issue is the emergence of multidrug-resistant organisms, posing challenging problems in therapy.[6,7]

Neonatal deaths in Lahore

Etiology

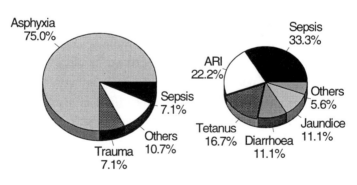

Based on ref 3

Figure 1 Aetiology of neonatal deaths in Lahore, Pakistan.[3]

Pathogenesis

Rational interventions require a close understanding of predisposing factors and pathogenesis of neonatal infections. Some infections such as syphilis[8] are acquired during pregnancy, whereas others, e.g. hepatitis B and HIV, are acquired during the process of birth.[9,10] For perinatal HIV infection the current evidence also suggests a comparatively higher risk of vertical transmission after vaginal delivery in comparison with cesarean births.[11-13]

Group B Streptococcus

Although vertically transmitted bacterial infections, especially group B Streptococcal (GBS) infections, are well described in developed countries, the situation in developing countries is far from clear. Early-onset GBS infections have been reported from Africa[14,15] and the West Indies.[16,17] However, other reports from Africa,[18] Turkey[19] and South Asia[20,21] attest to its relative rarity among newborn infants with sepsis. A number of factors may be responsible for these epidemiological differences, including varying rates of GBS carriage and virulence of prevalent strains. Despite this controversy, given the preventable nature of these infections, considerable emphasis should be given to prophylaxis and early recognition of GBS sepsis.[22,23]

Gram negative sepsis

In contrast to GBS infections, early-onset gram negative sepsis is commonly described from developing countries[24] and has been attributed to vertical transmission from the maternal genital tract.[25,26] It is also likely, given the high rates of microbial contamination, that a number of these early-onset infections also represent acquired infections from the environment. In a prospective study of Pakistani newborn infants from Lahore, Adlerberth *et al.*[27] described significantly greater and faster intestinal colonisation with pathogenic Enterobacteriacae in comparison with Swedish newborn infants. Interestingly, in the latter study, Pakistani infants delivered by cesarean section were more rapidly colonised than their vaginally delivered counterparts. Such early and rapid acquisition of pathogenic bacteria reflects the high degree of environmental colonisation with such bacteria, as well as inappropriate early feeding strategies. Indeed, in a case control study of neonatal sepsis in Lahore, an 18-fold higher risk of sepsis was seen in non-breastfed infants.[28]

Nosocomial infection

The importance of the environment and gastrointestinal tract is also underscored by the high rates of nosocomial sepsis reported among newborn infants admitted to nurseries and hospitals in developing countries. A common portal of entry for pathogenic bacteria in the newborn is the gastrointestinal tract[29] and epidemic diarrhoea in newborn nurseries has been frequently recognised as nosocomial infection.[30] Over a six-year period the rate of diarrhoea among newborn infants in a hospital in Rangoon was 15.4 per 1,000 live births with case fatality rates of 12%.[31] Interestingly, although neonatal diarrhoea was endemic in the hospital, diarrhoea rates among cesarean births were five fold higher than those born vaginally.

Given the general lack of resources and awareness of infection control procedures in developing country hospitals, even life-saving equipment can occasionally become the very source of fatal outbreaks of nosocomial infection.[32] With increasing recognition of the role of the gastrointestinal tract and bacterial translocation in neonatal sepsis,[33] it is imperative that preventive measures also focus on these factors.

Risk Factors

Recognition of important predisposing factors for perinatal/neonatal infections may allow institution of early remedial measures (see Figure 2). Of these there has been considerable interest in the risk factors for vertical transmission of maternal infections and early-onset neonatal infections.

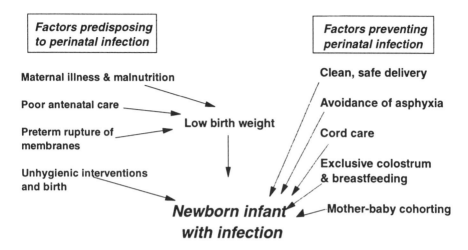

Figure 2 Risk factors for neonatal sepsis.

Prematurity and LBW

Clearly, a major predisposing factor towards neonatal infectious morbidity and mortality is prematurity and low birth weight.[2-4] Intra-amniotic infections were recognised as the most important cause of perinatal mortality in Ethiopia,[35] and in Nigeria 44% of deliveries with prolonged rupture of membranes were associated with neonatal sepsis.[36] The recent demonstration of the relationship of bacterial vaginosis with neonatal morbidity and a 40% increase in the risk of preterm birth[37] also supports the contention that infections and preterm deliveries are closely interrelated in developing countries.

Prolonged rupture of membranes

Although a view has been expressed that prolonged rupture of membranes is only associated with an increased risk of infection in combination with other independent factors,[38] others have found a significant association of neonatal infections with prolonged labour and rupture of membranes greater than 12 hours.[39] It is therefore crucial for health workers to recognise the high risk of intra-amniotic and early-onset neonatal infections with premature and prolonged rupture of membranes. It is also important in this situation to reduce the number of vaginal examinations and avoid internal monitoring, as these have been shown to increase the risk of ascending infection.[40]

Asphyxia

The association of sepsis with perinatal asphyxia is well described, and while this may represent intra-amniotic infection in such high risk pregnancies with prolonged labour,[41,42] in others the infection may be secondary to repeated interventions and handling in labour.[21]

Risk factors for perinatal HIV-1 transmission

There have been several recent advances in our understanding of the factors associated with the acquisition of perinatal HIV-1 infection. While almost three fold higher rates of intrauterine growth retardation and prematurity have been described among HIV seropositive mothers,[43] there may be no overt evidence of transmission of HIV infection at birth. Recent data on estimates of mother-to-child transmission rates of HIV-1 infection indicate that transmission rates are higher in developing countries and range from 25–48%.[9,44] Information based on DNA polymerase chain reaction[45] as well as Markov modelling,[46] indicate that one-third of the HIV-1 infections are acquired *in utero* in late pregnancy and two-thirds at birth. In a multivariate analysis of obstetric risk factors associated with increased risk of perinatal HIV-1 transmission were antenatal CD4+ count < 29% of total lymphocytes, low birth weight and the presence of ruptured membranes > 4 hours.[10] An almost two-fold increased risk of perinatal HIV-1 transmission was also noted with a maternal haemoglobin < 10 g/dl.[11] In contrast to industrialised country data, recent studies of breastmilk HIV-1 DNA and p24-antigen in infected Ugandan mothers suggest relatively low rates of HIV-1 transmission by breastmilk in chronically infected mothers.[47]

Diagnosis

The rapid diagnosis of perinatally acquired viral infections such as HIV-1 or cytomegalovirus infections requires advanced microbiological and serological diagnostic facilities, a difficult proposition for much of the developing world. In the developing world context, commonly the best one can hope for is basic microbial culture facilities; although in hyperendemic areas, such as sub-Saharan Africa, access to a referral centre for processing of HIV-1 samples is necessary.

Clinical signs

Given the high mortality of bacterial sepsis, it is important to make the diagnosis rapidly in a suspect situation. This is usually possible using a combination of clinical findings, suggestive adjunctive tests and confirmatory specific tests.[48] Given the ubiquitous features of neonatal sepsis, a diagnosis based on clinical criteria alone is difficult as findings may vary widely. To illustrate, while hypothermia may be a common feature of early-onset sepsis, even a pyrexial episode in the newborn must be looked upon with considerable suspicion.[49] Others have reported an axillary-core temperature difference of $\geq 2.2°C$ to be a sensitive early indicator of sepsis.[50] Singh *et al.* have found a scoring system based on the presence of different perinatal risk factors for sepsis, as a useful screening procedure for further laboratory evaluation.[51]

Laboratory tests

Notwithstanding the above clinical features, there is an urgent need for rapid supportive laboratory evidence of suspected infection. The common practice of obtaining body surface cultures in newborns with suspected sepsis is of fairly limited value in predicting the aetiology of sepsis,[52,53] although the importance of negative nasal swabs in excluding early-onset group B streptococcal sepsis has been recently highlighted.[54] While blood/CSF cultures are the gold-standard for diagnosing bacterial sepsis, they may also be negative in some advanced cases of fulminant sepsis or with maternal antibiotic therapy.[55] Haemostatic coagulation abnormalities have been well described in septicemic newborns,[56] but these require a larger volume of blood and are impractical screens. Similarly, other haematological parameters such as neutrophilia/neutropenia and thrombocytopenia are not invariable and may only be seen in severe cases of sepsis.[55] Other ancillary tests such as gastric aspirate examination[56] and acridine orange-stained buffy coat smears[57] may be sensitive early screening tests. Such clinical and laboratory screening tests have been shown to lead to decreased use of antibiotics in neonatal units.[58] Both single[59] and serial quantitative C-reactive protein (CRP)[60,61] concentrations have been shown to be sensitive indicators of neonatal sepsis. Although combined leukocyte parameters and CRP estimates may be sensitive early indicators of sepsis,[62,63] a recent critical review of available literature underscores the diversity and heterogeneity of results.[64] Despite these disparate data, two recent studies from India have highlighted the sensitivity and positive predictive value of a sepsis screen consisting of C-reactive protein, micro-ESR and gastric aspirate cytology in suspected cases of neonatal sepsis.[65,66]

Preventive and Management Strategies

Given the available information on diagnostic limitations and the rapid course of perinatal bacterial infections, it is important to initiate appropriate antimicrobial therapy at the earliest. A major problem in this context is the recent emergence of multidrug-resistant organisms, making effective therapy difficult and expensive.[67] It is imperative that our focus be mainly on preventive strategies targeted to both the community, where the majority of the births take place, as well as hospitals with newborn care facilities. A combination of approaches may be necessary, and the following discussion will focus on specific interventions and strategies that may prevent or reduce the severity of perinatal infections.

Maternal and intrapartal care

Surely the most important preventive strategy for perinatal infection in the developing world context is prevention of low birth weight (LBW).[68] This entails the provision of basic maternal antenatal care and recognition of high-risk pregnancies. The association of maternal genital tract bacterial colonisation with both preterm labour[69-71] as well as early-onset neonatal sepsis is well recognised[23] and may also be related to unhygienic antenatal or obstetric practices. A similar risk of LBW following maternal urinary tract infection is well known.[72] Estimates from endemic areas indicate that the population-attributable risk of LBW due to malaria in primiparous women ranges from 10–40%.[73] It is imperative in these settings that appropriate antimalarial therapy be used for effective control in susceptible women during periods of high malaria exposure.[74] The efficacy of antenatal tetanus toxoid administration in preventing neonatal tetanus has been demonstrated in several developing country settings and can be effectively administered by traditional birth attendants (TBAs).[75] It is thus important that TBAs be provided basic training for primary maternal antenatal care, screening for infections, and tetanus toxoid administration. Basic equipment such as delivery kits ensuring a clean hygienic birth and newborn cord care, must be available and can substantially reduce the morbidity associated with tetanus and early-onset neonatal sepsis.[76]

The enormous burden of perinatal HIV-1 infection in developing countries places a special responsibility on health workers. While antenatal zidovudine therapy and cesarean delivery have significantly reduced the risk of perinatal transmission of HIV-1 infection,[77,78] these strategies are impractical for most developing countries. However, in a theoretical model of short-course zidovudine therapy in a sub-Saharan African setting of 12.5% HIV-1 sero-prevalence, Mansergh *et al.* demonstrated that a 12% reduction in perinatal HIV-1 incidence would result in an average saving of almost $4000 per infant HIV-1 infection prevented.[79] Despite the above evidence, the optimal strategy for reducing the risk of perinatal HIV-1 transmission in developing countries remains uncertain. Given the increased risk of vertical HIV-1 transmission with prolonged rupture of membranes and the newborn's exposure to cervico-vaginal secretions,[80] there has been considerable interest in maternal vaginal chlorhexidine application during labour as a means of reducing HIV-1 transmission. Interestingly, although preliminary studies do not show a benefit of the latter approach in reducing HIV-1 transmission, a significant reduction in early neonatal bacterial infections is seen after vaginal chlorhexidine,[81,82] further underscoring the importance of vertically acquired bacterial infections in these settings. As an effective vaccine against HIV-1 remains elusive, the most important strategy for prevention is public education and awareness. The available evidence on the efficacy of hepatitis B vaccination in areas of high endemicity also makes this an extremely attractive preventive strategy.[83]

Postnatal care of the newborn

Apart from a clean, uncomplicated delivery with minimal intervention, the single most effective preventive strategy for preventing neonatal infections is exclusive breastfeeding and avoidance of prelacteal feeds. Breastmilk has potent antibacterial and antiviral properties[84] and has been shown to lead to reduced intestinal permeability[85] and intestinal bacterial overgrowth[86] in the newborn. The benefit of breastmilk feeding in reducing the incidence of neonatal infection in hospitalised newborns was amply demonstrated by Narayanan et al.[87] and subsequently also shown in relatively high risk LBW infants.[88,89] It thus appears that exclusive breastfeeding significantly reduces the likelihood of gastrointestinal colonisation and consequent bacterial translocation and sepsis in the newborn. Notwithstanding the recommendations for avoidance of breastfeeding among newborn infants of HIV-1 positive mothers,[90] recent data from Africa indicate that the risk of HIV-1 transmission from breastmilk in a chronically infected mother is relatively low,[47,91] thus supporting the current recommendations for continuing breastfeeding in chronically infected HIV-1 positive mothers in developing countries with high rates of environmental contamination and bacterial infections.

An important issue in neonatal care, even for hospitals in developing countries, is the paucity of nursing staff for the care of such infants. The pioneering work of maternal–infant skin-to-skin contact and care in Bogota, Colombia, indicated that mothers could be entrusted with the task of caring for their premature newborn infants.[92] Apart from comparatively improved survival among these infants, the so-called "kangaroo care" also resulted in significantly lower rates of infection, attributable in no small measure to improved rates of breastfeeding.[93] While there may be cultural differences in the mode of care, the important principle was that apart from maintenance of body temperature, mothers were capable of providing basic care to stablise very LBW newborns with resultant improved survival and lower rates of infection. Such maternal participation in the care of the newborn has also been shown to reduce rates of nosocomial sepsis and morbidity in both India[94,95] and Pakistan (Bhutta *et al.*, unpublished observations).

Strategies for control of neonatal infections in nurseries and hospitals

The control of nosocomial infections among hospitalised newborn infants in developing countries requires a combination of environmental control, cohorting, strict handwashing and periodic infectious disease surveillance.[96] While the latter may require laboratory resources and some knowledge of infectious disease epidemiology,[97] it is frequently the lack of attention to simple interventions such as handwashing,[98] which are most amenable to modification by focussed educational campaigns.[99] To illustrate, a combination of reduced congestion in the nursery, and reduced use of metallic needles and intravenous flushing with heparinised saline, was shown to reduce the incidence of neonatal sepsis almost two folds in a neonatal unit in India.[100]

An important consideration in neonatal nurseries is also the worrisome emergence of multidrug-resistant strains of bacteria, which not only produce fulminant inexorable infections but are also an enormous burden on limited health care resources.[32,33,67] The emergence of these multi-resistant organisms is frequently seen in the wake of indiscriminate antibiotic use.[101] The efficacy of periodic alterations in antibiotic protocols in order to reduce the likelihood of emergence of multidrug-resistant strains is well established[102] and should be part of nursery protocols.

In summary, most people in developing countries live in a delicate ecological balance with the environment and micro-organisms. The newborn infant, however, is extremely susceptible to infection in the perinatal period. Awareness of predisposing and preventive factors allows one to institute appropriate remedial measures such as environmental control, handwashing and exclusive breastfeeding. Given the vicious cycle of drug resistance and antimicrobial pressure, these measures are the only viable long-term measures for control of perinatal and neonatal infections in developing countries.

References

1. World Health Organization, "World Health Report 1995: Bridging the Gap," World Health Organization, Geneva (1995).
2. Bartlett AV, de Bocaletti MEP and Bocaletti MA, "Neonatal and early postneonatal morbidity and mortality in a rural Guatemalan community: The importance of infectious diseases and their management," *Pediatric Infectious Disease Journal* **10** (1991): 752–757.
3. Jalil F, Lindblad BS, Hanson LA, Khan SR, Yaqoob M and Karlberg J, "Early child health in Lahore, Pakistan. IX. Perinatal events," *Acta Paediatrical Supplement* **390** (1993): 95–107.
4. el-Nawawy A, Soliman AT, el-Azzouni O, Amer el S, Karim MA, Demian S and el-Sayed M, "Maternal and neonatal prevalence of toxoplasma and cytomegalovirus antibodies and hepatitis-B antigens in an Egyptian rural area," *Journal of Tropical Pediatrics* **42** (1996): 154–157.
5. Walraven G, Nicoll A, Njau M and Timaeus I, "The impact of HIV-1 infection on child health in sub-Saharan Africa: The burden on the health services," *Tropical Medicine & International Health* **1** (1996): 3–14.
6. Zaidi M, Sifuentes J, Bobadilla M, Moncada D and Ponce-de-Leon S," Epidemic of serratia marcescens bacteremia and meningitis in a neonatal unit in Mexico City," *Infection Control and Hospital Epidemiology* **10** (1989): 14–20.
7. Bhutta ZA, "Enterobacter sepsis in Karachi: A growing problem," *Journal of Hospital Infection* **34** (1996): 211–216.
8. Humphrey MD and Bradford DL, "Congenital syphilis: Still a reality in 1996," *Medical Journal of Australia* **165** (1996): 382–385.
9. Mulder DW, Nunn A, Kamail A and Kengerya-Kayondo JF, "Post-natal incidence of HIV-I infection among children in a rural Ugandan population: No evidence for transmission other than mother to child," *Tropical Medicine & International Health* **1** (1996): 81–85.
10. Rouzioux C, Costagliola D, Burgard M, Blanche S, Mayaux MJ *et al.*, "Estimated timing of mother-to-child human immunodeficiency virus type 1

(HIV-1) transmission by use of a Markov model," *American Journal of Epidemiology* **142** (1995): 1330–1337.

11. Bobat R, Coovadia H, Coutsoudis A and Moodley D, "Determinants of mother-to-child transmission of human immunodeficiency virus type 1 infection in a cohort from Durban, South Africa," *Pediatric Infectious Disease Journal* **15** (1996): 604–610.

12. Landesman Sh, Kalish LA, Burns DN, Minkoff H, Fox HE, Zorrilla C, Garcia Pat, Fowler MG, Mofenson L and Tuomala R, "Obstetrical factors and the transmission of human immunodeficiency virus type 1 from mother to child," *New England Journal of Medicine* **334** (1996):1617–1623.

13. Kuhn L, Bobat R, Coutsodis A, Moodley D, Coovadia HM, Tsai Wei-Yann and Stein ZA, "Cesarean deliveries and maternal-infant HIV transmission: Results from a prospective study in South Africa," *Journal of Acquired Immune Deficiency Syndromes and Human Retrovirology* **11** (1996): 478–483.

14. Nathoo KJ, Pazvakavamba I, Chidede OS and Chirisa C, "Neonatal meningitis in Harare, Zimbabwe: A 2-year review," *Annals of Tropical Paediatrics* **11** (1991): 11–15.

15. Haffejee IE, Bhana RH, Coovadia YM, Hoosen AA, Marajh AV and Gouws E, "Neonatal group B streptococcal infections in Indian (Asian) babies in South Africa," *Journal of Infections* **22** (1991): 225–231.

16. MacFaralane DE, "Neonatal group B Streptococcal septicaemia in a developing country," *Acta Paediatrica Scandinavica* **76** (1987): 470–473.

17. Robillard P-Y, Nabeth P, Hulsey TC, Sergent M-P, Perianin J and Janky E, "Neonatal bacterial septicemia ina tropical area. Four year experience in Guadelope (French West Indies)," *Acta Paediatrica* **82** (1993): 687–689.

18. Dawodu AH, Damole IO and Onile BA, "Epidemiology of group B Streptococcal carriage among pregnant women and their neonates: An African experience," *Tropical & Geographic Medicine* **35** (1983): 145–150.

19. Ayata A, Guvenc H, Felek S, Aygun AD, Kocabay K and Bektas S, "Maternal carriage and neonatal colonisation of group B streptococci in labour are uncommon in Turkey," *Paediatric and Perinatal Epidemiology* **8** (1994): 188–192.

20. Kishore K, Deorari AK, Paul VK, Singh M and Bhujwala RA, "Group B streptococcus colonization and neonatal outcome in north India," *Indian Journal of Medical Research* **84** (1986): 492–494.

21. Bhutta ZA, Naqvi SH, Muzaffar T and Farooqui BJ, "Neonatal sepsis in Pakistan: Presentation and pathogens," *Acta Paediatrica Scandinavica* **80** (1991): 596–601.

22. Walsh JA and Hutchins S, "Group B streptococcal disease: Its importance in the developing world and prospect for prevention with vaccines," *Pediatric Infectious Disease Journal* **8** (1987): 271–276.

23. Schuchat A, "Group B streptococcal disease in newborns: A global perspective on prevention," *Biomedicine and Pharmacotherapy* **49** (1995): 19–25.

24. Bhutta ZA, "Neonatal infections," *Current Opinion in Pediatrics* (1997) (in press).

25. Kishore K, Deorari AK, Singh M and Bhujwala RA, "Early onset neonatal sepsis — Vertical transmission from the maternal genital tract," *Indian Pediatrics* **24** (1987): 45–48.

26. Ayengar A, Madhulika and Vani SN, "Neonatal sepsis due to vertical transmission from maternal genital tract," *Indian Journal of Pediatrics* **58** (1991): 661–664.

27. Adlerberth I, Carlsson B, de Man P, Jalil F, Khan SR, Larsson P, Mellander L, Svanborg C, Wold AE and Hanson LA, "Intestinal colonization with enterobacteriacae in Pakistani and Swedish hospital-delivered infants," *Acta Paediatrica Scandinavica* **80** (1991): 602–610.

28. Ashraf RN, Jalil F, Zaman S, Karlberg J, Khan SR, Lindblad BS and Hanson LA, "Breastfeeding and protection against neonatal sepsis in a high risk population," *Archives of Disease in Childhood* **66** (1991): 488–490.

29. Levy J, "Enteral nutrition: An increasingly recognized cause of nosocomial bloodstream infection," *Infection Control and Hospital Epidemiology* **10** (1989): 395–397.

30. Yankauer A, "Epidemic diarrhea of the newborn, a nosocomial problem in developing countries," *American Journal of Public Health* **81** (1991): 415–417.

31. Aye DT, Sack DA, Wachsmuth K, Kyi DT and Thwe SM, "Neonatal diarrhea at a maternity hospital in Rangoon," *American Journal of Public Health* **81** (1991): 480–481.

32. Khan MA, Abdur-Rab M, Israr N, Ilyas M, Ahmad F, Kundi Z and Ghafoor A, "Transmission of *Salmonella worthington* by oropharyngeal suction in hospital neonatal unit," *Pediatric Infectious Disease Journal* **10** (1991): 668–672.

33. Leigh L, Stoll BJ, Rahman M and McGowan J Jr, "*Pseudomonas aeruginosa* infection in very low birth weight infants: A case-control study," *Pediatric Infectious Disease Journal* **14** (1996): 367–371.

34. Urrutia JJ, Mata LJ, Trent F, Cruz JR, Villatoro E and Alexander RE, "Infection and low birth weight in a developing country. A study in an Indian village of Guatemala," *American Journal of Diseases in Childhood* **129** (1975): 558–561.

35. Naeye RL, Tafari N, Judge D, Gilmour D and Marboe C, "Amniotic fluid infections in an African city," *Journal of Pediatrics* **90** (1977): 965–970.
36. Airede AK, "Prolonged rupture of membranes and neonatal outcome in a developing country," *Annals of Tropical Paediatrics* **12** (1992): 283–288.
37. Hillier SL, Nugent RP, Eschenbach DA, Hrohn MA, Gibbs RS, Martin DH, Farnces Cotch M, Edelman R, Pastorek II JG, Rao AV, McNellis D, Tegan JA, Carey JC and Klebanoff MA, "Association between bacterial vaginosis and preterm delivery of a low birth weight infant," *New England Journal of Medicine* **333** (1995): 1737–1742.
38. Bhakoo ON and Singh M, "Perinatal risk factors in neonatal bacterial sepsis," *Indian Journal of Pediatrics* **55** (1988): 941–946.
39. Raghavan M, Mondal GP, Bhat BV and Srinivasan S, "Perinatal risk factors in neonatal infections," *Indian Journal of Pediatrics* **59** (1992): 335–340.
40. Averbuch B, Mazor M, Shoham-Vardi L, Chaim W, Vardi H, Horowitz S and Shuster M, "Intra-uterine infection in women with preterm premature rupture of membranes: Maternal and neonatal characteristics," *Obstetrics and Gynecology* **62** (1995): 25–29.
41. Maberry MC, Ramin SM, Gilstrap III LC, Leveno KJ and Dax JS, "Intrapartum asphyxia in pregnancies complicated by intra-amniotic infection," *Obstetrics and Gynecology* **76** (1990): 351–354.
42. Meyer BA, Dickinson JE, Chambers C and Parisi VM, "The effect of foetal sepsis on umbilical cord blood gases," *American Journal of Obstetrics and Gynecology* **166** (1992): 612–617.
43. Taha TE, Dallabetta GA, Canner JK, Chiphangwi JD, Liomba G, Hoover DR and Miotti PG, "The effect of human immunodeficiency virus infection on birth weight, and infant and child mortality in urban Malawi," *International Journal of Epidemiology* **24** (1995): 1022–1029.
44. Dabis F, Msellati P, Dunn D, Lepage P, Newell ML, Peckham C and Van-de-Perre P, "Estimating the rate of mother-to-child transmission of HIV. Report of a workshop on methodological issues. Ghent (Belgium), 17–20 Feb 1992," *AIDS* **7** (1993): 1139–1148.
45. Dunn DT, Brandt CD, Krivine A, Cassol SA, Roques P, Borkowsky W, De Rossi A, Denamur E, Ehrnst A , Loveday C *et al.*, "The sensitivity of HIV-1 DNA polymerase chain reaction in the neonatal period and the relative contributions of intra-uterine and intra-partum transmission," *AIDS* **9** (1995): F7–11.
46. Rouzioux C, Costagliola D, Burgard M, Blanche S, Mayaux MJ *et al.*, "Estimated timing of mother-to-child human immunodeficiency virus type 1

(HIV-1) transmission by use of a Markov model," *American Journal of Epidemiology* **142** (1995): 1330–1337.

47. Guay LA, Hom DL, Mmiro F *et al.*, "Detection of human immunodeficiency virus type 1 (HIV-1) DNA and p24 Antigen in breast milk of HIV-1-infected Ugandan women and vertical transmission," *Pediatrics* **98** (1996): 438–444.

48. Gerdes JS, "Clinicopathologic approach to the diagnosis of neonatal sepsis," *Clinical Perinatology* **18** (1991): 361–381.

49. Voora S, Srinivasan G, Lilien LD, Yeh TF and Pildes RS, "Fever in full term newborns in the first four days of life," *Pediatrics* **69** (1982): 40–44.

50. Bhandari V and Narang A, "Thermoregulatory alterations as a marker for sepsis in normothermic premature newborns," *Indian Pediatrics* **29** (1992): 571–575.

51. Singh M, Narang A and Bhakoo ON, "Predictive perinatal score in the diagnosis of neonatal sepsis," *Journal of Tropical Pediatrics* **40** (1994): 365–368.

52. Evans ME, Schaffner W, Federspiel CF, Cotton RB, McKee KT and Stratton CW, "Sensitivity, specificity and predictive value of body surface cultures in a neonatal intensive care unit," *Journal of the American Medical Association* **259** (1988): 248–252.

53. Puri J, Revathi G, Faridi MMA, Talwar V, Kumar A and Prakash B, "Role of body surface cultures in prediction of sepsis in a neonatal intensive care unit," *Annals of Tropical Paediatrics* **15** (1995): 307–311.

54. Hall RT and Kurth CG, "Value of negative nose and ear cultures in identifying high-risk infants without early-onset group B streptococcal sepsis," *Journal of Pediatrics* **15** (1995): 356–358.

55. Squire E, Favara B and Todd J, "Diagnosis of neonatal bacterial infection: Hematologic and pathologic findings in fatal and nonfatal cases," *Pediatrics* **64** (1979): 60–64.

56. Alamelu V, Dutta AK, Narayan S and Saili A, "Hemostatic profile in neonatal septicemia," *Indian Journal of Pediatrics* **59** (1992): 249–253.

57. El-Radhi AS, Jawad M, Mansor N and Ibrahim M, "Sepsis and hypothermia in the newborn infant: Value of gastric aspirate examination," *Journal of Pediatrics* **103** (1983): 300–302.

58. Mathur NB, Saxena LM, Sarkar R and Puri RK, "Superiority of acridine orange-stained buffy coat smears for diagnosis of partially treated neonatal septicemia," *Acta Paediatrica* **82** (1993): 533–535.

59. Phillip AGS, "Decreased use of antibiotics using a neonatal sepsis screening technique," *Journal of Pediatrics* **98** (1981): 795–799.

60. Shabbir I, Hafeez A, Arif M, Ambareen, "C-reactive protein: A sensitive indicator of neonatal septicemia," *Pakistan Paediatrics Journal* **19** (1995): 23–25.

61. Pourcyrous M, Bada HS, Korones SB, Baselski V and Wong SP, "Significance of serial C-reactive protein responses in neonatal infection and other disorders," *Pediatrics* **92** (1993): 431–435.

62. Kawamura M and Nishida H, "The usefulness of serial C-reactive protein measurement in managing neonatal infection," *Acta Paediatrica* **84** (1995): 10–13.

63. Berger C, Uehlinger J, Ghelfi D, Blau N and Fanconi S, "Comparison of C-reactive protein and white blood cell count with differential in neonates at risk for septicaemia," *European Journal of Pediatrics* **154** (1995): 138–144.

64. Da Silva O, Ohlsson A and Kenyon C, "Accuracy of leukocyte indices and C-reactive protein for diagnosis of neonatal sepsis: A critical review," *Pediatric Infectious Disease Journal* **14** (1995): 362–366.

65. Chandna A, Rao MN, Srinivas M and Shyamala S, "Rapid diagnostic tests in neonatal septicemia," *Indian Journal of Pediatrics* **55** (1988): 947–953.

66. Sharma A, Kutty KCV, Sabharwal U, Rathee S and Mohan H, "Evaluation of sepsis screen for diagnosis of neonatal septicemia," *Indian Journal of Pediatrics* **60** (1993): 559–563.

67. Bhutta ZA, "Epdemiology of neonatal sepsis in Pakistan: An analysis of available evidence and implications for care," *Journal of College of Physicians and Surgeons Pakistan* **6** (1996): 12–17.

68. Victoria CG, Smith PG, Vaughan JP, Nobre LC, Lombardi C, Teixeira AM, Fuchs SM, Moreira LB, Gigante LB and Barros FC, "Influence of birth weight on mortality from infectious diseases: A case-control study," *Pediatrics* **81** (1988): 807–811.

69. Lamont RF and Fisk N, "The role of infection in the pathogenesis of preterm labour," In: *Progress in Obstetrics and Gynaecology*, Volume 10, Studd J, Ed., Edinburgh, Churchill Livingstone (1993): 135–158.

70. Hay PE, Lamont RF, Taylor-Robinson D, Morgan DJ, Ison C and Pearson J, "Abnormal bacterial colonisation of the genital tract and subsequent preterm delivery and late miscarriage," *British Medical Journal* **308** (1994): 295–298.

71. Hauth JC, Goldenberg RL, Andrews WW, DuBard MB and Copper RL, "Reduced incidence of preterm delivery with metronidazole and erythromycin in women with bacterial vaginosis," *New England Journal of Medicine* **333** (1995): 1732–1736.

72. Schultz R, Read AW, Straton JAY, Stanley FJ and Morich P, "Genitourinary tract infections in pregnancy and low birth weight: Case-control study in Australian Aboriginal women," *British Medical Journal* **303** (1991): 1369–1373.

73. Brabin B, "An assessment of low birth weight risk in primiparae as an indicator of malaria control in pregnancy," *International Journal of Epidemiology* **20** (1991): 276–283.

74. Steketee RW, Wirima JJ, Slutsker L, Roberts JM, Khoromana CO, Heymann DL and Breman JG, "Malaria parasite infection during pregnancy and at delivery in mother, placenta and newborn: Efficacy of chloroquine and mefloquine in rural Malawi," *American Journal of Tropical Medicine and Hygiene* **55**(Suppl 1) (1996): 24–32.

75. Galazka A, Gasse F and Henderson RH, "Neonatal tetanus and the global expanded programme on immunization," In: *Maternal and Child Care in Developing Countries*, Kessel E and Awan AK, eds., Thunn, Ott Publishers (1989): 109–125.

76. Awan AK, "Mobilizing TBAs for the control of maternal and neonatal mortality in Pakistan," In: *Maternal and Child Care in Developing Countries*, Kessel E and Awan AK, eds., Thunn, Ott Publishers (1989): 340–345.

77. Steer P, "Recent advances in obstetrics," *British Medical Journal* **311** (1995): 1209–1212.

78. Fiscus SA, Adimora AA, Schoenbach VJ, Lim W, McKinney R, Rupar D, Kenny J, Woods C and Wilfert C, "Perinatal HIV infection and the effect of zidovudine therapy on transmission in rural and urban counties," *Journal of the American Medical Association* **275** (1996):1483–1488.

79. Mansergh G, Haddix AC, Steketee RW, Nieburg PI, Hu DJ, Simonds RJ and Rogers M, "Cost-effectiveness of short-course zidovudine to prevent perinatal HIV type 1 infection in a sub-saharan Africa developing country setting," *Journal of the American Medical Association* **276** (1996):139–145.

80. Nielsen K, Boyer P, Dillon M, Wafer D, Wei LS, Garratty E, Dickover RE and Bryson YJ, "Presence of human immunodeficiency virus (HIV) type 1 HIV-1 specific antibodies in cervicovaginal secretions of infected mothers and in the gastric aspirates of their infants," *Journal of Infectious Diseases* **173** (1996): 1001–1004.

81. Biggar RJ, Miotti GP, Taha TE, Mtimavalye L, Broadhead R, Justesen A, Yellin F, Liomba G, Miley W, Waters D, Chiphangwi JD and Goedert JJ, "Perinatal intervention trial in Africa: Effect of a birth canal cleansing intervention to prevent HIV transmission," *Lancet* **347** (1996): 1647–1650.

82. Henrichsen T, Lindemann R, Svenningsen N and Hjelle K, "Prevention of neonatal infections by vaginal chlorhexidine disinfection during labour," *Acta Paediatrica* **83** (1994): 923–926.

83. Miel-Vergani G, "Hepatitis B virus," In: *Congenital, Perinatal and Neonatal Infections*, Greenough A, Osborne J and Sutherland S, eds., Edinburgh, Livingstone (1992): 85–94.

84. Hanson LA, Carlsson B, Jalil F, Hahn-Zoric M, Hermodson S, Karlberg J, Mellander L, Khan SR, Lindblad B, Thiringer K and Zaman S, "Antiviral and antibacterial factors in human milk," In: *Biology of Human Milk*, Hanson LA, ed., New York, Raven Press (1988): 141–157.

85. Crissinger KD and Burney D, "Intestinal oxygenation and mucosal permeability with luminal mother's milk in developing piglets," *Pediatrics Research* **40** (1996): 269–275.

86. Raibaud P, "Factors controlling the bacterial colonization of the neonatal intestine," In: *Biology of Human Milk*, Hanson LA, ed., New York, Raven Press (1988): 205–219.

87. Narayanan I, Prakash K and Gujral VV, "The value of human milk in the prevention of infection in the high-risk low birth weight infant," *Journal of Pediatrics* **99** (1981): 496–498.

88. Narayanan I, Prakash K, Verma RK and Gujral VV, "Administration of colostrum for the prevention of infection in the low birth weight infant in a developing country," *Journal of Tropical Pediatrics* **29** (1983):197–200.

89. Narayanan I, Prakash K, Murthy NS and Gujral VV, "Randomized controlled trial of effect of raw and holder pasteurized human milk and of formula supplements on incidence of neonatal infection," *Lancet* **ii** (1984): 1111–1113.

90. Committee on Pediatric AIDS, "Human milk, breastfeeding, and the transmission of the human immunodeficiency virus in the United States," *Pediatrics* **96** (1995): 977–979.

91. Van de Perre P, "Postnatal transmission of human immunodeficiency virus type 1: The breastfeeding dilemma," *American Journal of Obstetrics and Gynecology* **173** (1995): 483–487.

92. Sanabria ER and Gomez HM, "Management of premature infants in developing countries," *International Pediatrics* **1** (1986): 149–155.

93. Charpak N, Ruiz-Pelaez JG and de Calume ZF, "Current knowledge of kangaroo mother intervention," *Current Opinion in Pediatrics* **8** (1996): 108–112.

94. Narayanan I, Kumar H, Singhal PK and Dutta AK, "Maternal participation in the care of the high-risk infant: Follow-up evaluation," *Indian Pediatrics* **28** (1991): 161–167.

95. Mathur NB, Khalil A, Sarkar R and Puri RK, "Mortality in neonatal septicemia with involvement of mother in management," *Indian Pediatrics* **28** (1991): 1259–1263.
96. Siegel J, "Controlling infections in the nursery," *Pediatric Infectious Disease Journal* **4** (1985): S36–41.
97. Gupta AK, Anand NK, Manmohan, Lamba IMS, Gupta R and Srivastava L, "Role of bacteriological monitoring of the hospital environment and medical equipment in a neonatal intensive care unit," *Journal of Hospital Infection* **19** (1991): 263–271.
98. Larson E, McGinley KJ, Foglia A, Leyden JJ, Boland N, Larson J, Altobelli LC and Salazar-Lindo E, "Handwashing practices and resistance and density of bacterial flora on two pediatric units in Lima, Peru," *American Journal of Infection Control* **20** (1992): 65–72.
99. Berg DE, Hershow RC, Ramirez CA and Weinstein RA, "Control of nosocomial infections in an intensive care unit in Guatemala City," *Clinical Infectious Diseases* **21** (1995): 588–593.
100. Singh M, Paul VK, Deorari AK, Ray D, Murali MV and Sundaram KR, "Strategies which reduced sepsis-related neonatal mortality," *Indian Journal of Pediatrics* **55** (1988): 955–960.
101. Mason PR, Katzenstein DA, Chimbira THK, Mtimavalye L *et al.*, "Microbial flora of the lower genital tract of women in labour at Harare Maternity Hospital," *Central African Journal of Medicine* **35** (1989): 337–344.
102. Raz R, Sharir R, Shmilowitz L, Kenes I and Ephros M, "The elimination of gentamicin-resistant gram-negative bacteria in an newborn intensive care unit," *Infection* **15** (1987): 32–34.

Chapter 14

THE IMPORTANCE OF BREASTFEEDING AND STRATEGIES TO SUSTAIN HIGH BREASTFEEDING RATES

M. Q-K. Talukder

Professor of Paediatrics, Institute of Child and Mother Health, Matuail, Dhaka, Bangladesh

Introduction

Proper infant feeding is crucial for child nutrition, survival, and development. Breast milk is the gold standard for infant feeding, but sadly, erosion in breastfeeding practices has taken place worldwide. Since the 1980s there have been many global initiatives to promote breastfeeding such as UNICEF's child survival revolution,[1] the World Declaration on Children,[2] WHO's International Code for the Marketing of Breast Milk Substitutes,[3] the Innocenti Declaration for the protection, promotion and support of breastfeeding,[4] the Baby Friendly Hospital Initiative,[5] and the World Declaration in the International Conference on Nutrition.[6]

This paper attempts to review the benefits of breastfeeding, the associated threats to proper breastfeeding practices, and the strategies to sustain high breastfeeding rates with special reference to Bangladesh.

The Benefits of Breastfeeding

The Holy Quran, Sura Baqara, Ayat 233:

> *"The mothers shall give suck to their offspring for two whole years, if they desire to complete the term."*

Extensive research in the past decade in both developed and developing countries has shown many virtues to the ancient practice of breastfeeding. It is now clear that the beneficiaries of breastfeeding are not only infants but also the mothers, the family and society as a whole. Human milk not only supplies the full complement of nutrients that are necessary for the first six months of life,[7,8] but also acts as the child's "first vaccine"[9] because of its various immune properties. In the long run breastfeeding also protects from disease in later life.[10]

Nutritional aspects of breast milk

The balanced constituents of breast milk help in easy digestion and make for high bioavailability of most macro and micronutrients. Human milk contains less casein which forms softer curds and is easier to digest, and more whey protein than cow's milk, which contains mostly anti-infective protein. It also contains essential fatty acids that are not present in cow's milk or cow's milk products. The enzyme lipase in human milk helps to digest fat and its higher lactose content makes it more palatable. As Jelliffe points out the only similarity between human and cow's milk is that they are both white.

Though iron is present in equal amount in human and cow's milk, absorption is five times higher from human milk.[11] Different studies have confirmed the adequacy of iron from breast milk.[12,13] Bioavailability of zinc is greater for breast milk than for cow's milk and infant formula has been shown to adversely influence the selenium and copper status.[14] Although cow's milk contains four times more calcium than human milk, the infant fed on cow's milk may develop tetany because of its high phosphate load making the calcium less available. Breast milk contains vitamins A and C in greater amounts than cow's milk and so breastfed infants are protected from xerophthalmia and scurvy. Colostrum and hind milk are rich in vitamin K.[15] Hence, in order to avoid haemorrhagic disease of the newborn, the infant should be fed colostrum and allowed to empty the breast competely to obtain hind milk.

Growth factors

Various growth factors have been identified in human milk.[16,17] Although epidermal growth factor may have a general rather than specific role, most attention has been focussed on its ability to stimulate growth of the gastrointestinal tract. Nucleosides, essential in energy metabolism and enzymatic reactions, are found in significant quantity in breast milk.[18] Dietary nucleosides contained in breast milk are reported to be important in the growth and maturation of the developing gut and play several roles in immune function.[19,20] Experimental results in a group of infants of low socio-economic status in Peru suggested that nucleotide supplementation in formula fed infants decreased the incidence of diarrhoea.[21] These benefits have led to the speculation that nucleotides should be added to infant formula.[22]

Breast milk: Protection from infection

First immunisation from colostrum

Colostrum contains more immunoglobulins than mature milk and these provide protection to the newborn against infection. About 10% of protein in mature milk is secretory IgA, which is specific to pathogens commonly present in the mother's gastrointestinal or respiratory passages. This specific protection is obtained by migration of immunogen-triggered B-cells from Peyers patches and lymphoid centres in the bronchial tree to the lamina propria of the mammary gland.[23] Breast milk also contains lymphocytes, macrophages, protein with non-specific antibacterial activity, cytokines and complements whose actual functions are yet to be elucidated.

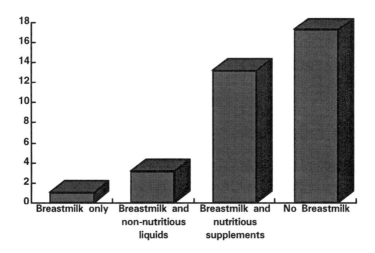

Figure 1 Risk of diarrhoea by feeding method (from WHO CDD programme).

Diarrhoea

Breastfeeding protects an infant from morbidity and mortality related to diarrhoea. The risk of diarrhoea is inversely related to the amount of breastfeeding. Exclusive breastfeeding has been shown to significantly reduce diarrhoea morbidity in the urban poor in both Dhaka, Bangladesh[24] and Lima, Peru.[25] Risk of mortality from diarrhoea is 25 times higher in infants aged 0–2 months who are not breastfed as compared to infants who are exclusively breastfed.[26] A study from Scotland showed specific protection from gastrointestinal and respiratory infection by breastfeeding up to 13 weeks or more.[27] Figure 1 shows the risk of diarrhoea by feeding method.[28]

The protection from diarrhoea with breastfeeding is mediated in two ways: directly, through specific and non-specific immune mechanisms, and indirectly, as no extra water is not needed in a breastfed infant[29] which may be the media of infection, particularly in a developing country. Secretory IgA, specific for most diarrhoeal agents, is found in breast milk.[30] Even antibody to Giardia has been found in breast milk which prevents the symptoms of diarrhoea produced by the flagellate.[31]

Neonatal infection

Clavano has shown that breastfeeding prevents infection in the term neonate.[32] A study in the UK in low birth weight infants suggests that the risk of necrotising enterocolitis (NEC) is six to ten times less in breastfed infants.[33] The risk attributable to formula feeding was greatest among the most mature, growth retarded infants. This protective effect of breast milk may be mediated through the presence of platelet activating factor (PAF)-acetylhydrolase. PAF is thought to be involved in the pathophysiology of NEC. Interestingly, the level of PAF-acetylhydrolase in breast milk is significantly higher in the earlier days of an infant's life and also more so in preterm milk when the chance of developing NEC is higher.[34] The levels of SIgA, lactoferrin and lysozyme are higher in preterm than mature milk and so human milk is essential for the preterm infant both for nutrition and protection against infection. It has also been reported that feeding of human milk is an independent predictor of decreased risk of re-hospitalisation in premature infants.

Acute respiratory infection (ARI)

Breastfeeding protects infants from ARI,[35] the most common cause of morbidity and mortality in developing countries. A study from Brazil has shown risk of death from severe pneumonia to be 3.6 times higher in artificial fed infants than in breastfed ones.[36] Figure 2 shows the risk of death from pneumonia by feeding method.

Effect on immunisation

Breastfeeding also influences the antibody response to conjugate vaccine.[37] The antibody level in the initial period may not differ but at 12 months the breastfed infant ultimately has significantly higher antibody titres than the formula fed infant.[38]

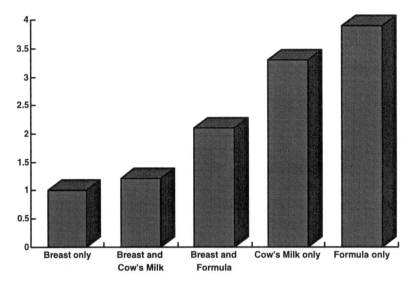

Figure 2 Risk of death from pneumonia by feeding method (from WHO CDD/ARI information).

Breastfeeding and neurological development

Breastfed infants are more intelligent, have less speech difficulties,[39,40] and achieve a higher score in vocabulary tests and design copying tests[41] than bottle fed children. They also achieve a higher Bayley score.[42] The difference in long chain fatty acid ratio (C22:6ω-3) and sensitiveness of the composition of lipids in the infant brain to dietary intake may be responsible for this.[43,44] Breast milk contains the full range of n-3 and n-6 polyunsaturated fatty acids (PUFA), including docosahexaenoic acid (DHA) and arachidonic acid, whereas infant formula contains only their precursors.[45] DHA has been implicated in neural development.[46-48] DHA helps in better early retinal response to light and better visual acuity. Breastfed infants accumulate DHA in the cortex for at least the first 40 weeks but not formula fed infants.[49] This has led to a recommendation for addition of DHA in infant formula in a concentration found in breast milk.[50,51] Human milk offers significant advantages to preterm and term infants in relation to visual and cognitive functions in comparison to standard infant formula.[52] Growth factors in breast milk may also be important in neurological development.

Breastfeeding and allergy

There is evidence that breast milk protects against allergic disease. A study in preterm infants showed that use of human milk significantly reduced the incidence of allergic disease in those with a family history of allergy but not in those without.[53] The lactoglobulin in cow's milk is responsible for allergy and is absent in human milk.

Breastfeeding and infant mortality

Many studies have demonstrated the positive impact of breastfeeding on infant mortality[54–57] in the developing world where high infant mortality is related to the complex interactions between malnutrition and infection. The risk of death increases by ten to 15 times for infants who are not breastfed during the first three to four months of life.[58]

Breastfeeding and disease in later life

A recent study strongly suggests a link between insulin-dependent diabetes mellitus (IDDM) and formula feeding. It was shown that the antibody to bovine albumin cross reacts with pancreatic islet β cell surface antigen p69.[59] An American study has shown that a baby who is breastfed for more than 12 months has half the risk of developing IDDM.[60] There are reports suggesting breastfed infants have a decreased risk of developing chronic inflammatory bowel disease.[61] A study from Denver on children with cancer showed the odds ratio increased for those artificially fed as infants.[62] No mechanism has been suggested and further study needs to be done to confirm this relationship.

Other benefits of breastfeeding

Sudden infant death syndrome (SIDS)

A study from New Zealand suggests that breastfed infants have a decreased risk of death from SIDS.[63] The Standing Committee on Nutrition of the British Paediatric Association suggests three possible mechanisms of this protection: (a) a decreased incidence of viral infection, (b) differences in sleep pattern between breast and bottle fed infants, and (c) the possible difference in neurological development attributed to dietary composition.

Family planning

On a population basis breastfeeding may contribute more to birth spacing than all family planning methods combined in many countries.[64] Lactational amenorrhoea and infertility result from decreased and disorganised ovarian follicular development through suckling and the hypothalamic-pituitary-ovarian feedback system. Family planning by breastfeeding is called the lactational amenorrhoea method (LAM). There is now consensus that women who use LAM, i.e. fully or nearly fully breastfeed, and amenorrhoeic had a less than 2% risk of pregnancy in the six months after delivery.[65,66] Studies from Bangladesh have shown that breastfeeding prevents an estimated 6.5 birth per woman.[67]

Psychological benefits

The seminal works[68] of Klaus and Kennell on mother–infant interaction or bonding have resulted in dramatic changes in maternity services worldwide. They have also opened up a whole new area of research on the multifarious aspects of mother-infant interaction.

Economic value

Breastfeeding also helps the family economically. It has been estimated that improper breastfeeding practices in Bangladesh result in the loss of approximately US$1 billion per year, which is about 2% of the country's gross national product.[69] It has been estimated that exclusive artificial feeding will cost about Taka 1,600–2,100 (US$33–43) per month per baby. If the cost of cleaning, bottle, nipple, sterilisation and time spent in doing these things are considered this will increase the cost further. Thus, the cost will be about the monthly pay of a lowly paid staff or a regular paid labourer which means it is unaffordable.

Threats to Achieving and Maintaining High Breastfeeding Rates

The WHO recommendation is to breastfeed the infants exclusively for six months and continue thereafter along with complementary feeding for at least two years. Although South Asian countries are regarded as traditionally breastfeeding regions, breastfeeding practices are far from ideal (Table 1). Despite various promotional programmes, there are many potential social, cultural and commercial threats to sustaining breastfeeding

Table 1 The breastfeeding scenario in South Asia.

Indicators of breastfeeding	Bangladesh (%)	Pakistan (%)	India, Rajasthan (%)	India, Andhra Pradesh (%)
Exclusive BF at 0–1 month	60	30	80	80
Exclusive BF at 4–6 months	20	15	10–15	30
BF at one year	98	85	90	90
BF at 2 years	75	30	60	50

Data sources: Bangladesh demographic health survey, 1993–1994; Pakistan demographic health survey, 1991; National Family Health Surveys in Rajasthan and Andhra Pradesh, 1992–1993.

which need consideration when planning appropriate interventions to promote breastfeeding.

Marketing of Breast Milk Substitutes (BMS)

Artificial infant milk is one of the fastest growing food industries in the world. World sales are estimated at over US$10 billion per year, with annual increases of up to 15%. Half of these sales are to developing countries.[70] Marketing methods include advertisements, labels, baby pictures, texts idealising bottle feeding, use of terms like 'humanised', 'maternalised', avoidance of local language, free samples, gifts, free or subsidised supply of powder milk discount coupons, promotion of BMS in health care facilities, posters, literature supply, financial and material inducements.

A randomised case-control study suggests that free infant formula samples to mothers may shorten the duration of breastfeeding and hasten the age at which solids are introduced.[71] Another study showed that mothers who received free formula stopped breastfeeding 1.4 months earlier than those who did not.[72]

In urban areas of Bangladesh, 80% of mothers feed their infants artificial milk (powder or infant formula). Because of the closeness of communities in this densely populated country, propaganda for formula feeding is reaching the villages. Bangladesh imports US$30 million worth of milk products a year, but since the price is beyond the reach of the majority of the people, they buy it and prepare it dilute thus contributing to malnutrition.[73]

Because existing marketing practices of Baby Food Manufacturers act as a detriment to successful breastfeeding, the World Health Assembly endorsed an International Code of Marketing of Breastmilk Substitutes in May 1981. The International Baby Food Action Network (IBFAN), a coalition of more than 140 breastfeeding promotion groups, monitors the implementation of the Code worldwide. IBFAN catalogues thousands of violations of the BMS Code in its report "Breaking the Rules 1994". The violations consist of promoting BMS to health workers, using labels describing a brand of formula in idealising terms, or not using labels stating in the local language that breastfeeding is the best feeding for infants.[74] IBFAN has also shown that milk companies have influenced medical school training, health care providers, UN and WHO policies, and governments of developing countries through advertising and tax income.[75]

The threat to breastfeeding has worsened because of the weakness of governments in implementing a law to protect the code. So far, 11 countries have passed legislation including all or almost all provisions of the International Code. Governments of 36 countries have passed legislation including only some provisions. In South Asia, only India and Nepal have a law with almost all provisions of the Code; Bangladesh and Pakistan has only some provisions, and others are lagging even further behind.[76]

A recently published report[77] enumerates violations of the International Code of Marketing of Breast Milk Substitutes in all four countries studied (Bangladesh, Poland, Thailand and South Africa). This was the first large, randomised and systematic survey of Code violations. A quarter of all mothers interviewed, and up to half of all facilities visited, had received free samples of milk, bottles or teats. None of these samples had been used for professional research. Sadly, health services were the most important source of free samples for mothers.

The Code also forbids gifts or inducements to health workers because those receiving gifts are more likely to promote a particular company product, and to remain passive in the promotion of breastfeeding. Nearly a fifth of health workers surveyed had received company gifts, three quarters of which bore a company brand name.

Many women interviewed in all four countries reported receiving information from a milk company which either promoted bottle feeding and, or discouraged breastfeeding. Mothers in all countries studied received samples of milk products within the health care facility. The company employees were found to have visited health facilities with the aim of giving information to mothers. Advertisement of products in the form of posters and displays were found in health facilities in all four countries. Code violations in Bangladesh were relatively low, perhaps because of national legislation and because breastfeeding campaign groups are very active.

This research proves that many companies are undertaking systematic activities that violate the code. It also clearly shows the danger of these violations in that women receive messages which endorse artificial feeding.

Unfavourable hospital policy and ignorance and apathy of health care providers

Health care facilities and maternity centres worldwide are often relatively unaware of the importance of breastfeeding. Health workers are rarely motivated or skilled to protect, promote and support breastfeeding.

One study in Metro Manila showed that most promotion of infant formula takes place in hospitals and health centres where milk companies are very active in providing samples and gifts to mothers, health personnel, and institutions. The hospital policies encouraged bottle feeding for newborns despite the positive attitude of the health care providers towards breastfeeding.[78]

In the Caribbean, breastfeeding is on the decline, partly because in hospitals (where 96% are born) the newborn infant is often separated from its mother after birth. The majority of hospital staff do not encourage and assist with breastfeeding, thus preventing the baby's consumption of colostrum. The hospital staff often prefer the convenience of substitution formula. At home or at work, women also face the objection of men who resent breastfeeding. In the office environment privacy for breastfeeding is rarely provided.[79]

In 1993 in Kanpur, India, a survey of seven private nursing homes showed that infant formula was given to most newborns (53%). Staff at five nursing homes gave prelacteal feeds (water, glucose water, and infant formula) to newborns when they were separated from their mothers. Staff at only two nursing homes gave the newborns to their mothers immediately after delivery. The longest period between delivery and giving the newborn to the mother was 24 hours. All but one of the nursing homes did not know about the government policy and the recent bill that bars free or low-cost infant formula supplies to hospitals. The administration of the nursing homes did not inform the procurement department, in writing, of the government policy. Four nursing homes bought low-cost supplies of infant formula from the companies. The companies sold the infant formula to the nursing homes at a price 48% to 87% lower than the market price. Medical stores inside or outside the nursing homes sold the infant formula to parents at the other three homes. The nursing homes used between two to 50 kg per month. Infant formula was in stock in five of the nursing homes, although none gave mothers free or low-cost infant formula at discharge. The physicians were frequently visited by company personnel. These results show that, despite government policy and the law, hospitals continue to use infant formula.[80]

In Indonesia, women who delivered at clinics or who were assisted by "modern" birth attendants weaned earlier (1.45 to 2.38 times) than women who delivered at home or who were assisted by traditional birth attendants.[81] In Lebanon, most educated and urban women reported having been delivered by a trained midwife or by a physician, but did not receive advice and support in the establishment of lactation.[82]

Rapid urbanisation and industrialisation, and rural to urban migration

The rapid urbanisation and radical changes in women's lifestyles that accompanied the Industrial Revolution led to an increase in artificial bottle feeding.[83] Data from the World Fertility Survey of four Arab countries demonstrated that urban living is most clearly associated with lower probabilities of ever breastfeeding or of continuing for a long period.[84]

Cultural diffusion

Bottle feeding culture began in the western world. There is a trend in developing countries to follow the fashion and culture of the west and formula feeding is regarded as a symbol of modernisation by the urban elite, who, in turn are copied by the rural poor.

Employment of women and unfavourable work place

With the urbanisation, more and more women are entering into jobs and thus has a negative influence on breastfeeding. There is no facility for feeding the baby in the work places. Mothers are not allowed adequate maternity leave. Many working women face obstacles such as long travelling distances to work, long or erratic working hours, few breaks, and unreliable infant caretakers.[85] Studies in North Sumatra and Chile showed that the cessation of or scanty milk secretion as well as mothers working were the main reasons for terminating breastfeeding in the urban areas. On average, a higher proportion of working mothers than their non-working counterparts had already introduced artificial milk both as a substitute for, as well as a complement to, breastfeeding when infants were three months old. Weaning foods were also introduced earlier in the diets of their infants.[86,87]

Low birth weight (LBW)

The high prevalence of low birth weight infants (31%) in South Asian countries[88] may be a threat to breastfeeding. Data from 3,080 mother–infant pairs from urban and rural communities of Metro Cebu in Philippines show the effects of LBW on feeding practices even after controlling for place of delivery (home, public, or private health facility); receipt of free infant formula samples; infant sex; urban residence; primiparity, educational level, and age of the mother; and family income and assets.

Birth of a LBW infant significantly decreased the likelihood that women would initiate breastfeeding. In a comparison of six-month feeding patterns, the authors also found that LBW increased the likelihood of not breastfeeding or of weaning before six months. Given the known health risks of LBW and the proven benefits of breastfeeding, these results emphasise the need for special efforts to promote breastfeeding of LBW infants born in clinical settings.[89]

Social taboos, misconceptions, and lack of information

Among mothers of 250 infants who were fed only commercial milk formula in an urban Indian community, most mothers could not understand the directions for use. They were also purchasing supplies from open tins on a daily or weekly basis as they could not afford the price of bulk purchase. The sterilisation of bottles was not prevalent. Many mothers used formula feeds because they were believed to be more digestible and nutritionally better. Many mothers perceived, erroneously, that there was a greater economy to using formula feeds. Others believed that breastfeeding caused liver trouble or recurring diarrhoea in their infants and therefore switched to formula milk. Most of the women were influenced primarily by health personnel with only 14% being influenced by advertising.[90]

There are other social taboos which threaten breastfeeding practice such as delay in initiating breastfeeding, prelacteal feeding, rejecting colostrum, giving water with breast milk, restricting a mother's diet, stopping breastfeeding during infant diarrhoea, or any maternal illness. In Guinea-Bissau, interviews were held with 20 elderly knowledgeable rural women. All the informants recognised colostrum but disliked its consistency. Depending on their ethnic background, they considered colostrum good, of no special value, or is harmful to the newborn baby. Further, all the informants held the belief that mature breast milk could turn bad, e.g. in the case of a mother's sickness or adultery.[91] Other common taboos were that infants should be given honey and other fluids after birth, that it takes three days for breastmilk to come in, and that mothers should be given dry food, but not certain fish, after delivery.

In Lima, Peru, a study evaluated the influence on mothers' decisions regarding breastfeeding. A lack of information about exclusive breastfeeding was common. Health workers knew to advise against other milks, but failed to advise mothers against the use of herbal teas and sweetened water as supplements. The women commonly believed they were unable to produce enough milk to feed their children because of their own undernutrition. Others believed exclusive breastfeeding would worsen their own health, while many experienced difficulties in breastfeeding which led to supplementation with other milks. Based on these findings, the project focussed educational efforts on providing better information to mothers. Educational activities, which continued for 12 months, included videos shown to small groups of mothers, posters, distribution of pamphlets, and messages broadcast over loudspeakers. A significant increase in the number of children aged 0–4 months being exclusively breastfed was observed.[92]

Use of hormonal contraceptives

It is well known that oestrogen-containing contraceptives reduce milk volume. World fertility survey data[85] supports the view that oral contraceptive use is the second most important variable associated with a decrease in the ever-breastfeeding rate and to an extent total duration.[93]

Policy makers not aware of the benefits of breastfeeding

Because of lack of communication from physicians or scientists, policy makers are neither fully aware of the benefits of breastfeeding and the risks of artificial feeding to child health. Nor are they aware that breastfeeding is a highly cost-effective health intervention.

Poor antenatal, delivery and postnatal care

In most South Asian hospitals antenatal, delivery and postnatal care are of poor quality. In Bangladesh, few hospitals have antenatal education sessions for mothers, consultation times are minimal, and the antenatal contact is not used for giving information on breastfeeding. Delivery room practices are also not supportive of breastfeeding. There is no awareness of the need for initial skin-to-skin contact between baby and mother, and no lactation counselling. In most cases mothers are not advised to come for routine postnatal check up. Exceptions to these practices are now found in those hospitals which have become Baby Friendly.

Maternal malnutrition

In South Asia, there is a high prevalence of maternal malnutrition. In some communities up to 50% of mothers have a body mass index less than 18.5. Breast milk output and quality varies to some extent with nutritional status. Though this variation is minimal in the case of mild to moderate malnutrition, severely malnourished mothers do produce less milk, which contains decreased nutrients, especially water soluble vitamins.

Strategies for Maintaining High Breastfeeding Rates

The Innocenti Declaration in 1990[4] (the first global initiative to protect, promote and support breastfeeding) recommends exclusive breastfeeding for all infants up to four to six months, and that breastfeeding should be continued for two years along with appropriate and adequate complementary feeding from four to six months. Committed, concerted and comprehensive programmes are essential in all countries to achieve these objectives.

A review[94] of the literature on breastfeeding promotion strategies indicates that the types of interventions which have been used and found to show positive results are:

- modification of hospital policies (Baby Friendly Hospital Initiative),
- use of social support,
- provision of incentives,
- education of mothers and health workers, and
- political action and legislation aimed at policy reform.

To get these policies into practice requires multifaceted strategies which will effectively promote, protect and support breastfeeding.

Formation of a national body as a campaign group

National body formation as a central campaign group in each country was recommended in the Innocenti Declaration. This group should play basically the co-ordinating role for the various breastfeeding activities described below.

It may be a government, semi-government or an independent organisation but should have the authority to work as the national body.

Baby Friendly Hospital Initiative (BFHI)[95]

BFHI is now in operation in most countries. This has proved to be an effective strategy establishing proper breastfeeding practices in hospitals. BFHI as an intervention programme demonstrates the model of primary health care within a hospital setting, and provides a base for teaching medical students, midwives, and other health care providers. The BFHI experience is varied in developed and developing countries. In 1996, there were about 5,000 baby hospitals in China, two in Japan, two in Australia, 1,000 in India, 1,000 in Thailand, and 133 in Bangladesh. Maintenance of Baby Friendly status will depend on the monitoring and evaluation of the local hospital BFHI Committee.

A mother friendly work place

Working mothers need special support to breast feed successfully.[96] Increasing numbers of women are now entering employment. Mothers can be provided support by:

* breaks for breastfeeding;
* being allowed to take the infant to the work place;
* day care or crèche facilities at the work place.

It has been found that mothers who are allowed to take their infants to work are more productive. Maternity leave (according to the ILO Provision of 1912) needs to be enhanced if we are to achieve successful exclusive breastfeeding for a period of six months.

Implementation of the Breast Milk Substitutes (BMS) Code

The marketing practices of milk companies must be controlled in line with the International Code for the Marketing of Breast Milk Substitutes (BMS).[97]

The International Baby Food Manufacturers Association in 1992 agreed with UNICEF and the WHO to stop supply of free or subsidised milk to hospitals. Violations of the code for the marketing of BMS are taking place in many countries. National legislation needs to be made and enforced effectively in order to curb violation, and monitoring for Code violations needs to be rigorous and systematic. So far only about 20 countries out of 118 who signed in favour have properly implemented the code.

Breastfeeding promotion during antenatal care[98]

Mothers are required to be counselled on breastfeeding at each visit during pregnancy. The health care providers should discuss with the mothers on the benefits and management of breastfeeding. The messages should be repeated at each visit. Mothers are very receptive during pregnancy and are likely to be highly motivated to breastfeed if proper counselling is given.

Use of news and electronic media[99]

In Guatemala, consistent promotion for breastfeeding in the electronic media over a decade resulted in high and sustained exclusive breastfeeding rates. News media also significantly contributes to the promotion of breastfeeding.

Training of health care providers

Helping mothers to breastfeed requires skill. Health care providers at all levels, particularly those who are associated with maternal and child health, should   receive training on the benefits and management of breastfeeding.[100,101] This includes obstetricians, paediatricians, teachers of community medicine, nurses, and basic health care workers. Medical students and nurses should be taught the benefits and management of breastfeeding in their undergraduate course, and efforts must be made to integrate breastfeeding teaching into their curricula.[102,103]

Lactation management centres

Mothers often encounter problems such as sore nipple, or "insufficient milk syndrome" during breastfeeding. Lactation management centres in major hospitals, clinics and health centres should be able to help these mothers. Ideally, the centres should be run by nurses who have been trained in lactation counselling.[104]

Breastfeeding as an intervention in Primary Health Care Programmes

Breastfeeding promotion must be integrated within Primary Health Care.[105] The basic health care providers, either as fixed or domiciliary services, should discuss with mothers the benefits and management of breastfeeding during antenatal visits or at childbirth and immunisation contacts.

Advocacy for political action

The campaign groups in all countries should try to sensitise politicians and administrators about the health and economic benefits of breastfeeding.[106,107] This is necessary, though not sufficient, for programme implementation.

Mother's breastfeeding support groups

Establishing mother's support groups to promote breastfeeding has been the strategy of many organisations such as La Leche League(LLL) in the USA, the Nursing Mothers Association of Australia (NMAA), Ammehjelpen of Norway, and Mother's group sub-programme in Brazil. The experience of these organisations is that mother's support groups bring positive change in breastfeeding practice.

Combined promotion of breastfeeding and Lactational Amenorrhoea Method (LAM)

Breastfeeding and LAM have a complementary effect. LAM, as a method of family planning, dictates that the mother is asked about three criteria:

- if she is amenorrhoeic,
- if she is fully or nearly fully breastfeeding, and
- if her infant is less than six months old.

If LAM is introduced as a regular family planning method in developing countries it will lead to optimum breastfeeding. On the other hand, full or nearly full breastfeeding will contribute to fertility control.[108,109]

Implementing Cost Effective Strategies for Maintaining High Exclusive Breastfeeding Rates in Bangladesh[110]

In 1989, when the Campaign for the Protection, Promotion and Support of Breastfeeding (CPPBF) began in Bangladesh, a great decline in the practices of breastfeeding was described.[111] Colostrum by tradition was largely discarded; prelacteal feeds were given to most newborn infants; initiation of breastfeeding by most mothers occurred only on the third or fourth day; exclusive breastfeeding for five months was almost non-existent; there was a high prevalence of bottle feeding even in the villages; unethical marketing of breast milk substitutes was widespread; health care providers often prescribed BMS; maternity centres' feeding practices were such that they indirectly promoted bottle feeding; complementary feeding practices were unsatisfactory; there was withdrawal of breastfeeding during illness, especially diarrhoea and ARI; and there was poor maternal nutrition.

The now renamed Bangladesh Breastfeeding Foundation (BBF) has the goal to significantly lower morbidity and mortality among children and women in Bangladesh through successful breastfeeding. It aims to achieve and sustain universal exclusive breastfeeding for the first six months ensuring colostrum for all infants; to improve complementary feeding practices and encourage the continuation of breastfeeding for two years or more; and to improve the nutritional status of pregnant and lactating mothers. To achieve these broad objectives, work has progressed in six areas, led by separate sub-committees: Baby Friendly Hospital Initiative (BFHI), research and monitoring, social mobilisation and communication, BMS code, working women, and primary health care.

Baby Friendly Hospital Initiative (BFHI)

A common national Hospital Breastfeeding Policy has been formulated and endorsed by the Ministry of Health and Family Welfare. 925 trainers have been trained, who have led training courses in 174 hospitals, Mother and Child Welfare Centres (MCWCs) and private clinics for over 3,500 staff members. 133 hospitals became Baby Friendly over a period of three years (1994–1996), and in most hospitals entry of formula milk representatives has been stopped. Four lactation management clinics have been set up, and three WHO/UNICEF lactation counselling courses held, each with 60 participants. Generally, in institutions there is now much greater awareness about breastfeeding. Nurses were found to be more enthusiastic than doctors; indeed lack of co-operation amongst the doctors in a facility affects the programme.

At primary health care level breastfeeding training for health and family planning workers in one district has been successfully piloted and is now being extended to 14 more districts. Breastfeeding is supposed to be promoted by the basic health care providers in the community through fixed centre service provisions at 108,000 outreach centres and 36,000 satellite clinics as well as during domiciliary visits.

Research and monitoring

Fourteen breastfeeding-related research studies have been completed. These included:

National breastfeeding survey

A national baseline survey was undertaken to assess the breastfeeding pattern in six divisions of Bangladesh. 3,026 mother–infant pairs from urban areas and 2,287 from rural areas were investigated. 27% of urban and 25% of rural newborns were immediately put to the breast. Colostrum was given to 75% of the infants; 80% in urban and 60% in rural areas. Mothers breastfeed 13 times a day on average. The exclusive breastfeeding rate was only 14% during the first four months of age.

Body weight in the first 14 days after birth

One study in 50 villages selected randomly in Trisal, Mymensingh, looked at body weight during the first 14 days of life. Mean birth weight of 100 newborns was 2.6 kg, and 90% lost weight in the first 24 hours. Prelacteal feeds were given to 69% of infants, and those that did not receive prelacteals lost less weight. All were breastfed yet exclusive breastfeeding was virtually non-existent even in the first 14 days.

Code violations

Violations of the BMS Code was surveyed in two hospitals and two markets from each division, in mid-1994. Among the 53% infants fed with powdered milk in 15 hospitals, just over half the parents were advised to purchase powdered milk. Low-cost free supplies were provided in 7%. Company representatives visited 87% of hospitals and offered gifts to 73% of hospital staff and to 20% of hospitals. None of the doctors or nurses advised mothers to breastfeed and none of the hospital staff were aware of the law. Companies distributed free samples to 60% of the hospitals. No writing on the labels of any brand was in Bangla. Pictures of infants were found on 35% of containers, no message of superiority of breast milk was found on 61% of them. Language aggressively promoting BMS was found on 85% of the labels, 66% had no statement that the infant formula was to be used only on doctor's instructions, no clear instructions were provided for use of the infant formula according to child's age in 68%, and 93% of labels used the picture of a bottle.

Factors influencing exclusive breastfeeding in rural villages

Factors influencing exclusive breastfeeding, studied in rural villages, were found to be:

- if the mother had more than one female child,
- if the mother owns a kutcha house,
- if she believes exclusive breastfeeding should be continued for more than five months,
- if she takes extra food during breastfeeding,
- if she has sufficient breast milk,
- if she does not restrict food during pregnancy,
- if the newborn is kept in touch with the mother, and
- if the mother has better nutritional status.

Colostrum feeding was associated with better economic status, if she or her husband had some education, if she was exposed to health workers during pregnancy, and if the deliveries were attended by relatives and neighbours.

Impact of BFHI training

The impact of BFHI training was evaluated by comparing trained hospital with untrained hospital staff. 48% of BFHI hospital staff had information about exclusive breastfeeding compared with 15% of control hospitals. 21% of Baby Friendly hospital staff took weight of the mother before and after delivery compared to 10% of control hospitals. Breastfeeding was not practiced in 10% of BFHI hospitals compared to 14% of control hospitals. 62% of BFHI mothers were giving exclusive breastfeeding compared to 49% of control hospitals. 70% of BFHI mothers continued breastfeeding their youngest child below three years of age compared to 59% of control hospital mothers. 64% of BFHI mothers suggested more coverage of breastfeeding in the mass media compared to 43% of control mothers. Other suggestions from mothers included campaigns in the rural community through regular group meetings on breastfeeding, publicity material on breastfeeding in all public places, and increased publicity about the bad effects of bottle feeding. Powdered milk, goat's or cow's milk, shuji, barley, and ground rice were found to be used by mothers as substitutes for breast milk.

Breastfeeding in private clinics

Factors influencing successful breastfeeding were studied in private clinics in Dhaka and Chittagong city. About 58% of doctors and 47% of nurses advised mothers to initiate breastfeeding within half an hour of delivery. 47% of doctors and 45% of nurses advised giving prelacteal feeds. 21% of mothers received antenatal advice for breastfeeding. None of the doctors advised demand feeding. There was no initiative from doctors and nurses to show mothers how to breastfeed infants properly and how to maintain lactation when the mother is separated from the baby. Advice on colostrum was given by all. 97% of doctors gave advice for postnatal breastfeeding. About 83% of mothers did not initiate breastfeeding within half an hour of delivery. 60% of mothers gave prelacteal feeds. 40% of mothers did not know about exclusive breastfeeding. About 95% of respondent mothers were aware of the merits of colostrum and 84% of mothers practiced demand feeding. 98% gave breast milk to their infants during diarrhoea or other illnesses.

BMS Code

Code legislation is being implemented and monitored by a 23-member advisory committee to the Ministry of Health and Family Welfare. Milk companies have pledged not to distribute low cost or free milk to any public or private maternity hospital. Systematic monitoring to detect violations of the Code has been proposed.

Working women

The ILO convention which recommends paid leave before and after childbirth is not in place in Bangladesh. Promotional materials, including a film, have been made to raise awareness on the existing laws on maternity benefits and how to apply them for working women. Creches have been set up in three garment factories, and seminars held with women's organisations on maternity leave and proper management of breastfeeding.

Social mobilisation

As a result of such a wide range of activities it does seem that there have been overall improvements during the past eight years in awareness about maternal nutrition during pregnancy and lactation, proper complementary feeding practices, a decrease in colostrum rejection, less delay in the initiation of breastfeeding. More mothers are now exclusively breastfeeding.

References

1. Grant JP, *The State of the World Children 1982*, Oxford University Press.
2. World Declaration on Child Survival and Development, UNICEF (1990).
3. International Code of Marketing of Breast Milk Substitutes, the WHO (1981).
4. Innocenti Declaration for the Protection, Promotion and Support of Breastfeeding, Florence, Italy (1990).
5. Baby friendly Hospital Initiative, the WHO, UNICEF (1991).
6. World Declaration at the International Conference on Nutrition, FAO/WHO, Rome, Italy (1992).
7. Talukder MQ-K and Kawser CA, "Growth patterns of exclusively breastfed infants," *Bangladesh Journal of Child Health* **10** (1986): 59–65.
8. Kumari S, Preethi PK and Mehra R, "Breastfeeding and physical growth during infancy," *Indian Journal of Pediatrics* **5** (1985): 73–77.
9. Editorial, "A warm chain for breastfeeding," *Lancet* **344** (1994): 1239–1241.
10. Standing Committee on Nutrition of the British Paediatric Association, "Is breastfeeding beneficial in the UK?" *Archives of Disease in Childhood* **71** (1994): 376–380.

11. Lawrence RA, "Biochemistry of human milk," In: *Breastfeeding. A Guide for the Medical Profession*, Fourth Ed., Mosby Year Book Inc., St. Louis (1994): 123–124.

12. Duncan B, Schifman RB, Corrigan JJ, "Iron and the exclusively breastfed infant from birth to six months," *Journal of Pediatric Gastroenterology and Nutrition* **4** (1985): p. 421.

13. Schulz-Lell G, Buss R, Oldigs HD, "Iron balances in infant nutrition," *Acta Pediatr. Scand.* **76** (1987): p. 585.

14. Lonnerdal B and Hernell O, "Iron, zinc, copper and selenium status of breastfed infants and infants fed trace element fortified milk-based infant formula," *Acta Pediatr. Scand.* **83** (1994): 367–373.

15. Woolridge MW and Baum JD, "Breastfeeding," In: *Recent Advances in Paediatrics*, David TJ, ed., Churchill Livingstone (1993).

16. Carpenter G, "Epidermal growth factor is a major growth-promoting agent in human milk," *Science* **210** (1980): p. 198.

17. Moran JR, Courtney ME, Orth DN *et al.*, "Epidermal growth factor in human milk: Daily production and diurnal variation during early lactation in mothers delivering at term and at premature gestation, *Journal of Pediatrics* **103** (1983): p. 402.

18. Leach JL, Baxter JH, Molitor BE, Ramstack MB and Masor ML, "Total potentially available nucleosides of human milk by stage of lactation," *American Journal of Clinical Nutrition* **61** (1995): 1224–1230.

19. Uauy R, Stringel G, Thomas R and Quan R, "Effect of dietary nucleosides on growth and maturation of the developing gut in the rat," *Journal of Pediatric Gastroenterology and Nutrition* **10** (1990): 497–503.

20. Carver J, "Dietary nucleosides: Cellular immune, intestinal and hepatic system effects," *Journal of Nutrition* **129**(Suppl) (1994): 144S–148S.

21. Brunser O, Espinoza J, Araya M, Cruchet S and Gil A, "Effect of dietary nucleotide supplementation on diarrhoeal disease in infants," *Acta Paediatrica* **83** (1994): 188–191.

22. Quan R, Barness LA and Uauy R, "Do infants need nucleotide supplemented formula for optimal nutrition?" *Journal of Pediatric Gastroenterology and Nutrition* **11** (1990): 429–437.

23. Goldman AS, Chheda S, Keeney SE, Schmalstieg FC and Schanler RJ, "Immunological protection of the premature newborn by human milk," *Seminars in Perinatology* **18** (1994): 495–501.

24. Kawser CA, "Growth of exclusively breastfed infants from 0–5 months," Dissertation submitted as part of FCPS Examination. Bangladesh College of Physicians and Surgeons, Dhaka (1983).

25. Brown KH, Black Re, de Romana GL and de Kanashiro HC, "Infant feeding practices and their relationship with diarrhoeal and other diseases in Huascar (Lima), Peru," *Pediatrics* **83** (1988): 31–40.

26. Victora CG, Vaughan JP, Lombardi C, Fuchs SMC, Gigante LP, Smith PG, "Evidence for protection by breastfeeding against infant deaths from infectious diseases in Brazil," *Lancet* **2** (1987): 319–322.

27. Howie PW, Forsyth JS, Ogston SA, Clark A and Florey du V, "Protective effect of breastfeeding against infection," *British Medical Journal (BMJ)* **300** (1990): 11–16.

28. *Breastfeeding Counselling — A Training Course.* Trainer's Guide. WHO CDD Program (1993).

29. Almroth S and Bidinger PD, "No need for water supplementation for exclusively breastfed infants under hot and arid conditions," *Transactions of the Royal Society of Tropical Medicine and Hygiene* **84**(4) (1990): 602–604.

30. Goldman AS, Chheda S, Keeney SE, Schmalstieg FC and Schanler RJ, "Immunological protection of the premature newborn by human milk," *Seminars in Perinatology* **18** (1994): 495–501.

31. Walterspiel JN *et al.*, "Secretory anti-Giardia lamblia antibody in human milk: Protective effect against diarrhoea," *Pediatrics* **93** (1994): 28–31.

32. Clavano NR, "Mode of feeding and its effect on infant mortality and morbidity," *Journal of Tropical Pediatrics* **82**(6) (1982): 287–293.

33. Lucas A and Cole TJ, "Breast milk and neonatal necrotising enterocolitis," *Lancet* **336** (1990): 1519–1523.

34. Moya FR *et al.*, "Platelet activating factor acetylhydrolase — A preliminary report," *Journal of Pediatric Gastroenterology and Nutrition* **19** (1994): 236–239.

35. Pisacane A, Graziano L, Zona G, "Breastfeeding and acute lower respiratory infection," *Acta Paediatrica* **83** (1994): 714–718.

36. Victora CG, Vaughan JP, Lombardi C, Fuchs SMC, Gigante LP, Smith PG *et al.*, "Evidence for protection by breastfeeding against infant deaths from infectious diseases in Brazil," *Lancet* **2** (1987): 319–322.

37. Pabst HF and Spady DW, "Effect of breastfeeding on antibody response to conjugate vaccine," *Lancet* **336** (1990): 269–270.

38. Zoric-Hahn M, Fulconis F, Minoli I, "Antibody responses to parenteral and oral vaccines are impaired by conventional and low protein formulas as compared to breastfeeding," *Acta Pediatr. Scand.* **79** (1990): p. 1137.

39. Broad FE, "The effect of infant feeding on speech quality," *New Zealand Medical Journal* **76** (1972): 28–31.

40. Broad FE, "Further studies of the effects of infant feeding on speech quality," *New Zealand Medical Journal* **82** (1975): 373–376.

41. Taylor B and Wadsworth J, "Breastfeeding and child development," *Developmental Medicine and Childhood Neurology* **26** (1984): 73–80.

42. Morrow-Tlucak M, Haude RH and Ernhart CB, "Breastfeeding and cognitive development in the first two years of life," *Soc. Sci. Med.* **26** (1988): 635–639.

43. Uauy RD, Birch DG, Birch EE, Tyson JE and Hoffman DR, "Effect of dietary ω-3 fatty acids on retinal function of very low birth weight neonates," *Pediatric Research* **28** (1990): 485–492.

44. Farquharson J, Cockburn F, Patrick AW, Jamieson EC and Logan RW, "Infant cerebral cortex phospholipid fatty acid composition and diet," *Lancet* **340** (1992): 810–813.

45. Makrides M, Simmer K, Neumann M and Gibson R, "Changes in the polyunsaturated fatty acids of breast milk from mothers of full-term infants over 30 weeks of lactation," *American Journal of Clinical Nutrition* **61** (1995): 1231–1233.

46. Carlson SE, Werkman SH, Rhodes PG and Tolley EA, "Visual acuity development in healthy preterm infants: Effect of marine-oil supplementation," *American Journal of Clinical Nutrition* **58** (1993): 35–42.

47. Makrides M, Simmer K, Goggin M and Gibson RA, "Erythrocyte docosahexaenoic acid correlates with the visual response of healthy, term infants," *Pediatric Research* **33** (1993): 425–427.

48. Makrides M, Neumann MA, Simmer K and Gibson RA, "Dietary docosahexaenoic acid (DHA) and the development of visual acuity in term infants," *Journal of Paediatrics and Child Health* **30** (1994): A2 (Abstr).

49. Makrides M, Neumann MA, Byard RW, Simmer K and Gibson RA, "Fatty acid composition of brain, retina and erythrocytes in breast and formula fed infants," *American Journal of Clinical Nutrition* **60** (1994): 189–194.

50. Uauy R, "Are omega-3 fatty acids required for normal eye and brain development in the human?" *Journal of Pediatric Gastroenterology and Nutrition* **11** (1990): 296–302.

51. ESPGAN Committee on Nutrition, "Comment on the content and composition of lipids in infant formulas," *Acta Pediatr. Scand.* **80** (1991): 887–896.

52. Cockburn F, "Breastfeeding and the infant human brain," In: *Nutrition in Child Health*, Davies DP, ed., Royal College of Physicians, London (1995).

53. Lucas A, Brooke OG, Morley R, Cole TJ and Bamford MF, "Early diet of preterm infants and development of allergic or atopic disease: Randomised prospective study," *British Medical Journal (BMJ)* **300** (1990): 837–840.

54. Scrimshaw NS, Taylor CE and Gordon JE, "Interaction of nutrition and infection," WHO Monograph, No. 29, World Health Organization, Geneva (1968).

55. Puffer RR and Serrano CV, "Patterns of mortality in childhood," Scientific Pub. No. 262, Washington DC, Pan American Health Organization (1973).

56. Victora CG, Smith PG, Barros FC, "Risk factors for death due to respiratory infections among Brazilian infants," *International Journal of Epidemiology* **18** (1989): p. 918.

57. Thapa S, Short RV and Potts M, "Breastfeeding, birth spacing and their effects on child survival," *Nature* **335** (1988): 679–682.

58. *Take the Baby-Friendly Initiative*, Unicef Publication (1992).

59. Karjalainen J, Martin JM, Knip M, "A bovine albumin peptide as a possible trigger of insulin-dependent diabetes," *New England Journal of Medicine* **327** (1992): 302–307.

60. Mayer EJ, Hamman RF, Gay EC, Lezotte DC, Savitz DA and Klingensmith GJ, "Reduced risk of IDDM among breastfed children," *Diabetes* **37** (1988): 1625–1632.

61. Koletzko S, Sherman P, Corey M, "Role of infant feeding practices in development of Crohn's disease in childhood," *British Medical Journal (BMJ)* **298** (1989): 1617–1618.

62. Davies MK, Savitz DA and Graubard BI, "Infant feeding and childhood cancer," *Lancet* **2** (1988): 365–368.

63. Mitchell EA, Taylor BJ, Ford RP, "Four modifiable and other risk factors for cot death: The New Zealand study," *Journal of Paediatric and Child Health* **28**(Suppl 1) (1992): S3–S8.

64. Labbok MH, Perez A, Valdes V, Sevilla F, Wade K, Lankanan VH, "The lactational amenorrhoea method (LAM): A post partum introductory family planning method with policy and programme implications," *Advances in Contraception* **10** (1994): 93–109.

65. van Look PFA, "Lactational amenorrhoea method for family planning," *British Medical Journal (BMJ)* **313** (1996): 893–894.

66. Kennedy KI, Labbok MH and van Look PFA, "Concensus statement: Lactational amenorrhoea method for family planning," *International Family Planning Journal of Gynaecology and Obstetrics* **54** (1996): 55–57.

67. Ford K and Huffman S, "Nutrition, infant feeding and post-partum amenorrhoea in rural Bangladesh," *J. Biosoc. Sci.* **20** (1988): 461–469.

68. Klaus M and Kennell J, "Parent to infant bonding: Setting the record straight," *Journal of Pediatrics* **102** (1983): p. 575.

69. Bangladesh, Unicef Report.

70. Clement D, "Commerciogenic malnutrition in the 1980s," In: *Programmes to Promote Breastfeeding*, Jelliffe DB and Jelliffe EFP, eds., Oxford, England, Oxford University Press (1988): 348–359.

71. Bergevin Y, Dougherty C and Kramer MS, "Do infant formula samples shorten the duration of breastfeedings?" *Lancet* **1**(8334) (1983): 1146–1151.

72. Adair LS, Popkin BM and Guilkey DK, "The duration of breastfeeding: How is it affected by biological, sociodemographic, health sector, and food industry factors?" *Demography* **30**(1) (1993): 63–80.

73. Muttalib MA, "Decline of breastfeeding — A socio economic catastrophe," *In Touch* **12**(89) (1988): 30–34.

74. *Breaking the Rules 1994*, "A worldwide report on violations of the WHO/UNICEF International Code of Marketing of Breastmilk substitutes. IBFAN International Baby Food Action Network. Published by Baby Milk Action.

75. Allain A, "IBFAN: On the cutting edge," *Development Dialogue* **2** (1989): 5–38.

76. *State of the Code by Country 1994*, IBFAN, ICDC, Penang, Malaysia.

77. "Cracking the Code: Monitoring the International Code of Marketing of Breastmilk Substitutes," Published by The Interagency Group on Breastfeeding Monitoring, London (1997).

78. Simpson-Hebert M, "Infant feeding in Metro Manila: Infant formula marketing and health institution policies," Manila, Philippines, Ramon Magsaysay Award Foundation, RMAF Research Report Volume II (1986): xiii, 116 p.

79. Anonymous, "Breastfeeding … back in fashion?" *Children In Focus* **4**(3) (1992): p. 1, p. 7.

80. Mathur GP, Pandey PK, Mathur S, Mishra VK, Singh K, Bhatt OP, Loomba RK, Luthra C, Taneja S and Kapoor R, "Breastfeeding status and marketing

practices of baby food manufactured in nursing homes," *Indian Pediatrics* **30**(11) (1993): 1333–1335.

81. Joesoef MR, Utomo B and Lewis GL, "Breastfeeding practices in metropolitan Indonesia: Policy considerations," *Journal of Tropical Pediatrics* **34**(6) (1988): 270–274.

82. Zurayk HC and Shedid HE, "The trend away from breastfeeding in a developing country: A women's perspective," *Journal of Tropical Pediatrics and Environmental Child Health,* **27**(5) (1981): 237–243.

83. MacIntyre UE and Walker AR, "Lactation — How important is it?" *Journal of The Royal Society of Health,* **114**(1) (1994): 20–28.

84. Akin JS, Bilsborrow RE, Guilkey DK and Popkin BM, "Breastfeeding patterns and determinants in the Near East: An analysis for four countries," *Population Studies* **40**(2) (1986): 247–261.

85. Wade KB, "Assisting working women toward optimal breastfeeding," Washington, DC, Georgetown University Medical Center, Institute for Reproductive Health, Sep. 22, [1] p. Institute Monograph Paper (1993).

86. Saat R, Yoel C, Meliala R, Noeriman AJ and Tambunan S, "A study of breastfeeding practices in some population in north Sumatra, Indonesia," *Paediatrica Indonesiana* **25**(1–2) (1985): 33–38.

87. Vial I, Muchnik E and Mardones F, "Women's market work, infant feeding practices, and infant nutrition among low-income women in Santiago, Chile," In: *Women, Work, and Child Welfare in the Third World,* Leslie J and Paolisso M, eds., Westview Press, Boulder, Colorado (1989): 131–159. AAAS Selected Symposium 110.

88. Anonymous, "The incidence of low birth weight: An update," *Mother and Child* **22**(1) (1985): 21–31.

89. Adair LS and Popkin BM, "Low birth weight reduces the likelihood of breastfeeding among Filipino infants," *Journal of Nutrition* **126**(1) (1996): 103–112.

90. Shrivastava DK, Sahni OP and Kumar A, "Infant feeding with commercial milk formula in an urban community of central India," *Indian Pediatrics* **24**(10) (1987): 889–894.

91. Gunnlaugsson G and Einarsdottir J, "Colostrum and ideas about bad milk: A case study from Guinea-Bissau," *Social Science and Medicine* **36**(3) (1993): 283–288.

92. Fukumoto M and Creed Kanashiro H, "Congratulations to the mothers. Breastfeeding," *Dialogue on Diarrhoea* (59) (1995): p. 4.

93. Akin JS, Bilsborrow RE, Guilkey DK and Popkin BM, "Breastfeeding patterns and determinants in the Near East: An analysis for four countries," *Population Studies* **40**(2) (1986): 247–261.

94. Wilmoth TA and Elder JP, "An assessment of research on breastfeeding promotion strategies in developing countries," *Social Science and Medicine* **41** (1995): 579–594.

95. Ramsay S, "UNICEF-WHO baby-friendly initiative," *Lancet* **341** (1993): p. 430.

96. Wade KB, "Assisting working women toward optimal breastfeeding," Institute Monograph Paper, Institute of Reproductive Health, Georgetown University Medical Center, Washington DC (1993) Sep. 22, [1].

97. Anonymous, "Breastfeeding in developing countries — Our challenge," [Amning i U-land — var utmaning.] *Jordemodern* **100**(6) (1987): 172–173.

98. Anonymous, "Breastfeeding ... back in fashion?" *Children In Focus* **4**(3) (1992): p. 1, p. 7.

99. Hernandez O, Marquez L and Parlato M, "Assessment of the impact of a national intervention to promote exclusive breastfeeding in Honduras," Tegucigalpa, Honduras, Ministry of Public Health (1995); xi, 68: [35].

100. Winikoff B, "Technical Working Group A report: Breastfeeding promotion and support in hospitals and maternity care institutions," In: *Proceedings of the Interagency Workshop on Health Care Practices Related to Breastfeeding*, December 7–9 (1988), Leavey Conference Center, Georgetown University, Washington, DC.

101. Valdes V, Perez A, Labbok M, Pugin E, Zambrano I and Catalan S, "The impact of a hospital and clinic-based breastfeeding promotion programme in a middle class urban environment," *Journal of Tropical Pediatrics* **39**(3) (1993): 142–151.

102. al-Nahedh NN, "Infant feeding practices and the decline of breastfeeding in Saudi Arabia," *Nutrition and Health* **10**(1) (1994): 27–31.

103. Ysunza-Ogazon A, "The decline of breastfeeding in Mexico: An example of medical-academic deformation," In: *Advances in International Maternal and Child Health*, Vol. 4, Jelliffe DB and Jelliffe EF, eds., Oxford University Press, Oxford, England (1984): 36–52.

104. Queenan JT, "The role of physicians in breastfeeding promotion. In: *Lactation Education for Health Professionals*, Rodriguez-Garcia R, Schaefer LA and Yunes J, eds., Washington DC, Pan American Health Organization (PAHO) (1990): 189–191.

105. Jelliffe EF, "Breastfeeding promotion around the world: Newer approaches and innovative programs," In: *Proceedings of the Workshop on Breastfeeding and Supplementary Foods*, Valyasevi A and Baker J, eds., Bangkok, Thailand, 17–18 November 1979. Mahidol University, Ramathibodi Hospital, Institute of Nutrition and Department of Pediatrics (1980): 23–29.

106. "The immediate need for breastfeeding promotion," In: *Proceedings of the Interagency Workshop on Health Care Practices Related to Breastfeeding*, December 7–9, 1988, Leavey Conference Center, Georgetown University, Washington, DC, edited by Miriam Labbok and Margaret McDonald with Mark Belsey, Peter Greaves, Ted Greiner, Margaret Kyenkya-Isabirye, Chloe O'Gara, James Shelton. Washington, DC, Georgetown University Medical Center, Institute for International Studies in Natural Family Planning (1988): p. 2.

107. Baer EO, "Promoting breastfeeding: A national responsibility," *Studies in Family Planning* **12**(4) (1981): 198–206.

108. Perez A, Labbok M and Queenam J, "Clinical study of the lactational amenorrhoea method for family planning," *Lancet* **339** (1992): 968–970.

109. Kazi A, Kennedy KI, Visness CM and Khan T, "Effectiveness of the lactational amenorrhoea method in Pakistan," *Fertility and Sterility* **64** (1995): 717–723.

110. Talukder MQ-K, "Protection, promotion and support of breastfeeding in Bangladesh," *Regional Health Forum* **1**(1) (1996): 18–24.

111. Talukder MQ-K, "Infant feeding practices in Bangladesh and the recent dangerous trends towards bottle feeding," *Bangladesh Journal of Child Health* **8** (1984): 84–90.

Commentary

IMPROVING BREASTFEEDING SUPPORT IN THE COMMUNITY

Shameem Ahmed
Health Scientist, Operations Research Project,
International Centre for Diarrhoeal Disease Research,
Bangladesh (ICDDR,B)
Dhaka, Bangladesh

Although important progress has been made in many countries through the Baby Friendly Hospital Initiative, the goal of enabling all women to breastfeed optimally will only be achieved when there is a more supportive environment both at work and in the community.

Community Support

Although a woman's choice about how best to feed her child is a personal one, whether she breastfeeds successfully or not depends partly on the attitude of other people in the community — fathers, grandmothers, relatives, friends, employers, community leaders, etc., — and partly on the mother's knowledge and understanding of breastfeeding.[1]

Every woman needs full support from those around her to enable her to initiate and sustain breastfeeding. It is the responsibility of the community to see that the best possible nutrition and health is available to all its members, especially children.[2]

To promote breastfeeding effectively requires an understanding of the attitudes and practices of the community. How to communicate, to whom, and through whom, needs to be a collective decision.

Health Service Support

Health services should also be more supportive of breastfeeding. It is essential to ensure that health service practices support breastfeeding: in maternity units, outpatient departments, EPI centres, and in MCH and family planning clinics. Any mother coming to a health facility should be given advice and support about initiation and duration of breastfeeding, especially exclusive breastfeeding. She should also be given practical support in the technique of breastfeeding. At the same time, mothers should be encouraged to share this information with other mothers. If she has been counselled in a health facility she can herself act as a "peer counsellor" in the community. Counselling breastfeeding mothers, and encouraging them to do so for peers, is an important activity of the "Breastfeeding Corners" set up in four large hospitals in Dhaka, Bangladesh.[3] Messages about the advantages of breastfeeding and up-to-date information are provided for mothers and health workers. The traditional birth attendants (TBAs), having an important influence in the community, should also be included in awareness raising. If there is a TBA training programme in the area, breastfeeding should be incorporated into the curriculum. Teaching sessions for health care workers and school teachers about the basics of breastfeeding, how to combine work (including school) and breastfeeding, and how to help women overcome early difficulties, can be arranged.

Women's and Mothers' Groups

It may also be very useful to incorporate women's groups into the breast-feeding campaign. They can be encouraged to make breastfeeding promotion and counselling a part of their activities, and to form breastfeeding promotion groups to help educate the community.

Another way to enhance breastfeeding practices in the community may be through the formation of direct "mother-to-mother support groups", as this may be a most effective means of promoting breastfeeding support. Coordinating with a woman who is an expert in breastfeeding and helping her initiate a peer support group is a good first step. The group members can meet regularly, share experiences, and discuss ways to cope with the difficulties they might face. La Leche League International offers guidelines on mother support groups.

It is important not only to strengthen mother support groups in the community but, when appropriate, to provide resources for the establishment of these groups. Advocacy for a community approach to supporting breastfeeding can be started by mother who have successfully breastfed their babies and are members of mother support groups. They can work as resource persons and influence families, neighbours, and relatives, to restore a "breastfeeding culture". They can also be "influence agents" to change attitudes of religious leaders, who are very important in many developing countries.

Every sector of the community has a role and can join the campaign to support breastfeeding. School teachers, religious leaders, and agricultural and health workers can all network towards promoting breastfeeding.

Paediatric Training and Higher Education

The importance of breastfeeding along with its practical aspects must be included in the paediatric curriculum of medical education. Still, many paediatric textbooks lack up-to-date information on breastfeeding. Breastfeeding should also be included in curricula for secondary schools, especially in developing countries where girls marry early.

Non-Government Organisations

Non-government organisations (NGOs) can play a vital role in networking groups at grassroots level. The World Alliance on Breastfeeding Action (WABA) launched the Mother-Friendly Workplan Initiative in 1993 as a follow-up to the Baby Friendly Hospital Initiative. Part of this initiative is to create supportive working conditions, like creches and better transport, that enable women to successfully combine exclusive breastfeeding with paid work. Community leaders and NGOs are important in developing the social support needed for women in the informal and agrarian sectors to combine breastfeeding and work. This will involve educating the public about the rights of working women to breastfeed, and ensuring that national legislation to protect these rights is implemented.

To reach a larger public, there should be extensive media coverage. Film shows, dramas and role-plays at the village level can be useful. Educational programmes on television can regularly feature aspects of breastfeeding. Pamphlets and posters on breastfeeding, designed attractively, should be made available at schools, health facilities and market places. Community workers should be encouraged to check any inappropriate promotional activities which breach the WHO's Code of Marketing of Breastmilk Substitutes. In Bangladesh, mothers' support groups have organised fairs and exhibitions highlighting the importance of breastfeeding. In India, 'Chetna' organised camps to impart information on infant feeding and child care practices. This camp approach can be integrated with existing community level activities, but regular follow-up after camps is crucial.

Shopping malls, shops and restaurants can show their support by having sales and various offers for breastfeeding mothers. Libraries can also be made more "baby-friendly" so that women can use them by keeping their children in the library creche.

All these activities have a common aim — to restore a "breastfeeding culture" and to protect breastfeeding from the commercial pressures of the infant milk companies.

References

1. King FS, *Helping Mothers to Breastfeeding*, African Medical and Research Foundation, Nairobi, Kenya (1992).
2. Amin S, *Nurturing the Future. Our First Five Years*, World Alliance for Breast-feeding Action (WABA), Penang, Malaysia (1996).
3. Ahmed S, "Lactation management centres in hospitals," Special Article. *Bangladesh Journal of Child Health* **18**(4) (1994): 140–142.

Chapter 15

NEONATAL HYPOGLYCAEMIA

Anthony Costello
Reader in International Child Health,
Institute of Child Health

and

Deb Pal
Research Fellow, Institute of Child Health,
University College, London

The progress of the newborn from an intra- to an extrauterine environment is accompanied by many physiological and metabolic changes. In developing countries, newborn infants face greater risks during the process of adaptation because they may be nutritionally disadvantaged *in utero* and endure greater external social and environmental risk factors such as delayed breastfeeding, thermal stress or exposure to infection.

Neonatal Hypoglycaemia: The Risks

Ther term hypoglycaemia refers to a low blood glucose level. There is no generally accepted "normal range" for blood glucose. The level is influenced by factors such as gestation, age after birth, and timing of feeds. Neonatal hypoglycaemia is a potentially avoidable cause of mortality and neurodevelopmental impairment. Neonatal mortality accounts for 50–60% of all infant deaths in developing countries.[1] Many neonatal deaths in poor countries are unexplained, so hypoglycaemia as a cause or consequence of foetal malnutrition, birth asphyxia, postnatal hypothermia, or apnoea could be a significant aetiological factor in some of these early deaths. Neurodevelopmental impairment has been shown to be 3.5 fold higher in preterm infants with recurrent mild hypoglycaemia[2] and there is evidence that glucose levels less than 2.6 millimoles per litre lead to acute neurophysiological changes in newborns.[3] In developing countries, where classical risk factors such as low birth weight (LBW), hypothermia and delays in the onset of breastfeeding are common, hypoglycaemia could be a widespread problem in the newborn population. However, the prevalence and associations of hypoglycaemia in these settings are not well described.

Prevalence of Risk Factors for Hypoglycaemia

Table 1 shows the risk factors for hypoglycaemia described in most textbooks of neonatology. It should be noted though that these risk factors were derived from early studies which described small numbers of infants and did not quantify relative risk nor control for important confounding variables such as postnatal age.[4,5]

Table 1 Known risk factors for hypoglycaemia.

Maternal
Toxaemia
Diabetes
Malnutrition

Infant
Preterm
Small-for-gestational age
Large-for-gestational age
Haemolytic disease of the newborn
Hypothermia
Asphyxia
Polycythaemia
Starvation
Inborn errors of metabolism
Any serious illness, e.g. cardiac failure, respiratory distress, infection

---

In developing countries, growth retardation, hypothermia, late feeding practices and maternal nutritional factors are perceived to be the most prevalent risk factors.[6] Intrauterine growth retardation is common: in sub-Saharan Africa, reported rates for LBW births vary from 10–20%. In South Asia, rates are higher varying from 22% in Sri Lanka to 34% in Bangladesh.[7] These rates may double among the poorest mothers.

Even in countries with warm climate, ambient temperatures may fall below the WHO recommended minimum of 25°C[8,9] at night in the cold season or at higher altitude. A low ambient temperature is associated with a lower population glucose level.[10] In many traditional cultures restriction of colostrum feeds and use of pre-lacteals in the first two days is a common practice[11] and might contribute further to the risk of hypoglycaemia. Endocrine status may also affect the risk of hypoglycaemia. Laboratory studies suggest that in sheep impaired thyroid status of the mother predisposes the newborn to hypoglycaemia.[12] Clinical and sub-clinical hypothyroidism due to iodine deficiency is still widely prevalent in the developing world and might contribute to an increased risk of hypoglycaemia.

Prevalence of Hypoglycaemia

There is little published about the prevalence and associations of hypoglycaemia in any developing country. Comparing the prevalence of hypoglycaemia in different populations is made difficult by differing definitions, populations, labour room practices, age and technical methods. Table 2 compares the reported prevalence rates from various published studies noting the definition of hypoglycaemia, the type of population studied and the time at which blood sampling was performed.

Recent studies of neonatal hypoglycaemia in Nepal

A pilot study in Nepal using glucose test strips on heelprick samples showed that 38% of newborns during the first three days experienced a blood glucose of less than 2.6 mmol/L (this estimate adjusted for the tendency of glucose strips to under-read). This compares with a reported prevalence of 18% of

Table 2 Comparison of hypoglycaemia prevalence in different studies.

Author	Definition	Population	Time	Frequency
Sexson, 1984	< 2.2 mmol/L	not specified, US	5 hours age	21%
Lucas, 1988	< 2.6 mmol/L	preterm, UK	0–9 weeks age	66%
Heck, 1987	< 2.2 mmol/L	term, US	first 48 hours	29%
Cole, 1994	< 2.2 mmol/L	term, US	2 hours age	37%
Holtrop, 1993	1.9–2.5 mmol/L	LGA/SGA, US	first 48 hours	8%/15%
Anderson, 1993	< 2.6 mmol/L	term, Nepal	first 50 hours	38%

For sources, see references.

Table 3 Prevalence (%) of hypoglycaemia in 578 newborns less than 48 hours of age born with an uncomplicated delivery in the maternity hospital in Kathmandu.

Definition of case	0–6 hrs n = 73	6–12 hrs n = 97	12–18 hrs n = 72	18–24 hrs n = 106	24–30 hrs n = 85	30–36 hrs n = 58	36–42 hrs n = 42	42–48 hrs n = 45	0–48 hrs n = 578
< 2.6 mmol/L	35 (48)	53 (55)	25 (35)	50 (47)	34 (40)	22 (38)	11 (26)	8 (18)	238 (41)
< 2.0 mmol/L	12 (16)	13 (13)	8 (11)	11 (10)	13 (15)	4 (7)	3 (7)	2 (4)	66 (11)

newborns in Newcastle, UK, studied during the same postnatal period and using the same definition of hypoglycaemia.[16,17]

In a more recent detailed study in the same maternity hospital in Nepal we aimed to measure precisely, using a standard laboratory glucose method, the severity and prevalence of hypoglycaemia among apparently healthy newborns, and to identify and evaluate the relative importance of maternal and infant (prenatal and postnatal) risk factors in order to design appropriate strategies for prevention.[10] 578 term newborns were studied and the results were as follows: 238 (41%, 95% CI: 37–45) newborns had mild (less than 2.6 mmol/L) and 66 (11%, 95% CI: 9–14) moderate hypoglycaemia (less than 2.0 mmol/L) (see Table 3).

Significant independent risk factors for moderate hypoglycaemia included postmaturity, (Odds Ratio (OR) 2.62, 95% confidence interval 1.00–6.86), birth weight < 2.5 kg (OR 2.11, CI 1.02–4.36), small head size (OR 0.59, CI

0.43–0.81), infant haemoglobin > 21 g/dl (OR 2.77, CI 1.15–6.67), and maternal TSH > 5 IU/l (OR 3.08, CI 1.55–6.13). Feeding delay increased the risk of hypoglycaemia at age 12–24 hours (OR 4.09, CI 1.45–11.53). The risks of moderate hypoglycaemia attributable to delay in feeding, low birth weight and raised maternal TSH were 43%, 25% and 18% respectively, and 21% of mild hypoglycaemia was attributable to low ambient temperature.

The results of this study suggest that neonatal hypoglycaemia is a surprisingly common problem in a developing country setting even among apparently healthy infants. Promotion of early feeding could reduce the occurrence of moderate hypoglycaemia mainly in the second 12 hours of life, but ambient temperature control may affect only the risk of mild hypoglycaemia. The significance of raised maternal TSH and maternal anaemia — newly identified prenatal risk factors for neonatal metabolic adaptation — requires further research.

The Role of Alternative Fuels

Acute hypoglycaemia may impair cerebral function, ultimately leading to cell death, but the full significance of a low blood glucose cannot be appreciated in the newborn infant without assessment of the availability of other cerebral metabolic fuels including ketone bodies, lactate, pyruvate, glycerol, and free fatty acids.[18,19] An increase in cerebral blood flow may also compensate for a low glucose level.[20]

Hawdon *et al.* in Newcastle, UK, observed in a cross-sectional study that the mean blood glucose of breastfed term infants up to one week in age was lower than formula fed infants, but ketone body concentrations were significantly higher on days two and three.[18] By contrast, small-for-gestational age infants have minimal fat and glycogen reserves as well as a reduced capacity for gluconeogenesis, and increased glucose utilisation. Hawdon and Ward Platt studied metabolic adaptation in 33 SGA infants longitudinally, and found a reduced ketogenic response in comparison to the data from appropriate-for-gestational age infants in their cross-sectional study. However, only 22 of their infants were term gestation, and most were receiving intensive feeding or intravenous fluids.

In the recent Nepal study described above we investigated whether apparently healthy but hypoglycaemic newborns in Nepal exhibited metabolic compensation by mobilisation of alternative fuels. We measured age profiles of levels of "alternative fuel" metabolites and blood glucose and examined the relationships between them. It has also been postulated that hyperinsulinaemia may contribute to the pathogenesis of hypoglycaemia in infants who are small-for-gestational age,[21] so we also looked for evidence of hyperinsulinaemia in a sub-group of hypoglycaemic infants. Table 4 compares the levels of various alternative fuels in infants with and without hypoglycaemia.

Interestingly, we found that there was no evidence for metabolic compensation in hypoglycaemic infants during the first 48 hours after birth. Alternative fuel levels, except free fatty acids, were significantly reduced in infants with lower blood glucose. Hypoglycaemic infants were also not hyperinsulinaemic. We also found that low ambient temperature and impaired infant thyroid function are potentially important and preventable risk factors for impaired ketogenesis after birth.

Table 4 Comparison of alternative fuel levels in infants with and without hypoglycaemia.

Alternative fuel	Mean fuel level		t test for difference	p value
	Glucose 2.6 mmol/L or above (sd)	Glucose < 2.6 mmol/L (sd)		
Lactate (mmol/L)	2.8 (1.0)	2.3 (0.9)	5.8	< 0.001
Pyruvate (umol/L)	156 (54)	133 (51)	5.3	< 0.001
Glycerol (umol/L)	485 (309)	417 (270)	2.74	0.006
Hydroxy-butyrate (umol/L)	219 (194)	167 (196)	3.12	0.002
Free fatty acids (mmol/L)	1.19 (0.55)	1.18 (0.53)	0.21	0.8

From these results we concluded that alternative fuels are important in the metabolic assessment of newborns, that hypoglycaemic newborns in Nepal were not hyperinsulinaemic, and that they did not exhibit metabolic compensation in the first 48 hours. However, caution must be exercised in interpreting these results. Are the lower levels of alternative fuels simply a reflection of increased consumption by the brain and other organs? The answer to this question would require dynamic longitudinal metabolic studies. And even if the levels are lower than in normoglycaemic infants, are these combined fuel supplies adequate for the metabolic needs of the newborn brain? We do not know the answer to this question. The most important message, however, is that early feeding is essential in order to avoid both hypoglycaemia and low levels of alternative brain fuels.

Public Health Implications

Screening and prevention

The public health implications are dependent on strategic aims, approaches and definitions. If the aim is to reduce the prevalence of infants with a low blood glucose, however defined, clinicians with limited resources might target screening and selective care to high risk groups such as premature, post-term and LBW newborns. More might be gained from a population approach to raising blood glucose levels in the newborn period, for example, by promoting early breastfeeding and raising the ambient temperature of postnatal hospital wards in winter might be relatively simple and cost-effective interventions.

The Baby Friendly Hospital initiative developed by UNICEF since 1992[22] has enjoyed considerable success in changing the culture of maternity hospitals so that early breastfeeding is promoted, assisted by changes in facilities and procedures to ensure continual contact between mothers and their newborns.

Clinical demands and the lack of equipment and trained personnel (even in capital city maternity hospitals) means that hypoglycaemia is rarely detected let alone treated. Improvements are needed in the reliability and availability of blood glucose screening methods. Many maternity hospitals are still without cotside methods for estimation of blood glucose or access to 24 hour laboratory analysis. Often, staff do not appreciate that hypoglycaemia is a major risk factor for death and brain damage.

The importance of early breastfeeding

Our study in Nepal confirmed that the largest population attributable risk[23] for moderate hypoglycaemia was a delay in feeding, which accounted for 43% of hypoglycaemia in the first two days. In view of this finding clinicians and midwives should pay the greatest attention to ensuring successful early breastfeeding and assisting mothers who have problems with lactation. Remember that the infant who is unwilling to feed or does not wake may be ill. Clinical observation and physical examination are more valuable than blood glucose testing in expediting the appropriate investigation and treatment of underlying disease. A useful guideline for health workers dealing with such infants is FEED–CHECK–REVIEW.

WHO recommendations for prevention and management of hypoglycaemia

Recent guidelines for appropriate blood glucose screening and management of neonatal hypoglycaemia in an excellent review of the literature edited by Williams for the Division of Child Health and Development and Maternal and Newborn Health and Safe Motherhood at the World Health Organization in Geneva.[24]

A synopsis of their most important recommendations are as follows:

1. Early and exclusive breastfeeding meets the nutritional needs of healthy term newborns.
2. Healthy term infants need not be screened for hypoglycaemia and need no supplementary foods or fluids.
3. Healthy newborns do not develop "symptomatic" hypoglycaemia as a result of simple underfeeding.
4. Thermal protection in addition to breastfeeding is necessary to prevent hypoglycaemia.

5. Breastfeeding should be initiated when the infant is ready, preferably within an hour of birth. The newborn should be dried and held against the mother's chest to facilitate breastfeeding and maintain temperature.

6. Breastfeeding should continue as the baby demands. Healthy term newborns show signs of hunger but the interval between feeds varies considerably, particularly during the first few days. There is no evidence that long intervals between feeds adversely affect healthy newborns.

7. Newborns at risk of hypoglycaemia include those who are preterm and/ or small-for-gestational age, those who suffered asphyxia or are sick, and those born to diabetic mothers.

8 . Hypoglycaemia is most likely to occur in the first 24 hours after birth. After this period, hypoglycaemia may indicate infection rather than under-feeding.

9. For newborns at risk, breast milk is the safest and nutritional most appropriate food. However, it may need to be supplemented with specific nutrients for some very low birth weight infants.

10. At-risk newborns of gestational age 32 weeks or more (or > 1,500 g at birth) may be able to breastfeed sufficiently and should be given the opportunity to breastfeed within one hour of birth like term infants.

11. At-risk newborns able to suckle should continue to breastfeed when they show signs of hunger but should not wait more than 3 hours between feeds, and should be kept warm.

12. At-risk newborns *not* able to suckle can be fed expressed breast milk, or of necessary an appropriate breast milk substitute by cup or gavage. Feeds should start within three hours of birth and continue three hourly.

13. For at-risk newborns the blood glucose concentration should be measured at around four to six hours after birth, before a feed, if reliable laboratory measurements are available. Measurements using glucose-oxidase based reagent paper strips have poor sensitivity and specificity in newborns, and should not be relied upon as an alternative.

14. For at-risk newborns who are asymptomatic the blood glucose concentration should preferably be maintained at or above 2.6 mmol/L (47 mg/100 ml). If the blood concentration is below 2.6 mmol/L the infant should be fed; the blood glucose should be repeated within the next three hours and treatment with intravenous glucose considered if it

remains low; if iv glucose is unavailable a supplementary feed might be given by cup or gavage; and breastfeeding should continue.

15. If reliable laboratory measurements of blood glucose are not available, at-risk newborns should be kept warm and breastfed. If breastfeeding is not possible they should be given supplements of EBM or an appropriate substitute by cup or gavage every three hours. The infant should continue to breastfeed as much as he or she is able.

16. If a newborn is unwell or shows signs of hypoglycaemia: apnoea, cyanosis, jitteriness, or convulsions ("symptomatic hypoglycaemia"), the above guidelines are superseded. Blood glucose should be measured urgently, and if it is below 2.6 mmol/l, intravenous glucose should be administered as soon as possible.

17. For management of "symptomatic hypoglycaemia", when intravenous treatment is indicated and feasible, give 10% glucose intravenously. Monitor the blood glucose, and adjust the rate of infusion accordingly. Continue normal feeding as soon as possible.

18. If reliable blood glucose measurement is not possible, intravenous glucose should be reserved for the treatment of major complications associated with hypoglycaemia (e.g. convulsions) and for situations in which enteral feeds are contra-indicated. Enteral treatment is otherwise preferable.

Sequelae

If mild-to-moderate hypoglycaemia is a preventable cause of neuro-developmental impairment — previous studies have shown both acute neurological effects[3] and longer term sequelae when newborns experience varying durations of blood glucose less than 2.6 mmols/L[2] — then raising newborn blood glucose levels would be of significant long-term social and economic value for developing countries. Preventive interventions exist that are potentially simple and cost-effective, for example, health education before and after childbirth, early suckling, swaddling or skin-to-skin contact to avoid hypothermia, promotion of early breastfeeding (known to reduce hypothermia as well[25]), and cotside blood glucose monitoring could all contribute to a significant reduction in hypoglycaemia and its sequelae, but further studies are needed to evaluate the cost-effectiveness of these approaches in different settings.

References

1. Ashworth A and Waterlow JC, "Infant mortality in developing countries," *Archives of Disease in Childhood* **57** (1982): 882–884.
2. Lucas A, Morley R and Cole TJ, "Adverse neurodevelopmental outcome of moderate neonatal hypoglycaemia," *British Medical Journal* **297** (1988): 1304–1308.
3. Koh TH, Aynsley-Green A, Tarbit M and Eyre JA, "Neural dysfunction during hypoglycaemia," *Archives of Disease in Childhood* **63** (1988): 1353–1358.
4. Cornblath J and Reisner SH, "Blood glucose in the neonate and its clinical significance," *New England Journal of Medicine* **273** (1965): 378–380.
5. Fluge G, "Clinical aspects of neonatal hypoglycaemia," *Acta Pediatrica Scandivanica* **63** (1974): 826–832.
6. "Child health and development: Health of the newborn," Report of the Director General. World Health Organization (1991), EB89/26: 15–172.
7. World Development Report 1996. Published for the World Bank by Oxford University Press.
8. Ellis M, Manandhar N, Shakya U, Manandhar DS, Fawdry A and Costello AM de L, "Postnatal hypothermia and cold stress among newborn infants in Nepal monitored by continuous ambulatory recording," *Archives of Disease in Childhood* **75**(1) (1996): F42–45
9. World Health Organization, "Thermal control of the newborn: A practical guide," In: *Maternal Health and Safe Motherhood Programme*, World Health Organization, Geneva (1993).
10. Pal D, Manandhar DS, Rajbhandari S, Land J, Patel, N and Costello AM de L, "Neonatal hypoglycaemia in Nepal: Prevalence and risk factors," submitted for publication (1998).
11. Bhargava SK, Singh KK and Saxena BN, eds., "A national collaborative study of identification of high risk families mothers and outcome of their offsprings with particular reference to the problem of maternal nutrition, low birth weight, perinatal and infant morbidity and mortality in rural and urban slum communities," An ICMR Task Force Study, Indian Council of Medical Research, New Delhi (1990).

12. Silver M, Fowden AL, Knox J, Ousey JC, Franco R and Rossdale PD, "Sympathoadrenal and other responses to hypoglycaemia in the young foal," *Journal of Reproduction and Fertility Supplement* **35** (1987): 607–614.

13. Heck LJ and Erenberg A, "Serum glucose levels in term neonates during the first 48 hours of life," *Journal of Pediatrics* **110**(1) (1987): 119–122.

14. Holtrop PC, "The frequency of hypoglycaemia in full-term large and small for gestational age newborns," *American Journal of Perinatology* **10** (1993): 150–154.

15. Anderson S, Shakya KN, Shrestha LN and Costello AM de L, "Hypoglycaemia: A common problem among uncomplicated newborn infants in Nepal," *Journal of Tropical Pediatrics* **39** (1993): 273–277.

16. Hawdon JM, Platt MP and Aynsley-Green A, "Neonatal hypoglycaemia-blood glucose monitoring and baby feeding," *Midwifery* **9** (1993): 3–6.

17. Hawdon JM, "Early neonatal hypoglycaemia levels from the Newcastle study," *personal communication* (1996).

18. Hawdon JM, Ward Platt MP and Aynsley-Green A, "Patterns of metabolic adaptation for preterm and term infants in the first neonatal week," *Archives of Disease in Childhood* **67** (1992): 357–365.

19. Nehliq A and de Vasconcelos AP, "Glucose and ketone body utilisation by the brain of neonatal rats," *Progress in Neurobiology* **40** (1993): 163–221.

20. Pryds O, Christensen NJ and Fris-Hansen B, "Increased cerebral blood flow and plasma epinephrine in hypoglycemic preterm neonates," *Pediatrics* **85** (1990): 172–176.

21. Collins JE and Leonard JV, "Hyperinsulinism in asphyxiated and small-for-dates infants with hypoglycaemia," *Lancet* **2** (1984): 311–313.

22. Grant J, ed., *UNICEF. State of the World's Children*, Oxford University Press (1995).

23. Bruzzi P, Green SB, Byar DP, Brinton LA and Schairer C, "Estimating the population attributable risk for multiple risk factors using case-control data," *American Journal of Epidemiology* **122**(5) (1985): 904–914.

24. Williams A, "Hypoglycaemia of the newborn: Review of the literature," Divisions of Child Health and Development and Maternal and Newborn Health and Safe Motherhood, WHO/CHD/97.1, WHP/MSM/97.1. World Health Organization, Geneva (1997).

25. Van den Bosch CA and Bullough CHW, "The effect of suckling on term neonates' core body temperature," *Annals of Tropical Paediatrics* **10** (1990): 347–353.

Chapter 16

NEONATAL HYPERBILIRUBINAEMIA IN DEVELOPING COUNTRIES

Therese Hesketh
Research Fellow, Institute of Child Health, London

The Importance of Neonatal Hyperbilirubinaemia

Clinically detectable neonatal jaundice $> 85umol/L$ occurs in 60–70% of term newborns and in virtually all preterm ones.[1] It is more common in breastfed babies and a higher incidence has been documented in babies of Chinese origin.[2,3]

Neonatal jaundice is of clinical importance for two reasons: it may signal serious potentially treatable illness, such as sepsis or galactosaemia, and it may lead to neurological damage. The classic picture of neurological damage is kernicterus which results in early death or leads to severe neurodevelopmental damage. In animal and human studies, the propensity to develop kernicterus seems to be a function of concentration and duration of bilirubin exposure.[4]

Bilirubin is bound by albumin and distributed to other tissues and organs besides the brain. It is the unbound form which is responsible for causing the neurological damage. The liver conjugates it into a soluble form which is excreted in the urine.

Biological variability exists at each stage of the defence, such as rate of excretion, binding, integrity of the blood-brain barrier, and sensitivity to bilirubin. These factors make it difficult to define a level at which bilirubin is universally toxic. Total bilirubin, the factor which is routinely measured, correlates only poorly with neurodevelopmental outcome.[1] Thus, it is still unclear at what level of bilirubin neurodevelopmental damage occurs. The precise role of other presumed predisposing factors, such as prematurity, acidosis, and infection, which are thought to interfere with the integrity of the blood-brain barrier, is also uncertain.[4]

How Were the Guidelines for Treatment Developed?

Until the early 1990s the management of neonatal jaundice was relatively aggressive. Guidelines were based on clinical studies carried out in the 1950s and 1960s on babies with haemolytic disease and criteria were established for exchange transfusion at a threshold bilirubin of 18–20 mg/dL (308–342 mmol/L).[5,6] These findings were extrapolated to all babies, irrespective of the aetiology of the jaundice, with lower thresholds for babies with other presumed risk factors such as prematurity and infection. In these early years exchange transfusion was the only treatment available. The development of phototherapy as a standard treatment came in the late 1950s. Its use, particularly in prophylaxis was a major advance and made for a non-invasive, relatively safe treatment.

Because of strict adherence to these guidelines and with the widespread use of prophylactic phototherapy, kernicterus became very rare in Western countries. But this led to the concern that many well babies, who were really not at risk of neurological damage, were receiving unnecessary and costly work-up and treatment.[7] In practice, treatment in premature babies means prophylactic phototherapy. The hospital stay is not affected, the increase in cost is small, and the treatment relatively benign. But term babies require frequent serum bilirubin levels, prolonged hospital stay or admission (common now with earlier discharge policies and more home deliveries) and frequent interruption or cessation of breastfeeding. This management is costly[7] and exacts an emotional toll for possible questionable benefits.[8] Despite questions being raised about overtreatment there was still an important unanswered question. Is hyperbilirubinaemia in the absence of kernicterus associated with smaller deficits in cognitive, neurologic or sensory function? A number of observational studies have been carried out but with conflicting results. However, the strength of evidence tends towards the view that no such deficits are caused by neonatal jaundice in the absence of kernicterus.[9-12] But these conclusions must be regarded with caution: because these studies were carried out at a time when the guidelines for treatment were strictly followed, they are hampered by very small numbers in the higher bilirubin ranges.[13] So this question remains essentially unanswered.

The New Guidelines

The issue of when to treat became highly controversial so the American Academy of Pediatrics convened a committee of experts to examine the evidence. This resulted in new guidelines published in October 1994.[14] The major change from previously published guidelines are that the serum bilirubin in healthy term babies should be kept below 25–27 mg/dL (428–462 mmol/L) as opposed to 18–20 mg/dL (308–342 mmol/L). But a heated debate has ensued. On the one hand, it is argued that the reason kernicterus has virtually disappeared in developed countries is precisely because the babies have been appropriately treated and that this is no reason to be complacent.[15] Concerns have centred around the fact that the new approach is supported by only two experimental trials, one in full-term infants and one in low birth weight infants.[16,17] Secondly, there have been a number of cases of kernicterus reported in healthy term babies who were allowed to attain high levels of bilirubin as a result of the new approach.[18] The fact that most of the cases reported were of breast milk jaundice is of particular concern since it was widely believed that breast milk jaundice was not deleterious to a well newborn.[19] It has even been suggested that the new guidelines could lead to a new mini-epidemic of kernicterus.[20]

A parallel has been made with the case of vitamin K therapy for the newborn in England, which was discontinued because no cases of haemorrhagic disease had been seen for years. Once the new policy was adopted there was a resurgence of cases of vitamin K-related cases of haemorrhagic diseases of the newborn.[21]

There are others who feel the new guidelines do not go far enough, and that there is never a case for intervention in a well newborn.[22]

In the Developing World

The new guidelines have been greeted with caution in many developing countries. In many of these countries kernicterus is not uncommon; the incidence of choreoathetoid cerebral palsy, deafness and mental retardation are high and risk factors such as asphyxia, sepsis, prematurity, and acidosis are common. A recent Indian study found very high levels of kernicterus in the cohort of newborns they studied: at a bilirubin level of 20 m/dL 10% were affected, at bilirubin of 25–30 mg/dL 50% and over 30 mg/dL 84%.[23]

There is an additional issue also since the two most accepted forms of therapy in richer countries — exchange transfusion and phototherapy — are rarely available. Phototherapy units are expensive and dependent on reliable sources of electricity. Exchange transfusion requires large quantities of donor blood and an intensive care type setting. Phenobarbitone and the new metalloprophyrins are possible alternatives, but they have not been sufficiently evaluated in randomised controlled trials. Phenobarbitone has been widely used in many developing countries and may have an important role in certain clinical situations. The metalloporphyrins decrease the production of bilirubin: much more research is needed to establish their efficacy and safety.[24] Maisels said of the metalloporphyrins that they "could be useful in developing countries where access to phototherapy and exchange transfusion is difficult or absent".[1]

Much also has been made of the importance of early feeding. Although important in the prophylaxis of physiological jaundice the precise role of early feeding in pathological jaundice remains uncertain.

Bilirubin Markers/Predictive Models

A further difficulty is the crudeness of the currently available measure, serum bilirubin, as a marker of risk of potential neurological damage. The important question is whether there is any clinically useful marker, for example, bilirubin-albumin binding, which would enable prediction of those at risk of kernicterus? Ahlfors has suggested the use of the bilirubin/albumin ratio to determine the level of unbound bilirubin concentration in the serum.[25] Taking this a step further, could a predictive model of bilirubin toxicity be developed that would take all potential causative factors of neurological damage into account and give them appropriate weight?[26] This would include factors such as gestational age, underlying illness, hypoxia, acidosis, and sepsis. What is needed is some kind of gold standard for bilirubin toxicity so that the treatment of neonatal jaundice can be more evidence-based and less pure guess-work.[27]

Policy Implications

There are important policy implications behind the whole debate. If we are overtreating, as has been suggested, there are important resource implications (physician, nurse time, costs of hospital stay) and emotional implications to parents, needless disruption of breastfeeding and large risks to babies who undergo exchange transfusion. But if we are undertreating, that is, if hyperbilirubinaemia has effects on neurodevelopmental outcome at levels below the threshold suggested by the American Academy of Pediatrics, then perhaps the new approaches are putting babies at risk.

The key commentators agree on one thing: that more information is necessary to settle the argument about what level of bilirubin must be treated.[28] In the meantime, it is agreed that caution should be exercised when treating high bilirubin levels.[26] The hypothesis that the new approach is safe and effective should be tested before it is accepted as a new standard of therapy.[20] Cashore has specifically stated that more can be learnt 'from our Asian colleagues, who defer phototherapy and exchange transfusion to higher levels then are generally seen in North America'.[29] We must not repeat the error of adopting a new standard of care without concurrent verification of its wisdom.[15]

Summary

Key questions about neonatal hyperbilirubinaemia in developing countries which remain essentially unanswered are:

- At what bilirubin level is treatment necessary?
- Is neonatal hyperbilirubinaemia associated with smaller deficits in cognitive function?
- Are there different thresholds of bilirubin toxicity in different populations according to gestational age, underlying illness and ethnicity, for example?
- What are the most effective and cost-effective interventions for neonatal hyperbilirubinaemia in developing countries? E.g. phenobarbitone, metalloporphyrins, early feeding.
- Is there any clinically useful marker (e.g. bilirubin-albumin binding) which would enable prediction of those at risk of kernicterus?
- Could a predictive model of bilirubin toxicity be developed that would take all potential causative factors into account and give them appropriate weight?

References

1. Maisels MJ, "Neonatal Jaundice," In: *Pathophysiology and Management of the Newborn*, 3rd ed., GB Avery Ed Philadelphia, JB Lippincott (1987).
2. Brown WR and Wong HK, "Ethnic group differences in plasma bilirubin levels of fullterm healthy Singapore newborns," *Pediatrics* **36** (1965): 745–751.
3. Linn S, Schoenbaum SC, Monson RR *et al.*, "Epidemiology of neonatal hyperbilirubinaemia," *Pediatrics* **75** (1985): 770–774.
4. Broderson R and Stern L, "Deposition of bilirubin acid in the central nervous system — A hypothesis for the development of kernicterus," *Acta Pediatrica Scandinavia* **79** (1990): 12–19.
5. Hsia DY and Gellis SS, "Studies on erythroblastosis due to ABO incompatibility," *Pediatrics* **13** (1954): p. 503.
6. Mollison PL and Cutbush M, "A method of measuring the severity of a series of cases of haemolytic disease of the newborn," *Pediatrics* **6** (1951): p. 777.
7. Newman TB, Easterling MJ and Goldman ES, "Laboratory evaluation of jaundiced newborns: Frequency, cost and yield," *American Journal of Diseases in Childhood* **144** (1990): 364–368.

8. Kemper K, Forsyth B and McCarthy P, "Jaundice, terminating breastfeeding and the vulnerable child," *Pediatrics* **84** (1989): 773–778.

9. Bjure J, Liden G, Reinand T *et al.*, "A follow-up study of hyperbilirubinaemia in full-term infants without isoimmunisation," *Acta Pediatrica Scandinavia* **50** (1961): p. 437.

10. Boggs T, Hardy J and Frazier T, "Correlation of neonatal serum total bilirubin and developmental status at age eight months," *Journal of Pediatrics* **71** (1967): p. 553.

11. Rubin R, Balow B and Fisch R, "Neonatal serum bilirubin levels related to cognitive development at ages 4 through 7 years," *Journal of Pediatrics* **94** (1979): p. 601.

12. Seidman DS, Paz I and Stevenson DK, "Neonatal hyperbilirubinaemia and physical and cognitive performance at 17 years of age," *Pediatrics* **88** (1991): 828–833.

13. Newman TB and Maisels MJ, "Does hyperbilirubinaemia damage the brain of healthy full-term babies?" *Clinical Perinatology* **17** (1990): 331–358.

14. American Academy of Pediatrics Practice Parameter, "Management of hyperbilirubinaemia in the healthy term newborn," *Pediatrics* **4** (1994): 558–565.

15. Wennberg RP, "Bilirubin recommendations present problems: New guidelines simplistic and untested," *Pediatrics* **89** (1992): 823–824.

16. Wishingrad P, "Prospective studies of non-haemolytic hyperbilirubinemia in premature infants," *Pediatrics* **36** (1965): p. 122.

17. Killander A, Michaelson M and Muller-Eberhard U, "Hyperbilirubinaemia in full-term infants without isoimmunisation," *Acta Pediatrica Scandinavia* **50** (1961): p. 437.

18. Maisels MJ and Newman TB, "Kernicterus occurs in fullterm healthy newborns without apparent haemolysis," *Pediatric Research* **35** (1994): p. 239A.

19. Grunebaum E, Amir J and Merlob P, "Breast milk jaundice: Natural history, familial incidence and late neurodevelopmental outcome of the infant," *European Journal of Pediatrics* **150** (1991): 267–270.

20. Merenstein GB, "New bilirubin recommendations questioned," *Pediatrics* **89** (1992): 822–823.

21. Loughnan PM and McDougall PN, "The efficacy of oral Vitamin K1: Implications for future prophylaxis to prevent haemorrhagic disease of the newborn," *Journal of Paediatrics and Child Health* **29** (1993): 171–176.

22. Watchko JF and Oski FA, "Bilirubin 20 mg/dl = vingtophobia," *Pediatrics* **71** (1983): 660–663.

23. Narang A, Conference presentation, National Neonatology Forum, Patna, India (1996).

24. Valaes T, Petmazki S and Henschke C, "Control of jaundice in preterm newborns by an inhibitor of bilirubin production: Studies with tin-mesoporphyrin," *Pediatrics* **93** (1994): 1–11.

25. Alhfors CE, "Criteria for exchange transfusion in jaundiced newborns," *Pediatrics* **93** (1994): 488–494.

26. Dennery PA, Rhine WD and Stevenson DK, "Neonatal Jaundice: What now?" *Clinical Pediatrics* **34** (1995): 103–107.

27. Poland RL, "In search of a gold standard for bilirubin toxicity," *Pediatrics* **89** (1992): 821–822

28. Newman TB and Klabanoff MA, "Neonatal hyperbilirubinaemia and longterm outcome: Another look at the collaborative perinatal project," *Pediatrics* **92** (1993): 651–657.

29. Cashore WJ, "Hyperbilirubinaemia: Should we adopt a new standard of care?" *Pediatrics* **89** (1992): 824–826.

Chapter 17

LOW BIRTH WEIGHT NEWBORNS — THE RISKS IN INFANCY AND BEYOND

Dipak K. Guha

Senior Consultant Neonatologist,
Sunderlal Jain Hospital, Delhi, India

Introduction

Universally, and in all population groups, the birth weight is the single most important determinant of the chances of the newborn to survive and experience healthy growth and development.[1] There is no indicator in human biology which will tells us as much about past events and the future trajectory of life as the weight of an infant at birth.[2] Birth weight is significantly affected by the health and nutritional status of the mother and therefore the proportion of infants born with low birth weight is a reliable index of the health status of the community.

What is LBW?

Infants with a birth weight of less than 2,500 g are designated as low birth weight (LBW) newborn infants.[3] They comprise infants born before 37 weeks of gestation, preterm LBW, and gestationally mature infants who have suffered intrauterine growth retardation or foetal malnutrition, called

IUGR-LBW. IUGR newborn infants are also termed small-for-gestational age (SGA) or small-for-dates (SFD) because of their subnormal position (below −2 SD of mean, or below 10th percentile) on an intrauterine growth chart.[4]

The size of the problem

Twenty-one million LBW newborn infants are born every year in developing countries and, of these, seven million are born in India. In a multicentric community based Indian Council of Medical Research study the prevalence of LBW ranged between 25.9–56.9% in urban slums and 35.2–40.8% in rural communities with an average of 41.4% and 38.1% respectively.[5] The prematurity rates were 12.7% and 14.4% in the rural and urban areas respectively. It can be deduced that the incidence of term LBW (IUGR) neonates were 27% in the rural population and 25.4% in the urban cohort. Thus, roughly two-thirds of LBW neonates in our country are small-for-dates and nearly one-third of Indian neonates have low birth weight, weighing less than 2,500 g at birth.[6,7]

The LBW rate in India is one of the highest in the world and contrasts with that of just 6% in China and Canada, 7% in USA, the UK and Egypt and 12–14% in Mexico, Indonesia and Iran.[3] Nearly 70% of all neonatal deaths and 80% of infant deaths in both the developed and developing countries occur among the LBW neonates.[8,9] Similarly, it is also estimated that over 70% of all perinatal deaths occur among LBW infants.[10,11] These outcomes are not unexpected as birth asphyxia, birth trauma, infections, hypothermia, and malformations are remarkably more common among LBW infants.[4]

48% of surviving LBW infants are malnourished at the age of one year compared to only 16% of those with birth weight of 2,500 g or more.[9] LBW infants are five times more likely to die in the perinatal period and three times more likely to die during infancy.[12] Birth weight is also a determinant of duration of breastfeeding,[13] a well known protective factor against infant death. LBW is also a risk factor for lower respiratory tract infections:[14] LBW infants have a two to three times higher risk of mortality due to infection than infants with normal birth weight.[15] LBW infants with birth asphyxia who survive the neonatal period develop neurodevelopmental sequelae three times more as compared to counterparts of normal weight.[16,17] Small-for-date infants may remain short and have impaired physical work capacity.[18]

A historical perspective on outcomes of LBW

Taking a historical perspective on current outcomes prior to and after the introduction of neonatal intensive care, it becomes apparent that developmental outcomes were the subject of concern and review as early as 1940 in the industrialised world.[19] Before 1960, the focus of attention was on infants with birth weight greater than 1.5 kg. With an increasing survival rate for LBW infants as a result of advances in neonatal intensive care attention shifted to infants less than 1,500 g in the 1960s and early 1970s,[20] less than 1,000 g in the late 1970s, and less than 750 g in the 1980s.[21] Even though gestational maturity is the predictor of outcomes,[22] studies have rarely been done on gestational age primarily due to the lack of accuracy of gestational age in mothers who have not received perinatal care.[23] Prior to the 1940s, care of LBW infants was conservative with very little intervention and the rate of neonatal mortality was high. Yet a review by Benton in 1940 demonstrated developmental retardation in these infants, and that the lower the birth weight, the greater the retardation.[19]

Between 1940 and 1960, various therapies were instituted, some of which like starving, use of oxygen, streptomycin and sulpha antibiotics had a devastating effect on later developmental outcome.[24,25] Lower IQ ratio and minimal brain dysfunction in children of normal intelligence including learning difficulties, hyperactive behaviour and neurological soft signs were also significantly higher in the LBW population.[26,27]

With the introduction of neonatal intensive care during the 1960s there has been significant improvement in the survival of LBW infants, accompanied by a marked decrease in the rates of cerebral palsy and neurodevelopmental handicaps.[20,28] Further technological and pharmacological improvement including surfactant therapy[29] introduced during 1970s, 1980s and 1990s survived and continued to improve, however, with few exception, rates of cerebral palsy and neurodevelopmental handicaps in early childhood among very LBW infants remained essentially unchanged.[20,30–34] As a result of these trends, there has been an increase not only in the absolute number of surviving children with normal development, but also in the number of children with handicapping conditions in a proportion of about 9:1.[35]

Outcomes of LBW Children

Advances in neonatal medicine have resulted in increased survival of infants at lower and lower birth weights though not necessarily so much in the developing countries as compared to developed countries. While these medical success stories highlight the power of medical technology to save many of the tiniest infants at birth, serious questions remain about how these infants will develop and whether they will have normal productive lives.

LBW newborn infants represent a heterogenous group of term and preterm infants with varying degrees of social and medical risks. Adverse outcomes include a broad spectrum of conditions ranging from normal growth and development to severe developmental abnormalities. The rate of abnormal outcomes increases as birth weight decreases. Recent reports on outcomes of low birth weight pertains to children who have reached 8–14 years of age. Adverse consequences of low birth weight continue to be apparent even in adolescence.[32,36–43]

Adverse outcomes of LBW vary in accordance with how it has been assessed, how the handicaps are classified and the method of exclusions from sample. The measurement of functional abilities includes ratings by the physician[30] or caretakers[43,44] of the child's ability to perform age-appropriate activities of daily living. Disabilities may be classified as mild, moderate and severe[14,38] or as suggested by the WHO.[39,116] Uniform definition of problems in school functioning or specific learning problems are lacking.[32,36,45–48] It is thus apparent that the outcomes[32,36,45–48] of children with low birth weight should be critically analysed.

Morbidity outcomes

Adverse health outcomes increase with decreasing birth weight. These include medical and surgical conditions, rehospitalisation and health related activities of daily living.[44,49–51] Common medical problems are respiratory infection, ear infection, asthma, and deranged pulmonary function tests. In India, diarrhoea and respiratory infections are common causes of morbidity and mortality in LBW newborn infants during the early months of life.[52] Common surgical problems are strabismus, ear tubes, adenoids, tonsils, tracheal complications, and orthopedic problems of cerebral palsy.[51] Although respiratory infections decrease after two years of age, health problems persist and contribute to excessive bed days, restricted activity, school absence, and poor school performances.[43,44,53] LBW children from poorer background do worse than socially advantaged children.[44]

Growth

The physical growth of LBW newborn infants is less than that of normal birth weight newborn infants. The mean weight, height, and head circumference is lower than the normal birth weight newborn infants.[50,54–57] This is noticeable both in term and preterm IUGR newborn infants as well as in preterm AGA newborn infants. The causes of growth failure in preterm are severe neonatal complications of prematurity such as chronic lung disease.[58] Although very little catching-up of head size occurs after one year of age, catching-up of weight and height can occur later.[56] One of the recent long-term studies from India,[59] showed that LBW boys significantly lagged behind their controls for all physical growth parameters untill 14 years, while the LBW girls had physical growth comparable to controls after 11 years. Preterms had comparable weight, height, and head circumference with their controls after 11 years. The SFDs, however, remained significantly handicapped in their overall physical growth even at 14 years. In comparison to controls, menarche occurred six months earlier in preterm and 12 months earlier in SFD girls. However, there was no change in sequence of pubertal changes in either preterm or SFDs children.

Neurosensory outcomes

The most common untoward outcomes of LBW are cerebral palsy, blindness, deafness, hydrocephalus, microcephaly, and convulsive disorders. The incidence is 20% in children with a birth weight less than 1,000 g,[49,60] 14–17% in the 1,000–1,500 g group, and 6–8% in the 1,500–2,499 g group as compared to 5% in the normal birth weight group.[43,50] The median incidence of cerebral palsy among all the cohort studies is 7.7% and the median incidence of disability is 25%.[32] Blindness is more common in children with birth weight less than 1,000 g to the extent of 5–6%. Deafness, which is found in 2–3% of LBW children, does not seem to specifically affect the smallest newborn infants.[36,43] In one recent three-year follow-up study from India on neurological sequelae in newborn infants weighing less than 2,000 g, the prevalence of cerebral palsy was 4.8%, mental retardation 5%, seizure disorder 3.9%, hearing impairment 1.5%, and cortical blindness 0.3%.[61] In yet another study from India in newborn infants below 1,500 g, 15% had mental retardation, 14% subnormal motor development, 1% microcephaly, 2% hearing loss, and 4% visual loss.[62]

The vast majority of LBW children are normal on neurological examinations, but the rates of neuromotor dysfunction are higher than in neurologically normal control groups. There is thus a spectrum of neurological disorders ranging from cerebral palsy to lesser and more subtle degrees of neuromotor abnormalities.

Cognitive and neuropsychological outcomes

Cognitive and neuropsychological functions of LBW children are compromised even when sociodemographic risk factors are taken into account. This compromise is again directly related to the degree of LBW at birth.[36,37,43,49,60,63,64] The incidence of deficient intelligent score (IQ < 70) and subnormal score (IQ 70–80) are significantly higher than among control group of children with normal birth weight even though the mean IQ score falls within the average range. This difference persists even when neurologically abnormal newborn infants are excluded.[37,63] Some cognitive skills are more compromised than others like mental arithmetic, visual motor and fine motor skills, spatial abilities, expressive language, and memory.[37,39,41,49,60,65] The verbal abilities are less compromised as compared to perceptical performance skills like motor functions and co-ordination.[42,49,66] In a prospective study from India psychomotor development was assessed for 18–24 months in preterm newborn infants (gestation less than 37 weeks) using corrected or post-conceptual age.[67] Preterm newborn infants, as a group, caught up with normal newborn infants between 18–24 months both on the motor and mental scale. The higher the birth weight, the better its mean motor development quotient at 18 months. Uncomplicated preterm newborn infants showed higher mean developmental quotients at 18 months than preterm newborn infants with additional complications. They also caught up earlier (12–18 months) than the latter group who caught up between 18–24 months. Similarly, preterm appropriate-for-gestational age (AGA) newborn infants showed earlier catching-up than preterm small-for-gestational age (SGA) newborn infants.

Academic achievement, social competence and behaviour problems

There is an increased risk of behaviour problem in LBW children especially among boys.[68–70] Brain injury is the cause of behavioural problems. They include conduct disorder,[71] hyperactivity,[45,72] and lack of concentration or attention-deficit hyperactivity disorder (ADHD).[73,74] The incidence of ADHD is 16% in newborn infants with birth weight less than 1,000 g as compared to 6.9% in the matched control group. These children are more shy, introverted, and unassertive.[74]

Children with low birth weight have poor school performances and more learning problems mainly in the field of reading, spelling and mathematics.[60,70] Even neurologically intact VLBW children of low IQ score less on tests of achievement.[39,46] They need special education assistance (34–50% vs 14% in normal birth weight children) and this rate increases as they progress to higher grades in school.[36,45–48]

Audiovisual outcomes

Hearing

The clinical significal sensorineural hearing loss can occur in 8–9% of VLBW survivors.[75] The incidence seems to be related to increased survival of hypoxic VLBW infants rather than to ototoxic medication or ambient noise levels.[76,77] The hearing loss is usually most marked in the high frequency range. Deafness should be suspected in all cases of delayed speech development. Unilateral hearing loss may not interfere with speech development but has been associated with significant impairment of school performance.[78] Hearing loss in Indian study varied from 1.5–2%.[61,62]

Vision

Visual disturbances constitute a major concern in the follow-up of a VLBW child. Refractive errors and ocular muscle imbalance account for the majority of the abnormalities that may be present in as many as 44% of the smallest of premature survivors.[79] Retinopathy of prematurity (ROP) accounts for a major proportion of visual defects in VLBW children. The incidence of ROP in the West has been reported to be 53–88.5% in < 1,000 g newborn infants.[80,81] In an Indian study of ROP was 73.3% among < 1,000 g newborn infants and 47.3% among < 1,500 g newborn infants.[82] This study also found that major risk factors for ROP were gestations < 32 weeks, oxygen administration, anaemia, apnea, and blood transfusions. Refractive errors are the other major causes of visual handicap in LBW children, the incidence of myopia and hyper metropia of 16% and 20% respectively has been reported. Birth weight had a significant positive correlation with astigmatism.[83] Strabismus is also contributed to visual handicap.[84]

Problems of term LBW children with IUGR

Prior to the 1960s, term LBW children were considered to have higher rates of major neurodevelopmental handicaps than normal birth weight children.

However, more recently, with the exception of children who have major congenital malformations or intrauterine infections, developmental outcomes for these children have been reported to be similar to those of their peers of normal birth weight.[85,86] This is considered to be due to improvement in perinatal care which minimises brain insult including optimal timing of delivery, cesarean section when indicated, prevention of birth asphyxia, optimal resuscitations and treatment of complications such as hypoglycaemia and polycythemia. Extended follow-up up to 9–11 years of age has, however, recently revealed learning deficits that were not identified prior to this age.[87]

Risk of cardiovascular disease in adulthood

Recent literature also suggests a relationship between an abnormal intrauterine environment associated with LBW and adult blood pressure, cardiovascular disease, poor pulmonary functions, and diabetes.[88–98] Thirty two studies worldwide have shown that low birth weight is associated with a raised blood pressure in childhood and adult life.[99] A recent study in South India has shown that as in other countries, low birth weight and coronary heart disease are linked.[100] Similarly, a study from western India showed that children with low birth weight had a higher plasma glucose and insulin concentration after oral glucose load independently of their current size.[92] The possibility that these new explanations for the origins of adult disease may have important implications for the epidemics of coronary heart disease and non-insulin dependent diabetes in India has not gone unremarked.[101,102] Clearly, these early findings in India need to be replicated and extended. A strategy to develop the initial epidemiological observations is now in places, and studies have begun in a number of centres in India.[103]

The concept of programming

Some of these newborn infants have low birth weights, some are small in relation to the size of placentas, some are thin at birth, and some are short at birth and fail to gain weight in infancy. The association of LBW at birth or during infancy and hypertension, cardiovascular disease, non-insulin dependent diabetes and poor pulmonary function in adult life has lead to the suggestion that these diseases are "programmed" by an inadequate supply of nutrients or oxygen *in utero* or immediately after birth. The phenomenon of "programming", whereby undernutrition in early life permanently changes body structure and function, is well documented in animals.[89,90] As yet we know very little about cellular and molecular changes which underlie it, but persisting changes in the secretion of hormones or in the sensitivity of tissues to them may be important in determining adult diseases.[89,90] However, there are also reports which do not substantiate or corroborate this hypothesis.[104-106]

Factors affecting long-term developmental outcome

Certain social and environmental factors are clearly known to affect the long-term developmental outcome of LBW newborn infants in terms of maternal education[26,43,107] race[26,108] or social class.[37-39,60,109,110] The social and environmental risk factors have a far greater risk on cognitive outcomes in LBW newborn infants and it becomes more pronounced over time.[49,110-112]

Despite speculation that VLBW infants are more susceptible to adverse environmental influences than are normal birth weight infants[26,109,113] evidence in support of an exaggerated effect of social factors among VLBW is scarce.[46] The combined effect of severe neonatal illness and a deprived environment can be devastating.[39,76,114]

Biological factors are more important influences on outcomes for children with severe neurological insult or extreme LBWB.[108,115] Medical and/or biological factors that contribute to the risk associated with LBW include birth defect,[116,117] male sex,[110] birth asphyxia, and neonatal complications of prematurity. IUGR in preterm VLBW does not seem to contribute to poor developmental outcomes over and above that resulting from prematurity and its complications. However, those with severe brain growth failure may have poorer outcomes. Specific neuropathologic brain lesions associated with adverse LBW outcome include periventricular leucomalacia and cerebral atrophy, which can result in cerebral palsy, non-specific hypotonia and cognitive and neuropsychological subnormality. Lesser degrees of brain damage are thought to be responsible for finer motor impairments, visuoperceptual and maths difficulties, and hyperactivity.[108,115]

The influence of biological genetic factors on outcomes such as intelligence and other cognitive abilities have rarely been examined in LBW.[63,118]

Recommendations and Strategies for Reducing LBW Births

Despite an increase in the survival of LBW infants during the last decade both in developed and developing countries, there have been no significant change in the neonatal and early childhood outcomes of the survivors.[32,119] Physicians and parents anticipating the delivery of LBW infants, in general in developing countries and extreme LBW in developed countries, must be aware of these outcomes in order to make an informed decision as to the advisability of aggressive care at birth and thereafter.[119] With the increasing number of LBW infants surviving and the high health care and educational costs involved in caring them, it is important that we understand fully the adverse outcomes, identify the families in need of monitoring and treatment, and recognise protective factors that may assist us in designing effective intervention.

Prediction of LWB

A large number of preconceptual maternal high risk factors can predict the birth of a LBW infant.[120] Table 1 outlines the preconceptional predictors of LBW newborn infants and appropriate corrective strategies. During the course of pregnancy, the adequacy of foetal growth can be assessed by monitoring maternal weight gain, uterine growth, and ultrasonographic dimension of foetus (Table 2). There is a need to develop optimal uterine growth, abdominal girth, and maternal weight gain chart during pregnancy by satisfactory community survey.[121,122]

Table 1 Preconceptional high risk factors associated with birth of LBW newborn infants and corrective strategies.

High risk factors	Corrective strategy
1. Low socio-economic and education status	Social welfare, female literacy, status of women.
2. Bad obstetrical history	Identify cause of previous obstetrical mishaps and LBW newborn infant.
3. Chronic systemic disease	Medical check-up and adequate treatment.
4. Unwed mother	Sex education.
5. Young mother (< 20 years)	Legal and social enforcement of child marriage act.
6. Short mother (< 145 cm)	Adequate female nutrition during childhood. Adolescene and pregnancy.
7. Light mother (< 40 kg)	Avoiding discrimination against female child.
8. Severe anemia (Hb < 8 g/dL)	Iron and folic acid during third trimester.
9. Primigravida	–
10. Gradmultigravida	Family planning and spacing.
11. Addictions	Public awareness.

Table 2 Predictors of foetal growth retardation during pregnancy.

1. Pregnancy induced hypertension.
2. Acute and chronic maternal infections.
3. Poor maternal weight gain (< 5 kg).
4. Poor uterine growth.
5. Slow increase in abdominal girth.
6. Slow foetal growth as assessed by ultrasonography.
7. Antepartum haemorrhage.
8. Placental dysfunction (urinary estriol).
9. Multiple pregnancy.

Prevention of LBW

The need for better data

The high LBW rate in developing countries is a multifactorial problem. On the one hand is a web of socio-economic problems which cannot be tackled simply, and on the other hand is a lack of good epidemiological data, which makes planning and decision making difficult.[12,123] Health care coverage continues to be poor especially in rural areas and urban slums. There is little information about long-term outcomes of LBW because of difficulties of tracking of families over many years and the lack of national commitment, a problem found even in developed countries like the USA.[32] Difficult to trace or untraced survivors may be equally as likely to be handicapped as those evaluated.[124,125] In contrast, in those countries that have practical and active health care systems where nationwide registration of health care users is mandatory, the implementation of long-term follow-up is easier. It is hoped that the development of a health care system based on epidemiological data, keeping in mind the local needs and problems, will facilitate long-term follow-up studies of LBW infants.[12,123]

Paediatric and obstetric co-operation

For too long paediatricians have been primarily concerned with newborn infants only and obstetricians with mothers alone. Instead of viewing each newborn infant separately as a foetus and then a neonate, they must be considered as one entity — the perinate. Working on this concept and providing minimal perinatal care with emphasis on risk approach, a reduction in the incidence of LBW and complication associated with LBW can be achieved and this in turn will improve the long-term health and developmental outcomes of LBW.[126–129]

The risk approach for frontline birth attendants

As short-term measures in developing countries traditional birth attendants (TBAs) and auxiliary nurse midwives should be properly trained and provided with simple guidelines to identify high risk pregnancy before 20 weeks of gestation.[121] Measures which might help improve birth weight are providing an additional 200 K cal and 20 g protein per day, supplementation of iron and folic acid, identification, and treatment of maternal infection and pregnancy-induced hypertension.[130-132] Complete physical rest[133] during last four to six weeks of pregnancy and motivation during pregnancy for breastfeeding will help salvage some of the problems of LBW. It should be mandatory to refer high risk mothers rather than the newborns to a centre with adequate infrastructure to take care of such mothers and their infants. It is important that health education should be imparted through available media for basic needs during pregnancy, the art of mother craft, and promotion of family welfare.[121]

Improving the social status of women

However, one must clearly understand that the adverse biological effect of malnutrition which has operated for generations cannot be reversed by crash programmes of supplementation of food during the third trimester of pregnancy. There is a need for long-term policy for improvement of socio-economic and environmental conditions, basic family welfare services, and recognition of the need for improvement of the status of women and functional literacy.[121] Educated and informed mothers can safeguard their own health needs and can optimally discharge her role and responsibilities towards her child. It is suggested that human nutrition, the art of child care, environmental safety, population control, family welfare, and sex education should be made compulsory subjects in school curricula. Similarly, available media resources should be utilised for spreading the messages of maternal nutrition and child care. The enhancement of female literacy will certainly yield more dividends as compared to *ad hoc* nutritional supplementation programs during pregnancy.[121]

Identification of LBW

In a health centre or hospital, LBW infants can be identified by recording birth weight on a reliable lever-type weighing scale. Where a reliable weighing scale is not available, mid-arm circumference measurement using simple tricolor tape has been found to be a reliable surrogate for low birth weight.[134,135] A mid-arm circumference of less than 9 cm is associated with birth weight of less than 2,500 g. Simple physical criteria incorporating scalp hair, ear cartilage, breast nodule, genitals and sole creases can be used to identify whether a newborn infant is term or preterm.

Management of LBW

95% of LBW newborn infants are above 1,500 g and, therefore, the effort should be concentrated to salvaging infants weighing more than 1,500 g. The principles of management[136] consist of adequate foetal monitoring during labour, effective management of infant at birth, prevention of hypothermia and infection, and provision of human milk for feeding. Newborn infants weighing more than 2,000 g may be managed at home under supervision, newborn infants between 1,500 g–2,000 g in district hospitals, and newborn infants below 1,500 g in apex institution with adequate infrastructure. It is of great importance to use equipment, therapy and drugs which are known to cause adverse effect with the utmost care. Newer modes of therapy like the use of antenatal steroid and surfactant have shown promising results in the survival rate of LBW infants.[137-140] Traditional birth attendants and auxiliary nurse midwives should be adequately trained to manage LBW asphyxiated newborn infants and identify the high risk mother and newborn infants. A well-coordinated referral system with suitable transport facilities should be mandatory to provide life support and prevent hypothermia during transport.

Early intervention and enrichment programmes

There is evidence to show that early intervention/enrichment programmes improve the developmental outcomes for LBW infants.[64,141,142] The gains in function were most pronounced in the domains of receptive language, visual-motor function, and special skills. The infants who benefit most from such programmes are those whose mothers have better educational background, greater understanding of the problem, heavier LBW, and have less medical problems.[64,141,142] Enrichment programmes should include in-hospital infant and parent support during infancy and early childhood.[141,142] At present, there are only few programmes designed specifically to meet the special health and developmental needs of these children and only in few selected institutions. Expanding the availability and accessibility of the enrichment programme has the potential to mediate some of the adverse developmental effect that confront LBW newborn infants.[141,142]

Future Research

We need to elucidate and better understand which pregnancy and perinatal factors affect brain development, how to prevent and/or treat identified neonatal complications of prematurity, and which component of enrichment programmes may best prevent and/or treat the developmental sequelae associated with both biological and social risk. This basic information will provide us with the tools needed to better serve LBW infants.[64]

References

1. "The incidence of low birth weight, a critical review of available information," *World Health Quarterly Statistics* **33** (1980): p. 197.
2. Ramalingaswami V, "The state of life," Report of the National Seminar on reducing incidence of low birth weight newborn infants in India. National Insurance of Public Cooperation and Child Development (1985).
3. World Health Organization, "The incidence of low birth weight: An Update," *Weekly Epidemiological Review* **59** (1984): 205–211.
4. Lubchenco O, *"The High Risk Infant. Major Problems in Clinical Pediatrics* (Vol. XIV), Philadelphia; WB Saunders (1976).
5. Indian Council of Medical Research, "A national collaborative study of identification of high risk families, mothers and outcome of their offsprings with particular reference to the problem of maternal nutrition, low birth weight, perinatal and infant morbidity and mortality in rural and urban slum communities," New Delhi (1990).
6. Ministry of Health and Family Welfare, "National Health Policy," *Indian Journal of Pediatrics* **53** (1986): 303–316.

7. Singh M, "Hospital based data on perinatal mortality in India," *Indian Pediatrics* **23** (1986): 579–584.

8. Villar J and Launer LJ, "The effect of maternal nutrition on infant health in developing countries," In: *Perinatal Determinants of Child Survival*, Mitra K, Berendes HW and Saxena BN, eds., ICMR (1988): 65–85.

9. Lal S, "Birth weight and survival during infancy," Paper presented at the National Seminar on Reducing LBW in India, NIPCCD, New Delhi (1985).

10. AIIMS perinatal data (1988–1991).

11. Shah M and Udani PM, "Analysis of vital statistics from the rural community. Palaghar II: Perinatal, neonatal and infant mortalities," *Indian Pediatrics* **6** (1969): 651–668.

12. Singh M and Paul VK, "Strategies to reduce perinatal and neonatal mortality," *Indian Pediatrics* **25** (1988): 499–507.

13. Barros F, Victoria C, Vaughan JP and Smith PG, "Birth weight and duration of breast feeding: Are the beneficial effects of breast feeding being overestimated," *Pediatrics* **78** (1986): 656–661.

14. McCall MG and Acheson ED, "Respiratory disease in infancy," *J Chr Dis* **21** (1968): 249–359.

15. Victoria CG, Smith PG, Vaughan JP and Nobre LC, "Influence of birth weight on mortality from infectious diseases. A case control study," *Pediatrics* **81** (1988): 807–811.

16. Hardy JMB, Draga JS and Jackson EC, "The first year of life: The collaborative perinatal study of the National Institute of Neurological and Communicative Disorders and Stroke," Baltimore, the Johns Hopkins University Press (1979).

17. Papile L-A, Munsick-Bruno G and Shaefer A, "Relationship of cerebral intraventricular hemorrhage and early childhood neurologic handicap," *Journal of Pediatrics* **103** (1983): 273–277.

18. Westwood M, "Growth and development of full term nonasphyxiated small for gestational age newborns: Follow up through adolescence," *Pediatrics* **71** (1983): 376–382.

19. Benton AL, "Mental development of prematurely born children," *American Journal of Orthopsychiatry* **10** (1940): 719–746.

20. US Congress, Office of Technology Assessment, "Neonatal intensive care for low birth weight infants: Costs and effectiveness," Health Technology Case Study 38, OTA-HCS-38. Washington, DC:OTA (1987).

21. Hack M and Fanaroff AA, "How small is too small? Considerations in evaluating the outcome of the tiny infant," *Clinics in Perinatology* **15** (1988): 773–788.

22. Johnson A, Townshend P, Yudkin P *et al.*, "Functional abilities at age 4 years of children born before 29 weeks of gestation," *British Medical Journal* **306** (1993): 1715–1718.

23. Hack M, Horbar JD, Malloy MH *et al.*, "Very low birth weight outcomes of the N.I.C.H.D. Neonatal Network," *Pediatrics* **87** (1991): 587–597.

24. Abramowicz M and Kass EH, "Pathogenesis and prognosis of prematurity," *New England Journal of Medicine* **275** (1966): 878–885.

25. Lubchenco LO, Horner FA, Reed LH *et al.*, "Sequelae of premature birth: Evaluation of premature infants of low birth weight at ten years of age," *American Journal of Diseases of Children* **106** (1963): 101–115.

26. Broman SH, Nichols SH and Kennedy WA, "Preschool IQ: Prenatal and early developmental correlates," Hillsdale NJ, Lawrence Erlbaum Associates (1975).

27. NIchols PL and Chen T, "Minimal brain dysfunction: A prospective study," Hillsdale NJ, Lawrence Erlbaum Associates (1981).

28. Rawlings G, Reynolds EOR, Stewart A and Strang LB, "Changing prognosis for infants of very low birth weight," *Lancet* **1** (1971): 516–519.

29. Bregman J and Kimberlin LVS, "Developmental outcome in extremely premature infants: Impact of surfactant," *Pediatric Clinics in North America* **40**(5) (1993): 937–953.

30. Saigal S, Rosenbaum P, Hattersley B and Milner R, "Decreased disability rate among 3-year-old survivors weighing 501–1,000 g at birth and born to residents of a geographically defined region from 1981 to 1984 compared with 1977 to 1980," *Journal of Pediatrics* **114** (1989): 839–846.

31. Shapiro S, McCormick MS, Starfield BH and Crawley B, "Changes in infant morbidity associated with decreases in neonatal mortality," *Pediatrics* **72** (1983): 408–415.

32. Escobar GH, Littenberg B and Etitti DB, "Outcome among surviving very low birth weight infants: A meta-analysis," *Archives of Disease in Childhood* **66** (1991): 204–211.

33. McCormick MC, "Has the prevalence of handicapped infants increased with improved survival of the very low birth weight infant?" *Clinics in Peritoniology* **28**(1) (1995): 255–277.

34. Wojtulewicz J, Alam A, Brasher P *et al.*, "Changing survival and impairment rates at 18–24 months in outborn very low birth weight infants: 1984–1987 versus 1980–1983," *Acta Paediatrica* **82** (1993): 666–671.

35. Bhushan V, Paneth N and Kiely JL, "Impact of improved survival of very low birth weight infants on recent secular trends in the prevalence of cerebral palsy," *Pediatrics* **91** (1993): 1094–1100.

36. Hack M, Taylor G, Klein N and Eiben R, "Outcome of < 750 g birth weight children at school age," *New England Journal of Medicine* **331** (1994): 753–759.

37. Hack M, Breslau N, Aram D *et al.*, "The effect of very low birth weight and social risk on neurocognitive abilities at school age," *Journal of Developmental and Behavioral Pediatrics* **13** (1992): 412–420.

38. Crowe TK, Deitz JC, Bennett FC and Tekolste K, "Preschool motor skills of children born prematurely and not diagnosed as having cerebral palsy," *Journal of Developmental and Behavioral Pediatrics* **9** (1988): 189–193.

39. Hunt JV, Bruce AB, Cooper DAB and Tooley WH, "Very low birth weight infants at 8 and 11 years of age: Role of neonatal illness and family status," *Pediatrics* **82** (1988): 596–603.

40. Klein NK, Hack M and Breslau N, "Children who were very low birth weight: Developmental and academic achievement at nine years of age," *Journal of Developmental and Behavioral Pediatrics* **10** (1989): 32–37.

41. Halsey CL, Colin MF and Anderson CL, "Extremely low birth weight children and their peers: A comparison of preschool performance," *Pediatrics* **81** (1993): 807–811.

42. Taylor HG, Klein N and Hack M, "Academic functioning < 750 g birth weight children who have normal cognitive abilities: Evidence for specific learning disabilities," *Pediatric Research* **35** (1994): p. 289A.

43. McCormick MC, Brooks-Gunn J, Workman-Denials K *et al.*, "The health and developmental status of very low weight children at school age," *Journal of American Medical Association* **267** (1992): 2204–2208.

44. Overpeck MD, Moss AJ, Hoffman HJ and Hendershot GE, "A comparison of the childhood health status of normal birth weight and low birth weight infants," *Public Health Reports* **104** (1989): 58–70.

45. McCormick MC, Gortmaker SL and Sobol AM, "Very low birth weight children: Behavior problems and school difficulty in a national sample," *Journal of Pediatrics* **117** (1990): 687–693.

46. Ross G, Lipper EG and Auld PAM, "Educational status and school related abilities of very low birth weight premature children," *Pediatrics* **88** (1991): 1125–1134.

47. Carran DT, Scott KG, Shaw K and Beydoun S, "The relative risk of educational handicaps in two birth cohorts of normal and low birth weight disadvantaged children," *Topics in Early Childhood Special Education* **9**(1) (1989): 14–31.

48. Vohr BR and Garcia Coll CT, "Neurodevelopmental and school performance of very low birth weight infants: A seven-year longitudinal study," *Pediatrics* **76** (1985): 345–350.

49. Teplin SW, Burchinal M, Johnson-Martin N *et al.*, "Neurodevelopmental, health, and growth status at age 6 years of children with birth weight less than 1,001 g," *Journal of Pediatrics* **118** (1991): 768–777.
50. Hack M, Weissman B, Breslau N *et al.*, "Health of very low birth weight children during their first eight years," *Journal of Pediatrics* **122** (1993): 887–892.
51. McCormick MC, Workman-Daniels K, Brooks-Gunn J and Peckham GJ, "Hospitalization of very low birth weight children at school age," *Journal of Pediatrics* **122** (1993): 360–365.
52. Das BK, Mishra RN, Mishra OP, Bhargava V and Prakash A, "Comparative outcome of low birth weight newborn infants," *Indian Pediatrics* **30** (1993): p. 15–21.
53. McGauhey PJ, Starfield B, Alexander C and Ensminger ME, "Social environment and vulnerability of low birth weight children: A social-epidemiological perspective," *Pediatrics* **88** (1991): 943–953.
54. Dunn HG, ed., "Sequelae of low birth weight: The Vancouver Study," *Clinics in Developmental Medicine series*, London: MacKeith (1986).
55. Low Birthweight Group, "The Scottish Low birth weight study: I. Survival, growth neuromotor and sensory impairment," *Archives of Disease in Childhood* **67** (1992): 675–681.
56. Ross G, Lipper EG and Auld PAM, "Growth achievement of very low birth weight premature children at school age," *Journal of Pediatrics* **117** (1990): 307–312.
57. Casey PH, Kraemer HC, Bernbaum J *et al.*, "Growth status and growth rates of a varied sample off low birth weight, preterm infants: A longitudinal cohort from birth to three years of age," *Journal of Pediatrics* **119** (1991): 599–605.
58. Hack M, Merkatz IR, McGrath SK *et al.*, "Catch-up growth in very low birth weight infants: Clinical correlates," *American Journal of Diseases of Children* **138** (1984): 370–375.
59. Bhargava SK, Ramji S, Srivastava U, Sachdeva HPS, Kapani V, Datta V and Satyanarayana L, "Growth and sexual maturation of Low Birth Weight: A 14 year follow up," *Indian Pediatrics* **32** (1995): 963–970.
60. Saigal S, Szatmari P, Rosenbaum P *et al.*, "Cognitive abilities and school performance of extremely low birth weight children and matched term controls at age 8 years: A regional study," *Journal of Pediatrics* **118** (1991): 751–760.
61. Choudhuri S, Kulkarni S, Barve S, Pandit AN, Sonak U and Sarpotdar N, "Neurologic sequele in high risk infants: A three year follow up," *Indian Pediatrics* **33** (1996): 645–653.

62. Paul VK, Radhika S, Deorari AK and Singh M, "Neurodevelopmental outcome of at risk nursery graduates," *National Neonatology Forum* (abstract) PGI, Chandigarh (1996).

63. Breslau N, DelDotto JE, Brown GG *et al.*, "A gradient relationship between low birth weight and IQ at age 6 years," *Archives of Pediatric and Adolescent Medicine* **148** (April 1994): 377–383.

64. Pandit A and Bhave S, "In: *Proceedings of Workshop on Developmental Assessment. Follow-up and Intervention in High Risk Neonates* (1990).

65. Ornstein M, Ohlsson A, Edmonds J and Asztalos E, "Neonatal follow-up of very low birth weight/extremely low birth weight infants to school age: A critical overview," *Acta Pediatrica Scandinavia* **80** (1991): 741–748.

66. Menyuk P, Liebergott J, Schultz M *et al.*, "Patterns of early lexical and cognitive development in premature and full-term infants," *Journal of Speech and Hearing Research* **34** (1991): 88–94.

67. Choudhari S, Kulkarni S, Pajnigar F, Pandit AN and Deshmukh S, "A longitudinal follow up of development of preterm infants," *Indian Pediatrics* **28** (1991): 873–880.

68. Petersen MB, Greisen G, Kovacs R *et al.*, "Status at four years of age in a 280 children weighing 2,300 g or less at birth," *Danish Medical Bulletin* **37** (1990): 546–552.

69. Breslau N, Klein N and Allen L, "Very low birth weight: Behavioral sequelae at nine years of age," *Journal of the American Academy of Child and Adolescent Psychiatry* **27**(5) (1988): 605–612.

70. Sommerfelt K, Ellertsen B and Markestad T, "Personality and behavior in eight-year-old, non-handicapped children with birth weight under 1,500 g," *Acta Paediatrica* **92** (1993): 723–728.

71. Ross G, Lipper EG and Auld PAM, "Social competence and behavior problems on mothers and premature and full-term infants," *Child Development* **54**(1) (1983): p. 209–217.

72. Brandt P, Magyary D, Hammond M and Barnard K, "Learning and behavioral-emotional problems of children born preterm at second grade," *Journal of Pediatric Psychology* **17** (1992): 291–311.

73. Szatmari P, Saigal S, Rosenbaum P *et al.*, "Psychiatric disorders at five years among children with birth weights < 1,000 g: A regional perspective," *Developmental Medicine and Child Neurology* **32** (1990): 954–962.

74. Klein NK, "Children who were very low birth weight: Cognitive abilities and classroom behavior at five years of age," *Journal of Special Education* **22** (1988): 41–54.

75. Bradford BC, Bandin J, Conway MJ *et al.*, "Identification of sensory neural hearing loss in very preterm infants by brainstem auditory evolved potentials," *Archives Disease in Childhood* **60** (1985): 105–109.

76. Slennert E, Schulte FJ and Wollrath M, "Incubator noise and hearing loss," *Early Human Development* **1** (1972): p. 113.

77. Finitro-Heber T, McCracken GH, Roeser RJ *et al.*, "Ototoxicity in neonates treated with gentamycin and kanamycin results of a four year controlled follow up study," *Pediatrics* **63** (1979): p. 443.

78. Bers FH and Tharpe AM, "Unilateral hearing impairment in children," *Pediatrics* **74** (1984): 206–216.

79. Pape RE, Bunus RJ, Ashby S *et al.*, "The status at two years of low birth weight infants born in 1974 with birth weight less than 1,001 g," *Journal of Pediatrics* **93** (1978): p. 253.

80. Fielder AR and Levene MI, "Screening for retinopathy of prematurity," *Archives of Disease in Childhood* **67** (1992): 660–867.

81. Clark DI, O'Brien C, Weindling AM and Saeed M, "Initial experience of screening for retinopathy of prematurity," *Archives of Disease in Childhood* **67** (1992): 1233–1136.

82. Swarna Rekha and Battu RR, "Retinopathy of prematurity: Incidence and risk factors," *Indian Pediatrics* **33** (1996): 999–1004.

83. Verma M, Chhatwal J, Jaison S, Thomas S and Daniel R, "Refractive errors in preterm newborn infants," *Indian Pediatrics* **31** (1994): 1183–1186.

84. Bennett Britton S, Fitzhardinge PM and Ashby S, "Is intensive care justified for infants weighing less than 801 g at birth," *Journal of Pediatrics* **99** (1981): 937–943.

85. Hawdon JM, Hey E, Kolvin I and Fundudis T, "Born too small — Is outcome still affected?" *Developmental Medicine and Child Neurology* **32** (1990): 943–953.

86. Winer EK, Tejani NA, Atluri VL *et al.*, "Four to seven year evaluation in two groups of small-for-gestational age infants," *American Journal of Obstetrics and Gynecology* **143** (1982): 525–529.

87. Low JA, Handley-Derry MH, Burke SO *et al.*, "Association of intrauterine foetal growth retardation and learning deficits at age 9 to 11 years," *American Journal of Obstetrics and Gynecology* **167** (1992): 1499–1505.

88. Barker DJP, ed., "The foetal and infant origins of adult disease," London: British Medical Journal Books (1992).

89. Barker DJ, "Outcome of low birth weight, " *Hormone Research* **42**(4–25) (1994): 223–230.

90. Barker DJ, Gluckman PD, Godfrey KM, Hayding JE, Owens JA and Robinson JS, "Foetal nutrition and cardiovascular disease in adult life," *Lancet* **341** (1993): 938–941.

91. Fall CH, Pandit AN, Low CH, Yajnik CS, Clark PM, Breier B, Osmond C, Sheill AW, Gluckman PD and Barker DJ, "Size at birth and plasma insulin like growth factor- 1 concentration," *Archives of Disease in Childhood* **73**(4) (1995): 287–293.

92. Yajnik CS, Fall CH, Vaidya U, Pandit AN, Bavdekar A, Bhatt DS, Osmond C, Hales CN and Barker DJ, "Foetal growth and glucose and insulin metabolism in four year old Indian children," *Diabetic Medicine* **12**(4) (1995): 330–336.

93. Barker DJ, Hales CM, Fall CH, Osmond C, Phipps K and Clark PM, "Type 2 (non insulin dependent diabete mellitus, hypertension and hyperlipidaemia (Syndrome X): Relation to reduced foetal growth," *Diabetologia* **36**(1) (1993): 62–.

94. Frankel S, Elwood P, Sweetnam P, Yarnell J and Smith GD, "Birth weight, adult risk factors and incident coronary heart disease: Caerphilly Study," *Public Health* **110**(3) (1996): 139–143.

95. Benediktsson R, Lindsay RS, Noble J, Seckl JR and Edward CR, "Glucocorticoid exposure *in utero*: New model for adult hypertension," *Lancet* **341** (1993): 339–341.

96. Barker DJP, Winter PD, Osmond C *et al.*, "Weight in infancy and death from ischemic heart disease," *Lancet* **338** (1989): 371–372.

97. Osmond C, Barker DJP, Winter PD *et al.*, "Early growth and death from cardiovascular disease in women," *British Medical Journal* **307** (1993): 1519–1524.

98. Barker DJP, Osmond C, Simmonds SJ and Wield GA, "The relation of small head circumference and thinness at birth to death from cardiovascular disease in adult file," *British Medical Journal* **306** (1993): 422–426.

99. Law CM and Shiell AW, "Is blood pressure inversely related to birth weight? The strength of evidence from a systematic review of literature," *Journal of Hypertension* **14** (1996): 935–941.

100. Stein CE, Fall CHD, Kumaran K, Osmond C, Cox V and Barker DJP, "Foetal growth and coronary heart disease in South India," *Lancet* **348** (1996): 1269–1273.

101. Bhatnagar D, Anand IS, Durrigton PN *et al.*, "Coronary risk factors in people from the Indian subcontinent living in West London and their siblings in India," *Lancet* **34** (1995): 405–409.

102. Indian Consensus for Prevention of Hypertension and Coronary Artery Disease: A Joint Scientific Statement of Indian Society of Hypertension

and International College of Nutrition. Indian Consensus Group," *Journal of Nutritional Environmental Medicine* **6** (1996): 309–318.

103. Fall CHD and Barker DJP, "Foetal origin of coronary heart disease and noninsulin dependent diabetes in India," *Indian Pediatrics* **34** (1997): 5–8.

104. Lucas A and Morley R, "Does early nutrition in infant born before term programme later blood pressure?" *British Medical Journal* (1994): 304–308.

105. Holland FJ, Stark O, Ades AE and Pekham CS, "Birth weight and body mass index in childhood, adolescence and adulthood as predictors of blood pressure at age 36," *Journal of Epidemiology and Community Health* **47** (1993): 432–435.

106. Vagero D and Leon D, "Ischaemic heart disease and low birth weight: A test of the foetal-origins hypothesis from Swedish Twin Registry," *Lancet* **343** (1994): 260–262.

107. The Infant Health and Development Program, "Enhancing the outcomes of low birth weight, premature infants: A multisite, randomized trial," *Journal of the American Medical Association* **263** (1990): 3035–3042.

108. Cohen S, Parmelee A, Sigman M and Beckwith L, "Antecedents of school problems in children born premature," *Journal of Pediatric Psychology* **13** (1988): 493–508.

109. Escalona SK, "Newborn infants at double hazard: Early development in infants at biologic and social risk," *Pediatrics* **70** (1982): 670–676.

110. Resnick MB, Stralka K, Carter RL *et al.*, "Effects of birth weight and sociodemographic variables on mental development of neonatal intensive care unit survivors," *American Journal of Obstetrics and Gynecology* **162** (1990): 374–378.

111. Ayhward GP, Pfeiffer ST, Wright A and Verhulst SI, "Outcome studies of low birth weight infants published in the last decade: A meta-analysis," *Journal of Pediatrics* **115** (1989): 515–520.

112. Collin JF, Halsey CL and Anderson CL, "Emerging developmental sequelae in the "normal" extremely low birth weight infant," *Pediatrics* **88** (1991): 115–120.

113. Sameroff AJ and Chandler MJ, "Reproductive risk and the continuum of caretaking casualty," In: *Review of Child development*. Vol. 4, Horowitz FD, Hetherington M, Scarr-Salapatet S *et al*, eds., Chicago: University of Chicago Press (1975): 187–244.

114. Leonard CH, Clyman RI and Piecuch RE *et al.*, "Effect of medical and social risk factors on outcome of prematurity and very low birth weight," *Journal of Pediatrics* **116** (1990): 620–626.

115. Hack M, Breslau N and Weissman B *et al.*, "Effect off very low birth weight and subnormal head size on cognitive abilities at school age," *New England Journal of Medicine* **325** (1991): 231–237.

116. Schreuder AM, Veen S and Ens-Dokkum MH *et al.*, "Standardized method of follow-up assessment of preterm infants at the age of 5 years: Use of the WHO classification of impairments, disabilities and handicaps," *Paediaric and Perinatal Epidemiology* **6**(3) (1992): 363–380.

117. McCormick MC, "Long-term follow-up of infants discharged from neonatal intensive care units," *Journal of the American Medical Association* **261** (1989): 1767–1772.

118. Aylward GP, "The relationship between environmental risk and developmental outcome," *Journal of Developmental and Behavioral Pediatrics* **13** (1992): 222–229.

119. Hack M, Friedman H and Fanaroff AA, "Outcomes of extremely low birth weight," *Pediatrics* **88** (1996): 931–937.

120. Chamberlin G, "The pregnancy clinic," *British Medical Journal* **281** (1980): 29–30.

121. Singh M, "Current perspective on low birth weight newborn infants in India," *Bulletin of the National Neonatology Forum* **2** (1988): 7–10.

122. Shah KP, "Low birth weight, maternal nutrition and birth spacing," *Assignment Children (UNICEF)* **61/62** (1983): 177–194.

123. Venkatesh A, "Perinatal mortality revisited," *Indian Pediatrics* **25** (1988): 497–498.

124. Tyson JE, Laskey RE, Rosenfield CR, Dowling S and Gant N, "An analysis off potential bias in the loss of indigent infants to follow-up," *Early Human Development* **16** (1988): 13–25.

125. Wariyar UK and Richmond S, "Morbidity and preterm delivery: Importance of 100% follow-up," *Lancet* **i** (1989): 387–388.

126. Shah U, "Perinatal mortality in India: Can it be reduced through primary health centre?" *Indian Journal of Pediatrics* **53** (1986): 327–334.

127. Kumar V, "Perinatal mortality in the community," In: *Proceedings of Workshop in Neonatology Update*, Menon PSN, ed., New Delhi, AIIMS (1986): 12–21.

128. Kapoor SK, Reddiah VP and Lobo J, "Antenatal care and perinatal mortality," *Indian Journal of Pediatrics* **52** (1985): p. 159–162.

129. Heins HC and Keane MWD, *High Risk Pregnancy: Prevention and Management*, Medical Examination Publishing Co. (1981).

130. Bergner L and Susser MW, "Low birth weight and prenatal nutrition: An interpretative review," *Pediatrics* **96** (1970): p. 946.

131. Iyengar I, "Influence of the diet on the outcome of pregnancy in Indian women," In: *Proceedings of 9th International Congress of Nutrition*, Mexico 1972, Vol. 2, Karger, Nutrition (1975): 48–53.

132. Sadka NL, *Integrated Child Development Services in India*, New Delhi, UNICEF (1984).

133. Tafaro M, Maeue R: Gpnezoe A/ Effects of maternal malnutrition and heavy physical work during pregnancy and birth weight," *British Journal of Obstetrics and Gynecology* **87** (1980): 222–226.

134. De Vaquera, Townsend JW, Arroyo OJW and Lechtig A, "The relationship between arm circumference at birth and early mortality," *Journal of Tropical Pediatrics* **29** (1983): 167–174.

135. Singh M, Paul VK, Deorari AK, Anandlakshmi V and Sunderam KR, "Simple tricolored measuring tape for the identification of low birth weight by community health workers," *Annals of Tropical Paediatrics* (accepted).

136. Guha DK, *Neonatology. Principles and Practice*, Jaypee Brothers, Delhi, India (1995).

137. Fanaroff AA, Wright LL, Stevenson DK *et al.*, "Very low birth weight outcomes of the NICHD Neonatal Network May 1991–Dec 1992," *American Journal of Obstetrics and Gynecology* **173** (1995): 1423–1441.

138. Schwartz RM, Luby AM, Scanlon JW and Kellogg RJ, "Effect of surfactant on morbidity, mortality and resource use in newborn infants weighing 500 to 1,500 g," *New England Journal of Medicine* **8330** (1994): 1476–1480.

139. National Institute of Health, "Effect of corticosteroids for foetal maturation on perinatal outcomes," NIH Consensus Statement, Bethesda, MD: National Institutes of Health **12** (1994): 1–24.

140. Jobe AH, Mitchell BR and Gunkel JH, "Beneficial effects of the combined use of prenatal corticosteroids and postnatal surfactant on preterm infants," *American Journal of Obstetrics Gynecology* **168** (1993): 508–513.

141. Bennett FC, "The effectiveness of early intervention for infants at increased biologic risk," In: *The Effectiveness of Early Intervention for At-Risk and Handicapped Children*, Guralnick MJ and Bennett FC, eds., Orlando FL: Academic Press (1987): 79–114.

142. The Infant Health and Development Program, "Enhancing the outcomes of low birth weight, premature infants," *Journal of the American Medical Association* **263** (1990): 3035–3042.

Chapter 18

DOES HEALTH EDUCATION IMPROVE NEWBORN CARE?

Alison Bolam, Dominique Tillen and Anthony Costello
Institute of Child Health, London, UK

Introduction

This chapter reviews the recent literature on health education in the perinatal period for mothers in developing countries, with particular reference to the evaluation and effectiveness of interventions. The importance of health education and definitions of health education are introduced. A description of potential target audiences and methods employed in imparting and evaluating health education is given. A randomised controlled trial of one-to-one health education for mothers about infant care and family planning practices recently conducted in Kathmandu is briefly described. We conclude that the effectiveness of many types of health education intervention remains to be proven and that there is a need for further randomised controlled trials with long-term follow-up to demonstrate efficacy.

The Alma Ata Declaration[1] proclaimed that "education concerning prevailing health problems and the methods of preventing and controlling them" is the first of the eight basic elements of primary health care. The primary health care approach, seen by the World Health Organization as the strategy for achieving Health for All by the Year 2000, is strongly promoted throughout the world. Most countries are signatories to the objectives. Health education is thus seen as a vital part of primary health care.

Infant mortality rates are high in developing countries for a variety of reasons including poor environmental conditions, inadequate housing, illiteracy, poor nutritional status, reduced access to health services, and a high incidence of illnesses such as diarrhoea, respiratory infection and the vaccine preventable diseases. High infant mortality rates lead to a rise in maternal morbidity and mortality as early neonatal or infant death commonly may lead to a rapid replacement pregnancy with all the risks to the mother this entails. Health education is potentially a cost-effective method for tackling some of the poor health outcomes arising from poor environmental and economic conditions.

This chapter reviews health education intervention strategies aimed at improving maternal and infant health in developing countries. Despite it being an integral part of primary health care programmes, especially those which focus on the needs of mothers and children, health education remains an ill-defined and poorly evaluated intervention.

Definitions and Models of Health Education

There are many different definitions of "health education" in the literature. It can be used to describe any effort to provide information and knowledge relating to health maintenance and promotion and therefore has both formal and informal aspects. Formal definitions imply planned and/or programmed efforts to bring about the promotion and continuation of health, and prevention of disease.

The WHO offers a *formal* definition of health education: "Health education concerns all those experiences of an individual, group or community that influence beliefs, attitudes and behaviour with respect to health as well as the processes and efforts of producing change when it is necessary for optimal health".[2] Thus, health education attempts not only to equip individuals, groups and communities with the wherewithal and means of making sound decisions, but also to influence the outcome in a desired direction by such decisions.

Informal aspects include the transmission of empirical knowledge about health from generation to generation and across families and societies.

In this paper we are concerned about health education in the formal sense.

Theoretical constructs

Some of the problems which have arisen in translating health education into practice relate to the theoretical constructs underpinning them. The *rational approach* to health promotion believes that giving people information will bring about change in health behaviour. Although this theory is now considered by social scientists as too limited, it underpins much of the programmatic thinking of policy makers. In contrast the *social cognitive theory* developed by Bandura and others in the 1970s suggests that experience rather than information is the key. Experiences from interactions within family, peer groups or communities is essential for successful health promotion.[3] Two important concepts which have arisen from this theory are *self-efficacy* and *life skills*.

Self-efficacy refers to a person's belief in their capability to organise and execute the course of action required to deal with prospective situations.[4] Self-efficacy judgements are specific to behaviours and the situations in which they occur. They have been shown to be an important causal mechanism in a wide range of health behaviours including smoking cessation, weight control, exercise, nutrition contraception and AIDS prevention.[5-7] For a fuller explanation of the self-efficacy construct in health promotion see Maibach and Murphy (1995).[8]

The concept of life skills is linked to self-efficacy: these are the actual skills needed to meet the demands of everyday life and which help to develop an enhanced sense of self-efficacy in relation to specific health behaviours. Measures of self-efficacy and life skills are specific to functions and populations. As Maibach and Murphy state "efficacy judgements are a function of both the specific behaviours and situational contexts in which they occur; these will vary from population to population". This makes evaluation of health education and promotion even more challenging because investigators need to identify appropriate competencies and challenges within the population they are working with, and then develop standardised and validated formats for the assessment of the self-efficacy in question.

Factors affecting success of health education programmes

Most investigators develop a *working* definition of health education in order to plan health education strategies with specific aims in mind. The following points have been described as crucial to the success of health education programmes:[9]

- Health education is more than the imparting of information, its focus is on changing and modifying behaviour.
- The health educator is therefore a change agent in a particular society and as such has to understand the structure and forces in that society.
- Understanding the society in question is essential because information and knowledge might not themselves lead to recognised changes in action, particularly if these conflict with existing motives, attitudes, beliefs and values and are not constant with social or group norms.
- Consequently, for success, it is essential that health education develops a two-angled stance to health behaviour and problems, as viewed by health professionals and the general public.
- Hence, there is also a need to recognise any differences in professionally defined problems and lay defined problems.
- Health education is a multisided and multidisciplinary activity bringing together health and social sciences in a educational setting.
- Of paramount significance is the need to have a scientific base for action which health education programmes may follow.

The challenge of health education is understanding how and when to intervene to maximum effect in order to produce a desire for positive health behaviour, a willingness to adopt and maintain this health behaviour and that this should, in turn, promote and encourage further positive health behaviour. In summary: *"Health education is about people, their behaviour and the process of change"*.

Intervention Strategies Used in Health Education

Health education intervention strategies can be divided into three groups; interventions at individual, community, and policy levels. Within these groups, different methods of health education can be employed.

Individual level health education interventions

This approach to health education focusses on behavioural change in the individual and has been widely used in medical care. In the context of improving newborn care many interventions have aimed to educate individual and groups of mothers about breastfeeding,[10] immunisation[11] and the care of the sick infant.[12] Evidence has mounted to support the efficacy of this intervention particularly in patients with chronic disease.[13]

The following factors facilitate the success of individual health education interventions:

- they are multi-component;
- the target audience is involved in planning and pilot testing the interventions;
- multi-professional teams are used in the design, implementation and evaluation of interventions; and
- there is intensive and ongoing contact with patients and family members.

Community level health education interventions

The most effective community health education interventions are those that raise the level of awareness and concerns for groups at risk of ill-health and enable them to devise their own strategies to reduce the risk.[13] Hence, from a practical point of view, changes in behaviour are more likely to occur when social and culture contexts are altered to support pro-health options thus creating a positive climate for health. Targets for community health interventions might include:

The whole community

Education via the mass media can target the whole community. A study in Jordan showed a positive impact from a TV/radio campaign about breast-feeding. The authors comment that information provided needs to be part of a programme supported by hospital policy and health worker practices.[14]

Linking agents

Persons who can connect the community with health education through existing social networks, for example grandmothers and lay health advisors. A study in Brazil in which traditional healers were taught about the use of oral rehydration solution showed an improvement in local mothers use of ORS.[15]

Community coalitions

For example, the mobilisation of key community leaders to effect community wide change.

Community empowerment strategies

Enabling people to have the ability to gain understanding and personal, social and economic and political forces in order to take action to improve their situation,[13] e.g. self help groups.

Policy level health education interventions

Health education interventions designed to influence individual and community health behaviour are often inadequate to alter the effects of policies that exert a powerful influence on environmental factors that influence health and shape behaviour.

The aim of policy-related health interventions is to make positive health behaviour "the easy choice", e.g. campaigns against the marketing of infant formula milks.

Methods Used in Health Education

Different health education methods may be used within each level of health education intervention strategy. Health education efforts can only be as successful as the methods and techniques that are used to disseminate the message, so the methods used must be appropriate to the situation. There are many methods of health education, each with its advantages and disadvantages, but whichever one is used the same focal objective remains — behavioural change on the part of the recipient.[9]

Methods of health education include:

- Working with people: one-to-one counselling, public meetings, lectures and story telling, group discussions, drama, role playing, demonstrations, and home visits.
- Working with mass media: radio, television, video film, film, news media, theatre, "enter-education" (a combination of entertainment and education, e.g. soap operas), wall newspapers, billboards, computer networks, and the telephone (e.g. for home-bound patients).
- Working with visual aids: leaflets, posters, pamphlets, booklets, comic books, film, slides, flannel graphs, and flip charts.
- For the future: CD-ROM, interactive video, video discs, and virtual reality programmes.[13,16]

Evaluation of health education

The importance of incorporating evaluation into health education programmes has been widely noted in the literature. It has been stated that "from the outset, a health promotion programme should be organised, planned and implemented in such a way that its operation and effects can be evaluated".[17] However, evaluation has often been lacking or inadequate. In a review of the literature about health education in developing countries spanning 20 years, only 67/542 (12%) of published articles described and evaluated the health education programme.[18] Of these 67, only three satisfied the authors' criteria for a rigorous evaluation. One of these related to newborn health care — a promotion of breastfeeding in South Africa.[19] There are good reasons for improving the quality of programme evaluations, particularly in developing country settings. Firstly, health education is often considered a low priority and thus the funds available are meagre. In some countries it constitutes as little as 0.01% of the health budget.[18] More money may be made available if rigorously evaluated studies can show the effectiveness and cost-benefits of health education.

Categories of evaluation

Evaluation can be divided into four categories:[20] needs assessment, process, impact, and outcome, each providing useful information about the overall programme. The focus of this chapter is on impact and outcome evaluation, so needs assessment and process evaluation will be mentioned only briefly. The methods of evaluation used vary according to the category. While it is considered that a comprehensive evaluation would include all four it is often only possible to pursue one or two.

(i) Evaluation of needs assessment

This involves feedback on knowledge, attitudes, risk behaviours, health status, and perceived needs of the target population and of the status of currently available health promotion programmes. The emphasis on context evaluation is particularly important when programme success individual behaviour is recognised as a function of community factors outside the influence of the intervention.

(ii) Evaluation of process

Process evaluation provides data to describe how a programme was implemented, how well the activities delivered fit the original design, to whom services were delivered, the extent to which the target population was reached, and factors external to the programme that may compete with the programme effects.

(iii) Evaluation of impact

This assesses the effectiveness of the programme in achieving changes in knowledge, attitudes, beliefs, and the behaviour of the target group.

(iv) Evaluation of outcome

Finally, this examines the effects of the programme on health status — the ultimate goal. Both impact and outcome evaluations are conducted when the purpose is to assess the effects of an intervention. The ultimate goal of health education intervention strategies is to positively influence health status. However, more proximal indicators of success are changes in intermediate outcomes (e.g. changes in knowledge, attitudes or behaviour, also known as impact). Because health education interventions work through these intermediate outcomes, the linkage to health status is often accepted at a conceptual or theoretical level.

Evaluation design

Historically, effective approaches to evaluating health education programmes have been primarily defined in terms of impact and outcome evaluations. Thus effective evaluations are considered to have the capacity to measure, with validity and reliability, the effects of a health education intervention and to separate such effects from similar effects produced by forces other than the health education programme. More recently, attention is turning to the importance of systematically documenting the processes involved in implementing an intervention. There remains disagreement on the effectiveness of less traditional evaluation approaches such as this.[20,21]

Impact and outcome evaluation

The classic evaluation design for measuring programme effect is the experimental model.[20] This model involves the use of intervention and control groups. In the randomised controlled trial, subjects (people, villages, schools, etc.) are randomly assigned to each group. This is the most efficient way to rule out the possibility that something other than the programme is associated with observed changes. For this reason results from such trials are generally accepted as providing credible evidence of programme effectiveness. However, in health education programmes it can be difficult to adhere to a strict experimental design. It may be unethical to withhold an intervention from certain groups or there may be contamination between groups. It may also be said that the trial conducted under true experimental conditions is cannot be generalised to the real world. For these reasons "quasi-experimental" evaluation designs have also been developed.[22,23] These methods involve non-randomised group assignment and often include sequential recruitment of control and intervention groups. It is more difficult to rule out other causes of any observed effect in such designs.

Needs assessment and process evaluation

Needs assessment evaluations aim to provide feedback on knowledge attitudes, behaviour, health status, and perceived needs of the target population. Process evaluations aim to provide a description of what programme staff and participants are doing. In both cases, multiple data collection methods including qualitative methods such as semi-structured individual interviews, focus group discussions, and participatory appraisal are employed. The perspectives of all groups involved are incorporated.

Effectiveness of Health Education Interventions

Does health education work? Different professional groups may apply different criteria for success: to an educationalist it may mean the successful transmission of a message, to a health worker a measurable improvement in morbidity or mortality, to the community it may mean the acquisition of knowledge on which to base informed choice (e.g. to breastfeed or not). Authors disagree about which outcomes confirm programme success. Loevinsohn considers that only objectively verifiable changes in behaviour, or better still in health status, are adequate to show programme effectiveness. However, other authors[20] consider that a change in knowledge is adequate.

Various studies[9,13,20,24,25] have reviewed the effectiveness of health education interventions and the methods used to evaluate them. The general consensus is that *the majority of evaluations of health education interventions to date have been methodologically unsound and do not allow firm conclusions to be drawn about the overall efficacy of health education.*

Health Education Intervention Study at the Maternity Hospital, Kathmandu

A study recently conducted at the maternity hospital, Kathmandu,[26] attempted to evaluate one-to-one health education using a rigorous study design. In this study the effects of postnatal health education for mothers on infant care and family planning practices was examined in a randomised controlled trial.

540 mothers were randomly allocated to one of four groups: health education immediately after birth and three months postpartum (group A), at birth only (group B), at three months only (group C), or not at all (group D). The mothers were followed-up by interview in the community at three and six months postpartum.

The intervention consisted of 20 minutes of one-to-one discussion which was designed to be interactive and supportive in style. Information was also given by the use of cloth flip chart pictures. The topics covered were infant feeding, diarrhoea and ARI, immunisation, and contraception after the puerperium. The main outcome measures were duration of exclusive breast-feeding, infant growth, immunisation of infant, knowledge of need to continue breastfeeding and use of ORS in diarrhoea, knowledge of infant signs suggestive of pneumonia, and postpartum family planning uptake.

Results showed some impact on knowledge of signs suggestive of pneumonia at three months, which had disappeared by six months, and a small impact on the uptake of family planning at six months but not on other health outcomes. In this study the recommended practice of individual health education for mothers in poor communities had minimal impact.

Conclusion

Overall, can we conclude that health education is effective? Reviews of the subject agree that for many areas of health education we do not have firm evidence demonstrating programme success.[18,24,25,27] An exception to this is the evidence that exists to support the efficacy of individual level interventions in the treatment and care of individuals with chronic disease in developed countries.[13] Further well-designed trials are required to provide an evidence base on which future health education interventions can be implemented.

The ultimate goal of health education interventions is to achieve an improvement in the health status of the individual or community. In evaluations this is often presumed to happen through the proxy indicators of either a change in knowledge and/or in behaviour. However, numerous studies have shown flaws in this linkage, with no change in behaviour of participants despite objectively verified improvements in knowledge. In addition, changes in behaviour will only result in improved health status if our understanding of the epidemiology of the disease in question is correct. Another problem highlighted by many studies is the lack of sustained improvement in outcomes, despite early success.[28,29] In addition, uncontrolled or poorly controlled trials may exaggerate the perceived effectiveness of an intervention, which will interfere with appropriate planning of health care.[30]

There is a need for further evaluation of health education interventions, especially trial designs which incorporate control groups and randomisation to the intervention, with adequate length of follow-up, so that a scientific basis for continuing health education interventions can be developed. In developing countries especially, the question of cost-effectiveness must also be considered because successful interventions on a small scale may not be feasible or sustainable when applied to the whole population.

Summary of Recommendations for Future Health Education Interventions and Their Evaluation:[18,20,31–34]

Programme planning with particular relevance to developing country settings

- Ensure that the desired changes in behaviour are realistic for the individual or community to implement. Consider economic, social, and cultural barriers. Interventions aimed at women must take into account their already heavy workload in the home and field.
- The new behaviour should accord with the values of the society and culture.
- Participants should have a clear understanding of the benefits to be derived from the new behaviour.
- Take into account the need for appropriate use of language in multilingual societies, the problems of working in areas with poor health infrastructure

and a lack of trained personnel, and the vast differences that can exist between rural and urban communities and different ethnic groups.

The intervention

- Use the results of evidence based reviews to design future interventions.
- Messages should be few, of proven benefit to this community, and repeated frequently in many forums.
- Pilot the intervention.

Programme effectiveness and evaluation

- A clear definition of aims should be provided.
- Number of participants in control and intervention groups should be provided.
- Pre- and post-intervention data for both groups should be presented.
- Attrition rates for both groups should be recorded.
- Findings for each outcome measure mentioned in the aims should be provided.
- Most authors consider that randomised controlled studies are the 'gold standard' study design. However, Israel[20] considers that although randomised and quasi-experimental designs have an important role to play particularly in small-scale individual level interventions these designs have limitations in other contexts. She proposes incorporation of multiple methods, including the use of qualitative data collection and analysis and a participatory model including the concerns and contributions of all important stakeholders to improve outcome evaluations.
- Include an adequate follow-up period to look at both short- and long-term effectiveness.

To allow others to review and learn from studies

- The target audience should be described to allow other workers to judge whether the population they work with is similar to the population studied.

- A description of the intervention sufficient to allow replication should be provided.

Funding and publishing

- Funding bodies should refuse to support studies with methodologically flawed designs.
- Journals should refuse to accept methodologically flawed papers. For guidelines on the journal requirements for publishing randomised controlled trials see the CONSORT statement.[34]

References

1. Alma Ata Declaration. World Health Organization (1978).
2. World Health Organization, "Research in health education: Report of a WHO scientific group," *World Health Organization Report* Series 432 Geneva (1969).
3. Bandura A, "Self-efficacy mechanism in physiological activation and health promoting behaviour," In: *Neurobiology of Learning, Emotion and Affect*, Madden J, ed., Raven Press, New York (1991): 229–269.
4. Bandura A, "Self-efficacy: Toward a unifying theory of behavioural change," *Psychological Review* **84** (1977): 191–215.
5. O'Leary A, "Self-efficacy and health," *Behaviour, Research and Therapy* **23** (1985): 437–451.
6. Stecher V, De Vellis BM, Becker MH and Rosenstock IM, "The role of self-efficacy in achieving health behaviour change," *Health Education Quarterly* **13** (1986): 73–91.
7. Yalow ES and Collins JL, "Self-efficacy in health behaviour change: Issues in measurement and research design," *Advances in Health Education and Promotion* **2** (1989): 181–199.
8. Maibach E and Murphy DA, "Self-efficacy in health promotion research and practice: Conceptualisation and measurement," *Health Education Research* **10**(1) (1995): 37–50.
9. Richards ND, "Methods and effectiveness of health education: The past, the present and future of social scientific involvement," *Social Science in Medicine* **9** (1975): 141–156.

10. Hoffman MN, Durcan NM and Disler PB, "Breastfeeding in an economically disadvantaged area of Cape Town," *South African Medical Journal* **66**(14) (1984): 66–67.

11. Zeitlyn S, Mahmudur Rahman AKS, Nielsen BH, Gomes M, Kofoed PL and Mahalanabis D, "Compliance with diphtheria, tetanus and pertussis immunisation in Bangladesh: Factors identifying high risk groups," *British Medical Journal* **304** (1992): 606–609.

12. Bhattacharya R, Kaur P and Reddy DCS, "Impact of education in the knowledge and practices of rural mothers and key family members on diarrhoea and its treatment at home," *Journal of Diarrhoeal Diseases Research* (1988): 15–20.

13. Steckler A *et al.*, "Health education intervention strategies: Recommendations for future research," *Health Education Quarterly* **22**(3) (1995): 307–328.

14. McDivitt JA, Zimiki S, Hornik R and Adulaban A, "The impact of the HEALTHCOM mass media campaign on timely initiation of breastfeeding in Jordan," *Studies in Family Planning* **24**(5) (1993): 298–308.

15. Nations MK, Auxiliadora de Sousa M, Correia LL and Niunes de Silva DM, "Brazilian popular healers as effective promoters of oral rehydration therapy (ORT) and related child survival strategies," *PAHO Bulletin* **22**(4) (1988): 335–354.

16. Walt G, "Community health education in developing countries: An historical overview and policy implications, with selected annotated bibliography," *EPC Publication* No. 1, London School of Hygiene and Tropical Medicine (1984).

17. American Public Health Association, "Work group on health promotion/disease prevention: Criteria for the development of health promotion and education programs," *American Journal of Public Health* **77** (1987): 89–92.

18. Loevinsohn BP, "Health education in developing countries: A methodological review of published articles," *International Journal of Epidemiology* **19**(4) (1990): 788–794.

19. Ross SM, Loening WEK and Van Middlekoop A, "Breastfeeding — Evaluation of a health education programme," *South African Medical Journal* **64**(3) (1983): 361–363.

20. Israel BA, Cummings KM, Dignan MB *et al.*, "Evaluation of health education programs: Current assessment and future directions," *Health Education Quarterly* **22**(3) (1995): 364–389.

21. McGraw SA, Stone EJ, Osganian SK, Elder JP, Perry CL, Johnson CC, Parcel GS, Webber LS and Luepker RV, "Design of process evaluation within the Child and Adolescent Trial for Cardiovascular Health (CATCH)," *Health Education Quarterly (Supplement)* **2** (1994): S5–26.

22. Cook TD and Campbell DT, *Quasi-Experimentation: Design and Analysis for Field Settings*, Houghton Mifflin, Boston (1979).
23. Campbell DT and Stanley JC, *Experimental and Quasi-Experimental Designs for Research*, Rand McNally College Publishing, Chicago (1963).
24. Gatherer A, "Is health education effective?" The Health Education Council, London (1979).
25. Oakley A *et al.*, "Sexual health education interventions for young people: A methodological review," *British Medical Journal* **310** (1995): 158–162.
26. Bolam A, Manandhar DS, Shrestha P, Ellis M and Costello AM de L, "The effects of postnatal health education for mothers on infant care and family planning practices in Nepal: A randomised, controlled trial," *British Medical Journal* **7134** (1998): 805–810.
27. Nutbeam D, Smith and Catford J, "Evaluation in health education. A review of progress, possibilities and problems," *Journal of Epidemiology and Community Health* **44** (1990): 83–89.
28. Hardy EE, Vichi AM, Sarmento RC, Moreira A and Bosquerio CM, "Breastfeeding promotion: Effect of an educational programme in Brazil," *Studies in Family Planning* **13**(3) (1982): 79–86.
29. Prasad B and Costello AM de L, "Impact and sustainability of a 'baby friendly' health education Intervention at a district Hospital in Bihar, India," *British Medical Journal* **310**(11) (1995): 621–633.
30. Sacks H *et al.*, "Randomised versus historical controls for clinical trials," *American Journal of Medicine* **72** (1982): 233–240.
31. Hubley JH, "Barriers to health education in developing countries," *Health Education Research* **1** (1986): 233–245.
32. Report of the Cochrane Collaboration. Oxford: Cochrane Centre (1994).
33. Altman DG, "Better reporting of randomised controlled trials: The CONSORT statement," *British Medical Journal* **313**(7057) (1996): 570–571.
34. Rennie D, "How to report randomized controlled trials: The CONSORT statement," *Journal of the American Medical Association* **276** (1996): p. 8, p. 649.

Chapter 19

COMMUNITY BASED STRATEGIES TO IMPROVE NEWBORN AND INFANT CARE PRACTICES

Fehmida Jalil

Professor (R) of Social Paediatrics,
King Edward Medical College, Lahore

Background

This chapter will describe the effects of interventions such as monthly visits from Lady Health Visitors, the use of trained Traditional Birth Attendants (TBAs), and the impact of health education on the health of mothers and infants in a large longitudinal study of poor families near Lahore, Pakistan. The baseline and post-intervention characteristics of mothers and infants are described, and conclusions drawn about the value of community-based interventions. For further details refer to the *Acta Paediatrica* 1993 supplement, volume 390, which is a collection of papers from this study.

The Lahore study (1984–94): Infant care practices and indicators of neonatal health within different social and economic groups

King Edward Medical College, Lahore, Pakistan, and a number of Swedish universities started a collaborative project where three birth cohorts were followed from 1984 to 1994 among 4,262 families in three geographically defined areas in and around Lahore. A village, a peri-urban slum, and an urban slum were included. An upper middle (UM) class group was selected as a control during the study of the first cohort. The economic conditions, social structure, and the quality of life were found to vary significantly among the four areas.[1]

The cohorts

The aim of the follow-up in the *first cohort* was to characterise child health determinants, to study maternal health and to examine its association with perinatal and neonatal health.

The study was conducted in two steps. An initial cross-sectional survey was aimed at collecting socio-economic and demographic background information. This was followed by a longitudinal study of 1,476 infants born alive out of 1,607 pregnancies identified and registered during the initial survey and in the subsequent surveys conducted every fifth month. Each pregnancy was followed through by home visits and the outcome was registered. The gestational age was determined by Dubowitz estimate for 65% of the newborns and from the history of the last menstrual period given by the mother using the calendar of local events or lunar/harvest months for 98% of the cases. The newborns were examined within 0–7 days (45% within 24 hours and 68% within 72 hours after birth) by a paediatrician. Body measurements were taken at or soon after birth and then during monthly home visits using standard equipment by trained health workers under the supervision of a community paediatrician. Each month information regarding illnesses and feeding was recorded. The infants were followed monthly for the first three years and then quarterly till the age of five. At 24 months of age 70% of the infants were still in the study, 11% had died before reaching that age, 13% had moved out, and 6% had refused to participate in the study.[1]

The *second cohort* of 889 newborns were registered and followed like the first one. The aim was to get answers to specific child health related questions arising out of the data analysis of the first cohort.

The *third cohort* of 1,906 newborns was planned to study the impact of certain interventions on the health and survival of the newborns and children. At the end of two years, 73% of the infants were still in the study, 7.8% had died, 8.9% had refused to participate in the study, and 10% had moved out of the area.

The Intervention Programme Introduced Between the First and Third Cohort Studies

The intervention programme included:

- Training and literacy of TBAs.
- Participatory health education of mothers, TBAs and teachers in breast-feeding, nutrition and child care.
- Promotion of adult female basic literacy.

TBA training

The first two components of the intervention were started together. The TBA is the only obstetrician, perinatalogist and social worker for over 70% of the population in Pakistan. The intervention programme aimed at education and skill based *training of TBAs* was introduced during 1990 to ensure good antenatal care, safe home delivery and basic care of the new born. It was fully functional during the study period of the third cohort. The TBAs in the project areas were made literate with the support of a non-governmental organisation (NGO), HEAL (Health Education and Adult Literacy), using the health education material developed by health professionals in the project. For their technical training help was sought from the experts working with the Family Planning Association of Pakistan (FPAP).

A card was developed for use by the TBAs. It required them to perform certain functions for each pregnant woman by themselves or with the help of the project health team at the 5th, 7th, and 9th month of pregnancy. It aimed at implementing both antenatal and obstetric care. It also included compliance for iron and folic acid supplements, and with vaccination against tetanus. TBAs were provided with an appropriate number of safe delivery kits each week. The TBAs were also responsible for quality obstetric and perinatal care, including timely referral of obstetric emergencies. For each function performed, a TBA was paid Rs 5 (about US$0.15). Thus, by paying the TBA Rs 30 per pregnancy, the provision of essential maternal care was ensured.

After delivery, the TBA was expected to perform key aspects of essential newborn care:

- clear airway passages;
- give mouth to mouth resuscitation;
- prevent hypothermia;
- initialise optimal breastfeeding practices; and
- encourage families to keep the newborn infant next to the mother.

Other duties included getting the newborn infant immunised, ensuring body measurements at birth and then every month, educating the families for effective use of available health services, particularly for immunisation, diarrhoea, acute respiratory infection (ARI), and referral to hospital when necessary. For this service also, the TBA was paid Rs 30 per child. Thus, Rs 60 were paid to provide essential minimum care to the mother–infant pair.

Health nutrition education and child care

During a campaign for *breastfeeding promotion*, mothers were contacted by Lady Health Visitors (LHVs) at the 5th, 7th and 9th month of pregnancy. The motivation package included a comedy play on a videotape in the local language, a flip chart, posters, and a pictorial book for mothers who could read.

Non-formal *health education for mothers* included topics such as immunisation, home management of diarrhoea and ARI, care of the sick newborn infant, and seeking timely medical help. The mothers of infants reaching the age of four months, or those whose infants had failed to gain weight during the past two months or height during the past three months, were advised to attend four to six *nutrition demonstrations* held weekly in the adult basic literacy schools. The mothers brought uncooked food from their homes and prepared the weaning recipes for feeding the group of infants attending the session. Mothers were also encouraged to participate in growth monitoring.

Adult female literacy

Two schools for non-formal education were started with the support of HEAL, and were sustained by raising funds locally. Mothers and young girls who had failed to attend formal schools were made literate in these schools through participatory methods. This activity was expanded later on.

Comparison of Findings from the Pre-Intervention First Cohort with the Post-Intervention Third Cohort

1. *Maternal and neonatal size and anthropometry*

In the first cohort, the mean weight for height standard deviation scores (SDS) of the mothers in the three poor areas was much lower than those in the upper middle class group by the 9th month of pregnancy: village –1.7, peri-urban –1.3, urban –0.8. The women from the UM class at this stage of pregnancy were similar to the Swedish reference group.[2] The correlation coefficient between maternal body size during the 9th month of pregnancy and the size of the newborn were between 0.08–0.23.[2]

The UM class infants showed a similar mean body size to the reference group of Swedish healthy newborns.[3] The mean size at birth for weight, length, weight for length, and head circumference as well as the proportion of babies with birth size < –2SDS in the first cohort compared to the third cohort is shown in Table 1. The difference in birth size between the two cohorts was not significant.

2. *Birth size and linear growth in early infancy*

A sub-study of birth length and postnatal linear growth with special emphasis on infants born short for gestational age was conducted. Infants examined within four days postnatally who were still under study at the age of six months were included. Such a study was impossible using birth weight because all newborns could not be weighed within the first 24 hours and, unlike length, the weight changes rapidly during the first three to four days after birth. Infants

Table 1 Birth size standard deviation scores by cohort and sex.

	Cohort 1		Cohort 3	
	Males (%) n = 203	Females (%) n = 191	Males (%) n = 206	Females (%) n = 212
Weight for age SDS				< −
2	13	12	15	9 −
1.9 to −1.0	30	29	31	35 > −
1.0	57	59	55	56
Length for age SDS				
< −2	8	12	4	10
−1.9 to −1.0	15	17	24	18
> −1.0	77	72	72	73
Weight for length SDS				
< −2	4	4	6	7
−1.9 to −1.0	24	29	30	42
> −1.0	72	67	64	50

born with length below −2SDS in the third cohort showed an early and significantly better catch-up growth at two months compared with a similar group from the first cohort ($p < 0.001$). This difference in length of the infants born short in the two cohorts remained significant at the age of 18 months ($p < 0.0037$).[4] Whether born short or > −2SDS, the length at 24 months had significantly improved in the third cohort: on average, the infants were taller by approximately 3 cm compared with the first cohort.[4]

3. Birth size and development

Preliminary analysis showed that infants with late onset in walking were shorter and lighter at birth. No such association was observed with body size at the start of walking.[5]

4. *Feeding practices*

In the first cohort, initiation of breastfeeding was delayed in all neonates. Colostrum was universally discarded. 65% of the urban slum mothers and 45% of the village mothers did not start breastfeeding by 48 hours after the birth of the infant. Prelacteal feeding, especially herb water, was the norm. At one month of age, exclusive breastfeeding was rare: 17.8% in the village, 10.4% in the peri-urban slum, 3% in the urban slum, while none of the mothers in the UM class group were practising exclusive breastfeeding. Partial breastfeeding was widely prevalent, being 80% in the village, 84% in the peri-urban slum, 88% in the urban slum, and 86% in the UM class group. In the partially breastfed group, water, buffalo milk, or formula were introduced in the poor areas. Commercial formula was preferred by the mothers from the UM class group. Water, in addition to any form of milk, was given to 73% of the babies in the peri-urban slum, 58% in the village, 45% in the urban slum, and 23% in the UM class group. 13% of UM class, 9% of urban slum, 5.6% of peri-urban slum, and 2.4% of the village babies were not fed any breast milk at the age of one month.[6] Bottle feeding was considered elite and preferentially given to the boys.[7]

In the *third cohort*, the median age of initiation of breastfeeding changed from 57 hours to 10 hours, and 29% of mothers initiated breastfeeding within the first couple of hours. Exclusive breastfeeding was practiced by 83% of the mothers during the first month of life, being highest in the village followed by the peri-urban and the urban slum.[8]

5. *Mortality and morbidity*

Significant changes were observed in the mortality and morbidity patterns between the first and third cohorts. Infant mortality in the first cohort was 103 per 1,000 live births (LB), where 32% (n = 45) died within the first week and 55% (n = 78) died within the first four weeks.[9] Of these, 30% (n = 21) died because of asphyxia or birth trauma, 21% (n = 17) of septicaemia, 18% (n = 14) of tetanus, 16% (n = 10) of diarrhoea, 7.7% of ARI, and the rest due to miscellaneous causes.[2,9] The relationship between neonatal mortality and

Table 2 Neonatal mortality in the first and third cohort.

	Village	Peri-urban slum	Urban slum	UM class
First cohort	67	87	44	4
Third cohort	26	21	5	na
Overall reduction	41	66	36	
Average annual rate of reduction	10	16	9	

size at birth was highest for short birth length ($p < 0.001$) and gestational age ($p < 0.001$).[2]

Mortality during the first four weeks declined from 59 per 1,000 live births (after excluding deaths in the UM class in the first cohort) to 19 per 1,000 LB in the third cohort ($p < 0.01$), giving an average annual rate of reduction (ARR) of 10 per 1,000 LB per year (Table 2).

There was an overall change in infant mortality rate (IMR) from 103 per 1,000 live births to 59 per 1,000 LB giving an annual rate of reduction in IMR of 11 per 1,000 LB per year. Mortality rates given here are non-adjusted.

The decline in neonatal mortality was due to a change in deaths of tetanus neonatorum from 14 to one, diarrhoea from ten to one, and sepsis from 17 to four (2, 9 and unpublished data).

Analysis of data from the village showed no significant change in morbidity or deaths due to asphyxia. The incidence of diarrhoea during the first month declined from 21% to 0.3% and of ARI from 22% to 0.8%.

6. *Inter-birth interval*

The inter-birth interval in the villages changed from a mean of 17.9 months (SD 8.6 months) in the first cohort to 27.3 months (SD 10.1 months) in the third cohort.[10]

7. *Health seeking behaviour during childbirth and the neonatal period*

Almost all women in the village and peri-urban slum and nearly 70% in the urban slum were delivered at home by a TBA or a relative in the first cohort. These figures were similar to the national figures.[11] Traditionally, due to the sanctity of the first 40 days, when women and newborn do not venture outdoors (the *chilla* period), the mother–infant pair would not be seen by any trained health professional. However, in the Lahore study medical assistance was extended to the mother and newborn during the first cohort as well. In the third cohort, practices of both the health care provider and the community changed as discussed below.

The Impact of Community Based Interventions in Pakistan

A number of governmental organisations and NGOs are providing community based health services for mothers and children mostly through home visits by health workers.

This section reviews the performance of two well established NGOs, working at national level compared to Lahore study. The first one compares the impact of community based interventions, including home visits on survival, and the second one on impart of training on the performance of TBAs.

Impact of home visits on maternal and neonatal health

During the study period of the third cohort the LHVs in the Lahore study paid at least three antenatal visits in collaboration with the TBAs to provide essential minimum antenatal and perinatal care with a well-defined protocol for each visit (Table 3). Monthly home visits were made to the infants after birth. Meanwhile, the families were encouraged to utilise health services provided by the field team and at a fixed health facility. In the NGO project, the LHVs paid up to 14 antenatal home visits during each pregnancy and then monthly home visits to the infants, together with service provision through a fixed health centre.

In the Lahore study the annual rate of reduction in mortality was 10 per 1,000 LB for neonates and 11 per 1,000 LB for infants, while it was only

Table 3 Antenatal services in the Lahore project.

Visit	
Survey conducted every 5th month	• To identify new pregnancies in the catchment population, often before 10 weeks, to confirm pregnancy • To provide nutritional advice and supplements • To provide first dose of tetanus toxoid • To give pictorial or written handout and counsel for warning signs.
First antanatal visit 20–24 weeks	• To detect and manage risk factors • To identify and refer cases with complications • To provide second dose of tetanus toxoid • To counsel for optimal breastfeeding practices
A second visit at 28–32 weeks	• To detect danger signs and provide management • Treat maternal illnesses/malnutrition • To counsel for optimal breastfeeding practices
A third visit at 36–37 weeks	• To confirm fetal position • To assess cephalopelvic disproportion • To detect and manage danger signs • To ensure preparedness for safe delivery/referral for obstetric complications • To counsel for optimal breastfeeding practices

2.5 per 1,000 LB for infants in the NGO project,[12] and 0.8 per 1,000 LB overall at national level.[13] It seems that it is possible to achieve better impact with fewer antenatal home visits.

Home visits may also improve the behaviour of the mother in relation to her own health and to the health of the new born in a high risk population, which is in agreement with other studies.[14]

The impact of TBAs

Another NGO providing contraceptive and Mother and Child Health (MCH) services through trained TBAs was evaluated for quality of service delivery

Table 4 Evaluation of TBA practices.

	Trained TBAs	*Untrained TBAs*
Deliveries conducted per year		
mean (range)	26 (2–125)	6 (0–20)
Antenatal visits		
Every month	3	1
Many visits	1	1
1–2 per pregnancy	4	1
When families call	7	3
None	85	94
Pregnant women with danger signs referred to hospital (%)		
Yes	100	–
Sometimes	–	99
If yes, where?		
LHV	87	–
Hospital	12	–
What kind of help is given to a woman in need of emergency obstetric care?		
Taken to hospital	3	6
Ask family to take to hospital	92	94
Help in arranging transport	2	–

Source: Family Planning Association of Pakistan.

by trained TBAs compared to an untrained control group.[17] The result is shown in Table 4.

Experience from the Lahore study and the NGO work has shown that families in the areas with poor education and meagre resources, or families tied to harmful cultural practices need support at their doorsteps by trained TBAs.[14] In the rural setting, doctors are not available, while TBAs are generally well integrated into village life. They conduct more than 70% of the deliveries and provide care for the newborn. They provide counselling and support to mothers in a familiar environment within known codes of behaviour. However, they lack knowledge and skills in modern obstetric and neonatal care, and cannot handle obstetric or neonatal emergencies. To improve the quality of home delivery and neonatal care by TBAs, it is important to upgrade their skills, provide appropriate training, means, supervision and back-up support by linking them to secondary and tertiary level health care facilities.

The compliance for referral is very poor in developing countries for a variety of reasons. Behavioural studies show that the reasons for this are lack of access to medical services, geographical and socio-cultural reasons. Mothers may fear indifferent or non-communicative care, the loss of security of a familiar environment at home, the lack of freedom to move around, not being pressed and massaged by the TBA or not receiving emotional support through prayers or traditional ceremonies.[16]

Impact of Health Education and Counselling

Health education as an intervention has very poor impact in countries with a low level of literacy, particularly if there is no back-up service provision. The results of health education vary depending on the strategy used (see Chapter 18).

The examples worth quoting are from programmes directed at breastfeeding and nutrition, immunisation, Control of Diarrhoeal Diseases (CDD), and Acute Respiratory Infections (ARI). Using mass media campaign and inter personal communication (IPC) in Pakistan, these programmes resulted in a coverage rate of 74% for immunisation and 60% for oral rehydration therapy in 1992.[11] Recent unpublished data from cities with hospitals accredited as Baby Friendly has shown a high prevalence of exclusive breastfeeding.

The health education was backed up by service provision which led to a signigicant reduction in neonatal tetanus. In the same study, participatory health and nutrition education was focused. A remarkable increase in optimal breastfeeding practices was followed by a decline in diarrhoea and respiratory infections in newborns and infants, a significant change in the inter-birth interval, and better postnatal linear growth. The increase in inter birth interval is shown by other studies also.[17]

A sub-study from the project area has shown high protection against neonatal sepsis in breastfed infants.[18] Health/nutrition education to mothers and supplementation with folic acid tablets resulted in a remarkable decline in neural tube defects. This is in agreement with other sudies.[19-20]

Conclusion

- TBAs are an important cadre of health workers who will continue to provide obstetric services and neonatal care in Pakistan in the foreseeable future. It is important to upgrade their skills, provide training, means, supervision and back-up support by linking them to secondary and tertiary level health facilities.
- Fewer but purposeful home visits can improve pregnancy outcome. However, to provide quality care, it is necessary to carefully design local protocols.
- It is important to develop local clearly written *guidelines* for health workers for neonatal resuscitation, breastfeeding, prevention of hypothermia and infection.
- Develop *neonatal care centres* within easy access for rural communities to improve referral.
- Stunting at birth and postnatal linear growth were significantly influenced by the intervention programme in the Lahore study.
- *Optimal Breastfeeding practices are* essential to impact survival and provide protection from diseases, e.g. diarrhoea, ARI and neonatal sepsis, and also as a contraceptive measure.
- Previous research and Lahore study have demonstrated a reduction in neural tube defects in infants of previously vitamin deficient mothers given folic acid. Folate and iron tablets are an essential component of antenatal and pre-pregnancy care.
- Above all, education and literacy bring about a positive change in the attitude and practices of mothers and families towards better health and survival.

References

1. Jalil F, Lindblad BS, Hanson LA, Khan SR, Ashraf RN and Carlsson B, "Early child health in Lahore, Pakistan: I Study design," *Acta Paediatr* **390**(suppl) (1993): 3–16.

2. Jalil F, Lindblad BS, Hanson LA, Yaqoob M and Karlberg J, "Early child health in Lahore, Pakistan: IX Perinatal events," *Acta Paediatr* **390**(suppl) (1993): 95–107.

3. Karlberg J, Ashraf RN, Saleemi M, Yaqoob M and Jalil F, "Early child health in Lahore, Pakistan: X1 Growth," *Acta Paediatr* **390**(suppl) (1993): 119–150.

4. Jalil F and Karlberg J, "Influence of birth length on early growth in a developing community over a decade," (Submitted).

5. Karlberg J and Jalil F, "Psychomotor milestone achievement and body size," *Acta Paediatr* **411**(suppl) (1994): p. 95.

6. Ashraf RN, Jalil F, Khan SR, Zaman S, Karlberg J, Lindblad BS and Hanson LA, "Early child health in Lahore, Pakistan: V Feeding Patterns," *Acta Paediatr* **390**(suppl) (1993): 47–61.

7. Hanson LA, Adlerbert I, Carlsson B, Jalil F, Karlberg J, Lindblad BS and Mellander L, "Breastfeeding in reality," In: *Human Lactation 2. Maternal and Environmental Factors*, Hamosh M and Goldman AS, eds., New York: Plenum Publication Corporation (1986): 1–12.

8. Ashraf RN, Jalil F, Zaman S and Hanson LA, "Promotion of breastfeeding in a traditional village and city slum population in Lahore, Pakistan: Effect on feeding practices," (Submitted).

9. Khan SR, Jalil F, Zaman S, Lindblad BS and Karlberg J, "Early child health in Lahore, Pakistan: Mortality. X," *Acta Paediatr* **390**(suppl) (1993): 109–117.

10. Jalil F, "Interbirth interval and birth length," Paper presented at International Perinatal Conference, Lahore, Pakistan (1995).

11. National Institute of Population Studies/Institute for Resource Development (1992) Pakistan Demographic and Health Survey 1990–1991. Islamabad (1992).

12. Maternity and Child Welfare Association of Pakistan. Annual Report, 1994.

13. World Health Organization; Economic and Social Commission for Asia and the Pacific (ESCAP). Mortality in South and East Asia: A review of changing trends and patterns, 1975–1995, Geneva, Switzerland, WHO (1992): 157–176.

14. Olds DL and Kitzman H, "Can home visiting improve the health of women and children at environmental risk?" *Pediatrics* **86** (1990): 108–116.

15. Family Planning Association of Pakistan. Participatory evaluation of TBAs trained by FPAP (1995).

16. Bughalho A and Bergstrom S, "Assessment and obstetric care quality in Mozambique by perinatal audit. Safe motherhood," *NU NYTT om U-Landshalsovard* **7**: 22–28.

17. Perez A, Labbok MH and Queenan JT, "Clinical study of the lactational amenorrhea method for family planning," *Lancet* (1992): 339–370.

18. Ashraf RN, Jalil F, Zaman S, Karlberg J and Lindblad BS, "Breastfeeding and protection against neonatal sepsis in a high risk population," *Archives of Disease Childhood*.

19. Holmes LB, "Prevention of neural tube defects," *Paediatrics* **6** (1992): p. 839.

20. MRC Vitamin Study Research Group, "Prevention of neural tube defects: Results of Medical Council on Vitamin study," *Lancet* **338** (1991): 131–140.

Section 4:

Improving Health Service Delivery

Chapter 20

SPECIAL CARE OF NEWBORNS AT THE DISTRICT HOSPITAL

Dharma Manandhar

Consultant Paediatrician, Executive Director,
Mother and Infant Research Activities (MIRA) project;
Visiting Professor, Institute of Medicine, Kathmandu, Nepal

Special Care of Newborns in District Hospitals

The need to invest in district hospital level-II care

The district hospital will be the first referral hospital for the care of most sick neonates. Lack of resources (personnel, equipment, and finance) is a problem in all developing countries particularly in the South Asia Association for Regional Co-operation (SAARC) region. Only limited services can be offered in some district hospitals, and in many others none at all. Investment in neonatal facilities and care at the district hospital is likely to be more cost-effective than simply investing in a few regional centres of excellence for the provision of intensive care. The key objective for governments should be to provide level-II care facilities in district hospitals so that most sick newborns are managed at an affordable cost.

Who needs special care?

Most newborn infants require only basic care, i.e. cleanliness, warmth, and breast milk which the mother herself can provide easily. However, 10–15%

will require special care and 1–3% intensive care. Admission figures in 1996 for the Special Care Baby Unit (SCBU) of the maternity hospital in Kathmandu, revealed that 1.1% of total admissions were newborn infants weighing < 1 kg and 5% of admissions were newborn infants weighing between 1 and < 1.5 kg. Similarly, 9.2% of admitted newborn infants were less than 32 weeks gestation. Most infants weighing < 1.5 kg and particularly those weighing < 1 kg needed intensive care facilities, whereas most newborn infants weighing over 1.5 kg can be managed by a low-cost special care newborn infant unit.[1]

Common Neonatal Problems

The common causes of neonatal admissions and early neonatal deaths in the SCBU of the maternity hospital are shown in Table 1. The information was derived from the analysis of routine data.

Basic Principles of Newborn Care

The basic principles of newborn care are essentially simple and were first described as early as 1905 by French obstetrician Pierre Budin. In summary, these principles are:

- a clean delivery,
- facilities for neonatal resuscitation,
- warmth,
- early and exclusive breastfeeding,
- maintenance of good hygiene,
- early recognition and appropriate management of any illness,
- referral to an appropriate centre when required, and
- keeping infants with their mothers whenever possible.

Management with limited resources

Using common sense and careful management good level-II neonatal care can be provided at low cost. Cost-effective management involves such

Table 1 Causes of neonatal admissions and early neonatal deaths (in order of importance) in the SCBU of the maternity hospital in Kathmandu in 1996.

Causes of admission	*Causes of death*
Low birth weight	Severe birth asphyxia
Birth asphyxia	Respiratory distress
Respiratory distress	Septicaemia
Neonatal jaundice	Extreme prematurity
Infections	Haemorrhages
Congenital anomalies	Congenital anomalies
Meconium aspiration	Aspiration
Poor sucking	Hypothermia
Diarrhoea/vomiting	Miscellaneous: hydops fetalis, severe
Miscellaneous — aspiration, hypothermia	diarrhoea, congestive cardiac failure, "cot death"

initiatives as the use of locally made, low-cost equipment; the training and employment of nursery aids to help nurses in the routine care of sick neonates; encouraging mothers to breastfeed and to be involved in the care of their sick newborn infants; and the continuing education of staff. The following are the basic requirements for providing special care for sick neonates in district hospitals:

1. *Room*

There should be a separate room for the care of sick neonates. This room should, if possible, be near the delivery room. The room should have facilities for hand washing: plastic buckets could be kept in the cubicle to encourage hand washing by staff and relatives. Autoclaved newspapers could be used to wipe the hands if disposable towels are unaffordable. Towels for drying hands should not be shared. The room should be kept warm (at about 28–30°C) with suitable heaters. The use of thick curtains and plastic sheets in windows will help reduce heat loss during winter. There should be adequate space for storing supplies.

Table 2 List of equipment and facilities for essential neonatal care in a district hospital.

Apparatus	Resuscitaire — or at least an improvised table with an overhead lamp or a heat source
	Self inflatable resuscitation bag made of silicon, e.g. Laerdal or Ambu bag
	Infant laryngoscope with a straight blade No. 0 and No. 1.
	Suction apparatus — electrical/foot operated or at least De Lee mucus trap or rubber bulb syringe
	Phototherapy unit
	Oxygen hood
	Infant warmer
	Incubators or open cots with overhead heat source or warm wooden cots
	Apnoea and heart rate monitors (desirable)
	Portable X-ray unit (desirable)
	Syringe infusion pump (desirable)
	Much of these equipments could be locally made.
Disposables	Feeding tubes Nos. 4, 5, 6,
	Endotracheal tubes Nos. 2.5, 3, 3.5
	Umbilical venous catheter (feeding tubes could used instead)
	Suction catheters
	Two-way or three-way stopcocks
	Cannula Nos. 22, 24
	Scalp vein needles Nos. 22, 24
	Neonatal face masks
	Disposable syringes — 1 ml, 2 ml, 5 ml, 10 ml, 20 ml
Sterile packs	Umbilical catherisation set: includes knife handle and a blade, needle and thread, probe, artery forceps, needle holder, dissecting forceps, steel bowls, cotton wool, gauze, towels.
	Exchange transfusion set: contains umbilical catheterisation set and one four-way or two three-way stopcocks.
Other supplies	Oxygen supply — supplied either from an wall outlet or a cylinder sterilisation facility
Laboratory facilities	Facilities for routine examination of blood, csf, urine and stool, plus micromethods:
	• Serum bilirubin estimation: total (by a bilirubinometer) and direct bilirubin
	• Glucose strips, e.g. BM stix and a glucometer
	• Urea and electrolytes
	• Prothrombin time and partial thromboplastin time

2. *Equipment*

The unit should be provided with essential equipment, as shown in Table 2. Most of the equipment could be made locally. Locally made low-tech pieces of equipment are cheap, easy to operate, and easy to maintain. Care must be taken to ensure quality control, especially for sources of heat to the infant such as incubators, but in our experience locally made overhead resuscitaires have provided a stable thermal environment and a more sustainable alternative to expensive foreign equipment for which spare parts are a real problem.

Resuscitation equipment and essential drugs should be kept in the delivery room. Oxygen cylinders, and electric or foot-operated suction units could be used instead of wall-fixed oxygen and vacuum units which are costly to install. In order to minimise cross infection, disposables like feeding tubes, suction catheters, and intravenous cannulae should not be reused. Cleaning of the equipment should be routine.

3. *Staff*

Recruiting well trained staff is a big problem. Most routine work, e.g. cleaning and feeding the newborn infant and cleaning the equipment, could be done by less skilled staff so that nurses can devote more time to caring for sick infants. Female health workers with seven years of school education were trained in the SCBU for six months and found to be quite capable of managing routine care of infants. The use of these health workers has made it possible to run the SCBU of the Kathmandu maternity hospital (which has 30 cots) with as few as seven nurses. One crucial worker is a competent electric technician who has to maintain various equipment.

4. *Unit policy*

Encouraging mothers to breastfeed their newborn infants

Newborn infants who cannot suck are given expressed breast milk either with a spoon or through a feeding tube. Bottle feeding is not allowed. This policy, along with the introduction of disposable towels for hand washing, has dramatically reduced neonatal deaths due to diarrhoea during the summer months in the SCBU. Mothers are also encouraged to feed and clean their newborn infants. This policy has not only saved nurses' time but also helped to develop in the mother enough confidence to handle small babies.

Procedures

Nurses need to be trained in taking blood samples and putting up intravenous drips even in tiny newborn infants. This will save a lot of a doctor's time and improve the feeling of involvement of nurses in the care of sick neonates.

Training

Regular training of doctors and nurses, particularly of the newcomers, in the proper technique of resuscitation and other procedures is very important (see Chapter 27 on continuous medical education programmes).

Other useful tips

- A simple manual like the one used in the SCBU of the maternity hospital in Kathmandu[2] for the management of sick neonates is a valuable help for the residents. One of the standard books on neonatal care[3–5] should also be kept in the unit.
- A chart showing a list of most commonly used drugs, their dosages in mg/dose and expressed in volume as well (particularly number of units of a 1 ml syringe which has 100 units per ml markings), the dilution if required, and their mode of administration is another valuable help for both residents and nursing staff. The charts used in our SCBU in Kathmandu are shown in Table 3.
- BM stix strips or dextrostix strips are useful for checking blood sugar in the unit itself.
- Digital electronic thermometers are useful as they record as low as 32°C, are sturdy, and are inexpensive.

Table 3 Most commonly used drugs in the SCBU of the maternity hospital in Kathmandu.

Name of the drug	Available	Dilution	Amount per kg per dose	Unit per kg per dose	Frequency	Route
Adrenaline	1 ml (1/1000)	10 times	0.1–0.3 ml of the diluted solution		stat and can be repeated	i.v., i.m., i.t.
Amikacin	100 mg/2 ml		7.5 mg	15	b.d.	i.v., i.m.
Aminophyline	250 mg in 10 ml		5 mg–stat 2.5 mg	20–stat 10	b.d/t.i.d	i.v. slowly
Ampicillin	250 mg vial	2 ml	30 mg	24	b.d./ t.i.d	i.v, i.m
Calcium gluconate (10%)	10 ml		0.2 ml–stat 400 mg/kg/day			i.v. slowly oral
Cefazoline	250 mg	2 ml	25 mg	20	b.d	i.v., i.m.
Cefotaxime	250 mg	2 ml	50 mg	40	b.d.	i.v., i.m.
Chloramphenicol	500 mg	10 ml	12.5/ 25 mg	25/ 50	b.d., t.i.d.	i.v.
Dexamethasone	4 mg/ml 2 ml vial	0.1 mg	2.5		t.i.d., q.i.d.	i.v., i.m.
Diazepam	10 mg/2 ml		0.25 mg	5	stat, can be repeated	i.v. slowly/ rectal
Dopamine*	40 mg/ml 5 ml vial		5–20 mcg/kg/min			continuous infusion
Gentamycin	40 mg/ml 2 ml vial		2.5 mg	6.2	b.d.	i.v., i.m
Hydrocortisone	100 mg	2 ml	10 mg	20	8 hourly	i.v., i.m.
Mannitol	350 ml bottle		5 ml		6 hourly for 8 doses	slow i.v.
Metronidazole	5 mg/ml 100 ml		15 mg 7.5 mg	3 ml/kg 1.5 ml/kg	loading dose b.d.	i.v.
Phenobarbitone	200 mg/ml		20 mg 5 mg	10 2.5	loading dose o.d.	i.v., i.m.
Sodium bicarbonate (7.5%)	10 ml	equal vol. of 5% DW	1 ml		can be repeated	i.v. slowly
Tobramycin	20 mg/ml		2 mg	10	b.d.	i.v., i.m.

N.B: i.v. = intravenous, i.m. = intramuscular, i.t. = intratracheal.
Lower dose for preterms; b.d. = dosage for infants < 7 days, t.i.d. = dosage for infants > 7 days
1 ml syringe with markings of 100 units (1 ml = 100 units)

$$* \text{ Dopamine infusion}: \frac{6 \times \text{wt(kg)} \times \text{desired dose (mcg/kg/min)}}{\text{desired fluid infusion rate (ml/hr)}} = \text{mg of dopamine in 100 ml of infusion fluid}$$

- Regular audit of the unit is important in order to identify problems and also show staff how the unit is performing.

Intensive care of the newborns has not been discussed because it is not possible to provide such a service in a district hospital of a developing country. The above suggestions have been based on the experience of running a 30-bed Special Care Baby Unit (SCBU) of the maternity hospital in Kathmandu which has very limited resources. The unit admits over 2,200 newborn infants per year and the majority of mothers who deliver in this hospital are from poor socio-economic strata of society. In spite of resource constraints the results of managing sick neonates in this unit have been satisfactory except for the extremely low birth weight newborn infants.

Conclusion

The majority of sick neonates can be managed in a low-cost special care newborn infant unit. Emphasis should be on expansion of such services in developing countries rather than on spending limited resources in one or two neonatal intensive care units with only a few beds. The development of low-cost special care newborn infant units will upgrade the skills of medical and nursing staff, who will then be able to provide intensive care services as well once the necessary equipment becomes available.

References

1. Manandhar DS and Costello AM de L, "A low-cost Special Care Baby Unit at the maternity hospital in Nepal," *Postgraduate Doctor Middle East* **18**(10): 362–368.
2. Manandhar DS, "Essential neonatal care," *Nepal Pediatric Society* (1996).
3. Guha DK, *Neonatology: Principles and Practice*, Jaypee Bros (1995).
4. Singh M, *Care of the newborn*, 4th ed., Sagar Publications, New Delhi (1991).
5. *Schaffer's Diseases of the Newborn*, Sagar Publications, New Delhi (1993).

Commentary

LESSONS FROM A NEONATAL DEATH

Sajid Maqbool

Professor of Pediatrics, Shaikh Zayed Medical Complex, Lahore

Case History

A 3.1 kg full term male baby was transferred to the neonatal unit of our hospital at the age of four hours. He was born to a gravida-3-para-2 mother and delivery was conducted by a *Dai* (untrained midwife). According to the aunt, the second stage of labour was prolonged to two hours due to difficulty in the delivery of the head and when delivered, the baby did not cry, was limp and was deeply blue. The mother had no antenatal care and may have been hypertensive. The baby was given vigorous tactile stimulation, wrapped in blankets, and then rushed to the district headquarter hospital where oxygen was given, ambubagging instituted and warmth provided. With the development of generalised seizures, a shot of phenobarbitone was given. The infant was then moved to our special care unit. Despite vigorous efforts to resuscitate and rehabilitate him, the neonate continued to convulse, developed disseminated intravascular coagulation and died within 24 hours of admission.

Lessons to be Learned

Political commitment

The fate of this neonate is inextricably linked to the dismal state of affairs of health in Pakistan. Poverty and illiteracy of the individual are undoubtedly compounded by the lack of commitment of the government to health, education, and social welfare. A population of 140 million, a population growth rate of 3.2%, a female literacy rate of below 20%, and less than 1% of the central budget allocation to health is indeed a recipe for disaster.[1]

Referral of high risk infants

That this neonate did make it to the district headquarter (DHQ) hospital speaks for the awareness of the referral channel and the fact that all DHQ hospitals have the services of an obstetrician, a paediatrician and the necessary technology (oxygen, ambubag, drugs) to resuscitate and stabilise sick neonates.[2] Despite required measures, the neonate did succumb to asphyxia, one of the commonest causes of mortality in the neonatal period in Pakistan. The infant mortality rate (IMR) is still hovering around 91/1,000 live births and for those of us interested in the welfare of the neonate, neonatal mortality contributes between 45–60% of these deaths. Other causes include sepsis, prematurity, birth trauma, congenital malformations, and tetanus.

The problem of birth asphyxia

Birth asphyxia is one of the commonest causes of the high neonatal and thus infant mortality in the developing world.[3] In Pakistan, the situation is no different.[4] Statistics, although hospital based, indicate an incidence of from 1%[3] to 6%.[5] It accounts not only for the commonest reason for admission to neonatal units[6] but also for the largest single cause of deaths (80% of all deaths in the first 24 hours).[7] Birth asphyxia is probably the single most important cause, with a case fatality of 71.4% in India,[8] 65% in Pakistan in a hospital based study,[6] and 55–80% in a community based study conducted near Lahore enrolling populations from a village, a peri-urban slum, an urban slum as well as, a middle class community.[9] A review of data even from the developed countries indicates mortality rates of between 4–61% for severe birth asphyxia.[10] Not only is asphyxia a cause of mortality, it is also responsible for significant morbidity and is a major cause of developmental disabilities in later life. Since the definition of asphyxia used in different studies is variable, the incidence of long-term sequelae related to brain damage caused by severe asphyxia varies between 4 to 57%.[11-13]

Since conditions contributing to asphyxia are generally present before a mother goes into labour;[14] these might have been recognised and documented (toxaemia, antepartum haemorrhage, abnormal presentation, prematurity, and low birth weight).

Community based interventions

In a recent survey of obstetric and neonatal services conducted by the National Neonatology Group of the Pakistan Pediatric Association, Pakistan, it was found that only about 25% of the deliveries took place in hospitals or private clinics with obstetricians in attendance.[2] The remaining 75% were conducted in the community (as in the case presented) and it is here that maximum attention needs to be focussed. Recognising this, a national programme of Lady Health Workers (LHWs) has been launched under the Social Action Program. It envisages the training of 100,000 such workers, each one responsible for a population of 1,000–1,200 or roughly 200–250 households. Half the required number have already been trained and their training includes recognition of the high risk pregnancy, the appropriate supervision of the conduct of delivery, and timely newborn resuscitation and stabilisation.

With an overwhelming number of deliveries taking place in the community, due emphasis needs to be given to prompt and early identification of these high risk mothers. Subsequent timely referrals or interventions can then help in reducing birth asphyxia. For this mother's pregnancy risk assessment to be effective, three conditions should have been fulfilled: first, the factors predisposing to risk should have been identified; second, this identification should have been made early; and thirdly, service use should have led to the reduction, reversal or elimination of the existing risk. The main purpose of assessment of risk in pregnancy is to prevent maternal and perinatal morbidity and mortality, not only by early identification but also by formulating appropriate intervention measures. An appropriate history and limited examination suffices for this purpose, but risks must be identified early at a time when efforts to intervene will be fruitful.[15]

For this mother and her baby the system was non-existent in her community, help was not forthcoming and the consequence was a death to be entered into the statistics. The mother was herself lucky to have survived and not be counted amongst the 340 who succumbed per 100,000 births representing the maternal mortality figures of the country.[1]

References

1. *The State of World's Children*. UNICEF, Oxford University Press (1997).
2. Maqbool S *et al.*, "A survey of neonatal services by the National Neonatology Group Pakistan," (unpublished data).
3. Rantakallio P, von Wendt L and Koivu M, "Prognosis of perinatal brain damage: A prospective study of a one year cohort of 12,000 children," *Early Human Development* **15** (1987): 712–716.
4. Maqbool S, Saeed M and Khan SRK, "Birth asphyxia," *Journal of the Pakistan Medical Association* **38** (1988): 217–219.
5. Molteno CD, Malan AF and Heese H de V, "Asphyxia neonatorum-assessment of the infant at birth," *South Africa Medical Journal* **48** (1974): 2139–2142.
6. Arif MA and Nizami SQ, "A study of 10,566 newborn babies," *Pakistan Paediatric Journal* **9** (1985): 20–25.
7. Haneef SM, Sofia T, Qureshi Z and Illahi S, "Pattern of neonatal disease," *Pakistan Paediatric Journal* **9** (1985): 42–48.
8. Scott H, "Outcome of very severe birth asphyxia," *Archives of Disease in Childhood* **51** (1976): 712–716.
9. Jalil F, Lindblad BS, Hansen LA, Khan SR, Yaqoob M and Karlberg J, "Early child health in Lahore, Pakistan: IX: Perinatal events," *Acta Paediatrica* **390**(suppl) (1993): 95–107.
10. Brann AW, "Factors during neonatal life that influence brain disorders," In: *Prenatal and Perinatal Factors Associated with Birth Disorders*. Freeman JM, ed., NIH Pub No. (1985): 85–1149.
11. Thomson AJ, Searle M and Russel G, "Quality of survival after severe birth asphyxia," *Archives of Disease in Childhood* **52** (1977): 620–626.
12. DeSouza SW and Richards B, "Neurological sequelae in newborn babies after perinatal asphyxia," *Archives of Disease in Childhood* **53** (1978): 564–569.

13. Nelson KB and Ellenberg JH, "Obstetric complications as risk factors in cerebral palsy or seizure disorders," *Journal of the American Medical Association* **252** (1984): 1843–1848.

14. Josten BE, Johnson TR and Nelson JP, "Umbilical cord blood pH and Apgar scores as an index of neonatal health," *American Journal of Obstetrics and Gynecology* **157** (1987): 843–848.

15. Scherger JE, "Assessing obstetrics risk: Commentary," *Journal of Family Practice* **27** (1988): 162–163.

Chapter 21

CURRENT CONTROVERSIES AND RECOMMENDATIONS FOR THE CARE OF HIGH RISK NEWBORN INFANTS

Meharban Singh

Professor and Head, Department of Pediatrics, WHO Collaborating Centre for Training and Research in Newborn Care, All India Institute of Medical Sciences, New Delhi, India

There have been tremendous advances both in our understanding and the availability of technology for effective management of high risk newborn infants. The focus has changed from mere survival to quality of life among survivors. The earlier passive nurse-dominated "neutral" approach in the care of premature infants has been replaced by more "positive" interventional strategies to enhance newborn survival. An aggressive approach, though often beneficial, has led to the emergence of many potentially avoidable iatrogenic disorders.

In order to practice rational evidence based medicine, we need to review relevant studies and debate controversies in order to identify the most effective, acceptable and safe therapeutic modality. Even meta-analysis of available studies of prophylactic and therapeutic procedures in the care of high risk infants may not provide ready answers because of methodological issues of bias, lack of precision, generalisability, and uniform applicability. In this chapter, an attempt is made to review some of the important controversies in the care of high risk newborn infants and recommendations are made for rational management at a district hospital having basic level-2 newborn care facilities.

High Risk Infants and Place of Their Care

Risk to a newborn infant at birth is best assigned by birth weight and gestation. There are no guidelines based on studies for deciding the placement of neonates at different levels of neonatal care. In view of available resources and expertise available at different levels of care, the birth weight and gestational age cut-offs for providing care to low birth weight infants (LBW) at different levels of MCH health care are shown in Table 1.[1] Based on this model of care, the necessary infrastructure, patient care and laboratory facilities, and expertise should be developed within the first referral units and district hospitals of a developing country. Some neonatal units restrict their care to infants weighing up to 1,000 g while more advanced centres may cater for infants with a birth weight up to 750 g.

Table 1 Birth weight and gestation cut-offs for providing care to newborn infants at different health care levels.

Level of Facility	Birth Weight	Gestation
Community Hospital or First Referral Unit (Level 1)	up to 1,800 g	up to 34 weeks
District Hospital (Basic Level 2)	up to 1,500 g	up to 32 weeks
Medical College Hospital or Good Level 2	up to 1,200 g	up to 30 weeks
Level 3 or Tertiary Newborn Unit	Any weight	Any gestation

Essential Newborn Care Facilities at a District Hospital

Essential antenatal care to all mothers, safe delivery practices, and optimal newborn care are crucial for enhancing newborn survival and improving the

Table 2 Community based criteria for identification of high risk mothers.

1. Primigravida
2. Too young (< 18 yr) or too old (> 35 yr) mother
3. Short (< 145 cm) or light mother (< 40 kg)
4. History of two or more previous foetal/neonatal deaths
5. History of previous LBW infant
6. Chronic systemic disease (tuberculosis, heart disease, asthma, hypertension, diabetes mellitus)
7. Severe anaemia
8. Pregnancy-induced hypertension

quality of life among survivors. High risk mothers should be identified early and referred to the district hospital for further management and confinement (Table 2). The mother is the safest transport incubator and it is preferable to transfer the high risk mother to the appropriate level, where she and her infant can get optimal care, rather than deliver the infant and cope with problems related to ensuring the safe transfer of a sick, unstable infant to the level-2 unit.

Essential care for infants below 1,500 g or 32 weeks gestation at a district hospital requires adequate infrastructure and infant care facilities (Table 3). Facilities should be available for the safe and effective management of hyper-bilirubinaemia with phototherapy and exchange blood transfusion.[2] Assisted ventilation facilities should not be developed in a district hospital, but attempts should be made to provide CPAP (Continuous Positive Airways Pressure) through nasal prongs with the help of an indigenous and affordable system. Even in a level-2 special care neonatal unit of a medical college, it is unwise to launch assisted ventilation facilities unless the neonatal mortality rate is brought down to less than 30 per 1,000 live births by other more effective and affordable strategies.

Minimum laboratory facilities (Table 4) should be provided at a district hospital for effective monitoring, early diagnosis, and prompt management of common neonatal disorders, e.g. sepsis, hyperbilirubinaemia, hypoglycaemia and polycythaemia or anaemia.

Table 3 Desirable infrastructural facilities at a district hospital.

1. Optimal care and resuscitation facilities at birth
2. Ensuring asepsis (hand washing facilities)
3. Provision of warmth (radiant warmers, room heaters)
4. Accurate administration of intravenous fluids, electrolytes and drugs (neoflon, microburette sets)
5. Effective management of hyperbilirubinaemia (phototherapy, exchange blood transfusion
6. Basic treatment of RDS (safe oxygen administration, indigenous CPAP facilities, apnea monitors, and pulse oximeter)
7. Ensuring feeding with human milk (gavage feeding, spoon and cup feeding, accurate weighing scales, etc.)
8. Oxygen concentrator

Table 4 Laboratory screening facilities at a district hospital.

1. Sepsis screen (total and differential leucocyte count, band cell count, micro-ESR)
2. Gastric aspirate cytology and "shake test"
3. Blood glucose (Dextrometer)
4. Serum total bilirubin (Icterometer, bilimeter)
5. Haematocrit (microcentrifuge)
6. Portable skiagrams
7. Blood bank facilities

Care at Birth

It is universally accepted that effective and optimal care of a newborn infant at birth by prevention and prompt management of hypothermia and birth asphyxia is associated with reduced neonatal morbidity, enhanced survival, and improved quality of life among the survivors.

Cord clamping

The issue of early versus late cord clamping is still unresolved. Early or immediate clamping of the cord is associated with an increased risk of intraventricular haemorrhage (IVH) and respiratory distress syndrome (RDS). When clamping is delayed beyond five minutes, the infant is at increased risk of developing polycythaemia, transient tachypnea of the newborn, jaundice, elevated blood pressure, and patent ductus arteriosus (PDA).[3] It is recommended that the obstetrician should follow a relaxed approach in clamping the cord, neither immediately nor with deliberate delay. Early clamping of the cord is indicated in situations such as the cord around the neck, severe foetal hypoxia and Rh-isoimmunisation. In normal circumstances, it would appear that delayed clamping (as late as the birth of the placenta in animal studies) does not lead to any adverse consequences as long as the infant and mother are placed at the same level. In developing countries with a high incidence of nutritional anaemia among pregnant women, delayed clamping of the cord may be beneficial in providing additional haemoglobin to the infant to boost compromised iron stores.[4]

Neonatal resuscitation issues

The birth of a high risk infant should be attended by a care-giver experienced in the art of neonatal resuscitation. The recommendations incorporated in the Neonatal Resuscitation Programme of the American Academy of Pediatrics and the American Heart Association have resolved most of the controversies pertaining to neonatal resuscitation.[5]

Meconium-stained infants

It remains controversial whether tracheal suctioning should be attempted in all meconium-stained infants or a selective policy should be adopted.[6] Early and thorough suction of the oropharynx and periglottic area with a 10 French catheter should be done as soon as the head is delivered in all meconium-stained infants. In infants who are vigorously crying at birth, intubation is associated with risk of trauma, hypoxia, bradycardia and even IVH in preterm infants. In infants who are depressed and covered with thick pea-soup meconium, endotracheal intubation and thorough suctioning of meconium is recommended. It is futile to insert a suction catheter inside the endotracheal tube; instead an ET tube should be directly attached to an intermittent source of suction and all traces of meconium should be sucked by applying negative pressure of up to 100 mm Hg. Oral suction of the ET tube should never be attempted due to the potential risk of transmission of HIV infection.[7] The meconium-stained infant should never be bagged till all traces of meconium have been sucked from the airways to prevent the occurrence of meconium aspiration syndrome.

Prevention of hypothermia should receive more urgent consideration than suctioning of the oral cavity in infants with clear amniotic fluid. Suctioning of the airways should be gentle and intermittent with minimal pharyngeal stimulation due to the potential risks of cardiac arrhythmia, bradycardia, laryngospasm, and pulmonary artery vasospasm.

Drugs for resuscitation

The aggressive approach of using drugs during resuscitation has been rationalised and the focus shifted to more efficient ventilation. Naloxone is recommended if the mother has received morphine or pethidine within four hours of delivery. The currently recommended intravenous dose of naloxone is 0.1 mg/kg (minimum of 0.5 mg). Epinephrine is a useful drug if there is severe bradycardia or asystole despite effective ventilation. It can be administered through an intravenous or intratracheal route, but an intracardiac route is strongly contraindicated because of the attendant hazards. There is no role for sodium bicarbonate, calcium, and atropine administration in the delivery room.[8]

After ensuring effective ventilation, if there is documented metabolic acidosis (or lack of spontaneous breathing at five minutes if blood gas facilities are not available) 7.5% sodium bicarbonate solution diluted in an equal volume of distilled water or double volume of 5% dextrose should be administered slowly intravenously at a dose of 2.0 mEq/kg. Bolus administration of sodium bicarbonate is dangerous because of the risk of development of intraventricular haemorrhage in preterm infants.

Administration of volume expanders is indicated if there are signs of shock with evidence of foetal haemorrhage or foeto-maternal transfusion. Ringer's lactate, physiological saline, and 5% albumin in aliquots of 5–10 ml/ kg are recommended until shock is corrected. Placental blood drawn in a 20-ml syringe containing 50 units of heparin can be safely administered without any cross-matching through a blood transfusion set provided with a filter.

Eye prophylaxis

A routine policy for eye prophylaxis should be replaced by a selective policy depending upon the incidence of gonorrhoea in the region. Administration of 1% silver nitrate drops, even when dispensed in single use ampoules, is associated with the risk of chemical conjunctivitis.[9] Erythromycin 0.5% ophthalmic ointment, or drops, and tetracycline 1% ophthalmic ointment are as effective as 1% silver nitrate for affording protection against gonococcal ophthalmia and they are without any side effects.[10] Erythromycin and tetracycline have the additional benefit of providing protection against chlamydial conjunctivitis, though the incidence of chlamydial pneumonia is unaffected.[11,12]

Care of the umbilical cord

It is generally agreed that the umbilical cord should be kept open without any dressing to prevent the growth of anaerobic organisms. There is no need to keep the cord moist for any anticipated umbilical vessel catheterisation. A large number of antiseptics (gentian violet, triple dye, methylated spirit, absolute alcohol, etc.) and antibacterial agents (neomycin, bacitracin) for topical application have been found to be equally effective in reducing colonisation and infection of the cord. When environmental conditions are satisfactory and aseptic routines are strictly followed, there is no need to apply any antiseptic dye or antibiotic to the cord stump without any risk of umbilical sepsis. However, in a developing country, it is recommended to routinely apply antiseptic dye or methylated spirit to the base and tip of the cord at least once daily.

Vitamin K prophylaxis

The American Academy of Pediatrics recommends that vitamin K in a dose of 0.5–1.0 mg should be administered to all neonates to prevent haemorrhagic disease of the newborn (HDN). The risk of HDN is higher among breastfed infants because of the lower content of vitamin K in breast milk.[13-15] Despite this recommendation vitamin K is not routinely administered to all newborn infants in many centres in both developed and developing countries. All neonatal units do, however, recommend prophylactic administration of vitamin K to all high risk neonates admitted to special care neonatal units.

Naturally occurring vitamin K is safe and effective in preventing HDN. Concerns about a higher risk of lymphoreticular malignancy following neonatal use of injectable vitamin K have not been substantiated. Nevertheless, it seems unlikely that a healthy breastfeeding mother can meet all the nutritional requirements of her healthy term infant except for vitamin K. We know that milk is not only species-specific but also infant-specific, with unique nutritional and immunological properties. Is it really deficient to meet the physiological requirements of vitamin K of healthy term infants? Recent data suggest that the incidence of classical HDN among breastfed infants is around 0.1% compared with earlier estimates of 0.25–0.5%. With the prevalent practice of prelacteal feeds in many developing countries, despite subsequent exclusive breastfeeding, the gut is rapidly colonised with bacteria capable of endogenous synthesis of vitamin K. To prevent one case of HDN, 1,000 intramuscular injections of vitamin K are needed with the attendant risks of local abscess, hepatitis B, HIV, and overdosage. Oral administration of 2.0 mg of vitamin K can prevent classical HDN, but does not prevent late-onset HDN.[16,17] Unfortunately, there is no suitable oral preparation of vitamin K, and untill such time it may be prudent to restrict the prophylactic administration of vitamin K to high risk neonates.

Infant baths

The practice of bathing infants in the delivery room must be condemned. The bath should be deferred to the next day when the infant's temperature has stabilised. It is preferable to avoid dip baths till the cord has fallen. During the hospital stay the skin of the infant should be sponge-bathed gently, avoiding scrupulous cleaning of the vernix caseosa. Special attention should be paid to cleaning the skin creases in the axillae, groin, and neck area, which are predisposed to develop pyoderma. Routine application of hexachlorophene to the skin is not recommended as it carries the risk of serious toxic effects to the infant. Medicated soap may be too irritating for the delicate skin and should be avoided. High risk and LBW infants should not be given a bath.

Prophylactic Therapy During the Perinatal Period

Corticosteroids

Antenatal administration of betamethasone or dexamethasone to the mother who goes into premature labour before 34 weeks of gestation is universally accepted as an effective intervention for the prevention of hyaline membrane disease (HMD). It can be administered in a dose of 12 mg intramuscularly in two doses 24 hours apart or 6.0 mg every 12 hours for four doses. There is no absolute contraindication for its administration. It is essential that all attempts should be made to universalise antenatal administration of corticosteroids as a cost-effective strategy to reduce the incidence of HMD in developing countries, because surfactant is neither readily available nor affordable. Postnatal administration of corticosteroids for prevention of HMD has not been prospectively studied and is not recommended. There is no role for corticosteroids either in the prevention or management of hypoxic-ischaemic encephalopathy. Corticosteroids are useful for preventing laryngeal edema after taking infants off a ventilator and for attenuation of inflammatory damage in neonates with bronchopulmonary dysplasia. The recommended dosage regime and protocol should be followed.

Indomethacin

Indomethacin is a global inhibitor of prostaglandin synthesis and reduces perfusion of all organs. It is an effective and useful tocolytic agent but its duration of administration should be restricted to 48 hours because of the potential risk of patent ductus arteriosus (PDA) and periventricular leucomalacia (PVL) in premature infants. It has also been used for the treatment of polyhydramnios as it causes foetal oliguria.

Several double-blind controlled trials have been conducted to study the prophylactic utility of indomethacin for prevention of IVH. The meta-analysis of available studies show that incidence of grade three and four IVH is significantly reduced among treated infants. However, the risk of prophylactic indomethacin in the causation of PVL and retinopathy of prematurity (ROP) has not been carefully studied. It is administered intravenously in a dose of 0.1 mg/kg in three doses 12 hours apart; the first dose is given around 6–12 hours of age. Parenteral indomethacin is not available in most developing countries. Because of the potential toxicity of indomethacin, ibuprofen has been tried prophylactically and found to be useful for prevention of PDA.[18]

Intravenous immunoglobulins

Prophylactic and therapeutic administration of IVIG in preterm infants for the prevention and treatment of bacterial infections have given variable results. On the basis of a meta-analysis of available studies it seems there is no utility of prophylactic administration of IVIG to prevent neonatal sepsis. Ideally, we need specific monoclonal antibodies or harvested immunoglobulins from the sera of a local maternal population which is likely to yield a high concentration of specific antibodies against the locally prevalent pathogens.

Antibiotics

There is no place for prophylactic administration of antibiotics to newborn infants. They are not only useless but dangerous both to the infant and to the community due to the emergence of resistant bacteria. Prophylactic antibiotics can never replace strict house-keeping routines for the prevention of nosocomial infections. A lack of disposables and poor asepsis policy implementation means that prophylactic antibiotics are often administered if a infant is likely to have multiple exchange blood transfusions (more than two) or prolonged (> 72 hr) assisted ventilation. Several studies have documented that there is no need to administer prophylactic antibiotics to infants who develop meconium aspiration syndrome.[19]

In the rare event of an epidemic of thrush or diarrhoea in the nursery, all contacts should be given a topical application of gentian violet/clotrimazole or oral colistin sulfate respectively for five to seven days.

Thermo-Regulation and Temperature Monitoring

Newborn infants, especially those prematurely born or small-for-dates, need a warm micro-environment to maintain skin temperature of 36.5°C. The survival of preterm infants has been improved by the singular awareness that they must be nursed in a thermoneutral environment so that energy and oxygen are not wasted on endogenous thermogenesis due to cold stress (see Chapter 9).

Room warmers and radiant heaters without servo control are suitable and affordable in a district hospital. Effective covering of the infant with cap, blanket and stockinets are useful to prevent thermal and evaporative losses. Effective clothing or covering of a infant with a plastic blanket reduces insensible water loss and oxygen consumption.[20] The covered and clothed infants are more comfortable, sleep well, and grow better. Application of liquid paraffin to the skin can reduce insensible water loss by 40–60%.[21]

Low reading clinical thermometers (temperature range 30–40°C) are mandatory for monitoring the temperature of high risk infants; otherwise the severity of hypothermia may be overlooked. It has been shown that nurses and doctors can be trained to accurately assess the core and peripheral skin temperature of the infants with their hands for making an early diagnosis of hypothermia and cold stress.[22] Thermocole boxes have been found to be useful for keeping infants warm in a district hospital and they need to be standardised and popularised by using indigenous technology.[23] Skin-to-skin contact, reported as the Kangaroo method, is apparently a simple and effective method to keep the infants warm.[24] However, Gragge *et al.*[25] observed that at an operative environmental temperature of 20–30°C, the mean skin temperature of a clothed adult ranges from 34–35°C, which is below the temperature required for conducting heat to the infant. Moreover, its effectiveness, safety and cultural acceptability in Asia needs further study before it can be recommended. At present, early skin-to-skin contact in the labour room can be promoted to improve maternal–infant bonding, enhance lactation, and promote breastfeeding.

Feeding and Nutrition

Expressed breast milk and fortifiers

Earlier studies recommended initial starvation followed by use of energy and protein dense formula for feeding LBW infants to enhance growth velocity.[26,27] The current recommendations universally promote early enteral feedings with human milk for its unique properties. It reduces the risk of sepsis and necrotising enterocolitis. The milk of a mother who delivers prematurely has a higher protein and electrolyte content, so is most suitable to serve the nutritional and immunologic needs of her own infant.

Concern has been raised that mature human milk may not provide enough calories, protein, calcium, phosphorous, and micronutrients to serve the nutritional needs of LBW infants. Milk fortifiers (whey protein, medium chain triglycerides, and glucose polymers) are commonly used in developed countries to fortify the expressed breast milk (EBM). It has been documented that infants fed with fortified EBM show rapid initial weight gain velocity, but their subsequent physical and mental growth is similar to infants fed with unfortified EBM.[28,29] Infants fed with unfortified EBM require larger volume of feeds to meet their caloric needs: After 10–14 days most LBW infants demand 200–250 ml of EBM per kg every day. No attempt should be made to establish facilities for total parenteral nutrition at a district hospital.

Mode of feeding

The mode of feeding is determined by the gestational maturity, birth weight, and health status of the infant. The infant on oro-gastric feeds of EBM is gradually weaned to direct breastfeeding with an intervening transitional phase of feeding with the help of cup and spoon or *paladay*. Infants with a gestational maturity between 32–34 weeks have co-ordinated sucking and swallowing movements and effectively drink with the help of a spoon or *paladay*. It is advocated that bottle feeding should be completely eliminated in developing countries in order to avoid nipple confusion and risk of infection. In developing countries, non-nutritive sucking should be provided on the mother's breast rather than a pacifier to reduce the potential risk of infection and to enhance lactation.

Supplements

Nutritional supplements of calcium, phosphorous, vitamin E, and folic acid are recommended in infants with a birth weight of less than 1,500 g. Supplements are not required and can be stopped in infants who are self feeding directly from the breast. It is unwise to express breast milk in these infants for administration of nutritional supplements.

Oxygen Therapy

Oxygen is life saving when used judiciously, and useless and even toxic when administered indiscriminately. Routine administration of oxygen to all preterm infants is a dangerous practice fraught with the risk of development of ROP and blindness.[30] It is difficult to judge the need for oxygen therapy in newborn infants on clinical grounds alone without having facilities for monitoring arterial oxygen saturation. Goldman *et al.*[31] demonstrated that circumoral cyanosis has a sensitivity of 96% to detect oxygen desaturation (SaO_2 less than 85%) but a specificity of only 25%.

A head box is ideal for administration of oxygen to newborn infants. Depending upon the size of the head box and flow of oxygen, FiO_2 concentrations can be deduced for clinical purposes.[32] Oxygen can also be effectively administered with minimal wastage using a catheter with nasal cannulae or twin-holes aligned in front of the nostrils.[33] Oxygen should be given in the lowest concentration necessary to maintain satisfactory arterial oxygenation, and stopped immediately when no longer indicated. When free flow 100% oxygen cannot achieve normoxia, facilities should be available in a district hospital to administer oxygen with the help of a locally made CPAP system using nasal prongs. The infant should be closely monitored for development of ROP and, if present, early referral to an ophthalmologist is advised.[34,35]

Discharge Policy

The policy of discharging infants when they weigh 2 kg has been gradually replaced by earlier discharge. Early discharge reduces overcrowding in the nursery and rationalises the use of resources. The infant should be discharged if he has:

- regained birth weight,
- a daily weight gain velocity of at least 1%,
- remained stable and is free from any illness,
- maintained satisfactory body temperature without any evidence of cold stress, and
- is sucking directly from the breast.

The mother is the best primary health worker and she must be provided with information, knowledge, and skills needed to handle her infant with ease and confidence. She should be trained to identify the earliest evidence of illness in her infant so that medical help is sought without any delay. Home conditions must be assessed before the infant is discharged and the infant ideally should be closely followed to ensure that exclusive breastfeeding is continued at home.

References

1. Singh M, "Recommendations for creation of modest level-2 neonatal care facilities in India," *Indian Pediatrics* **29** (1992): 891–894.

2. Singh M and Paul VK, "Organisation of neonatal services in developing countries," *Indian Journal of Pediatrics* **62** (1995): 139–144.

3. Spears RL, Anderson GV, Brotman S, Farrier J, Kwan J, Masto A *et al.*, "The effect of early versus late cord clamping on signs of respiratory distress," *American Journal of Obstetrics and Gynecology* **95** (1966): 564–568.

4. Colozzi AE, "Clamping of the umbilical cord; its effect on the placental transfusion," *New England Journal of Medicine* **250** (1954): 629–632.

5. American Heart Association and American Academy of Pediatrics, *Textbook of Neonatal Resuscitation*, Dallas, Texas (1987).

6. Gregory GA, Gooding CA, Phibbs RN and Tooley WH, "Meconium aspiration in infants — A prospective study," *Journal of Pediatrics* **85** (1974): 848–852.

7. Ballard JL, Musial MJ and Myers MC, "Hazard of delivery room resuscitation using oral methods of endotracheal suctioning," *Pediatric Infectious Diseases* **5** (1986): 198–200.

8. American Academy of Pediatrics Committee on Drugs, "Emergency drug doses for infants and children," *Pediatrics* **81** (1988): 462–465.

9. Nishida H and Risemberg HM, "Silver nitrate ophthalmic solution and chemical conjunctivitis," *Pediatrics* **56** (1975): 368–373.

10. Mathieu PL, "Comparison study: Silver nitrate and oxytetracycline in newborn eyes," *American Journal of Diseases of Children* **95** (1958): 609–611.

11. Bernstein GA, Davis JP and Katcher ML, "Prophylaxis of neonatal con-junctivitis," *Clinical Pediatrics* **21** (1982): 545–560.

12. Hammerschlag MR, Cummings C, Robin PM, Williams TH and Delke I, "Efficacy of neonatal ocular prophylaxis for the prevention of chlamydial and gonococcal conjunctivitis," *New England Journal of Medicine* **320** (1989): 769–772.

13. Motohara K, Matsukura M, Matsuda I, Iribe K, Kondo Y *et al.*, "Severe vitamin K deficiency in breastfed infants," *Journal of Pediatrics* **105** (1984): 943–945.

14. Vietti T, Murphy TP, James JA and Pritchard JA, "Observations on the prophylactic use of vitamin K in the newborn infant," *Journal of Pediatrics* **56** (1960): 343–346.

15. Sutherland J, Glueck J and Gleser G, "Hemorrhagic disease of the newborn. Breastfeeding as a necessary factor in the pathogenesis," *American Journal of Diseases of Children* **113** (19679): 524–533.

16. O'Connor ME and Addiego JE, "Use of oral vitamin K_1 to prevent hemorrhagic disease of the newborn infant," *Journal of Pediatrics* **108** (1986): 616–619.

17. Bakhshi S, Deorari AK, Roy S, Paul VK and Singh M, "Prevention of subclinical vitamin K deficiency based on PIVKA II levels: Oral versus intramuscular route," *Indian Pediatrics* **33** (1996): 1040–1043.

18. Vavarigou A, Bardin CL, Behary K, Chemtob S, Papageorgiou A and Arande JV, "Early ibuprofen administration to prevent ductus arteriosus in premature newborn infants," *Journal of the American Medical Association* **275** (1996): 539–544.

19. Shankar V, Paul VK, Deorari AK and Singh M, "Do neonates with meconium aspiration syndrome require antibiotics?" *Indian Journal of Pediatrics* **62** (1995): 327–331.

20. Baumgart S, "Reduction of oxygen consumption, insensible water loss and radiant heat demand with use of plastic blanket for low birth weight infants under radiant warmers," *Pediatrics* **74** (1984): 1022–1028.

21. Rutter N and Hull D, "Reduction of skin water loss in the newborn I. Effect of applying topical agents," *Archives of Disease in Childhood* **56** (1981): 669–672.

22. Singh M, Rao G, Malhotra AK and Deorari AK, "Assessment of newborn infant's temperature by human touch: A potentially useful primary care strategy," *Indian Pediatrics* **29** (1992): 449–452.

23. Malhotra AK, Deorari AK, Paul VK, Bagga A and Singh M, "A new transport incubator for primary care of low birth weight infants," *Indian Pediatrics* **29** (1992): 587–593.

24. Fardig J, "A comparison of skin-to-skin contact and radiant heaters in promoting neonatal thermoregulation," *Journal of Nurse-Midwifery* **25** (1980): 19–28.

25. Gragge AP, Winslow CEA and Herrington LP, "The influence of clothing on the physiological reactions of the human body to varying environmental temperatures," *American Journal of Physiology* **124** (1938): 30–50.

26. Babson SG and Bramhall JL, "Diet and growth in the premature infants. The effect of different dietary intake of ash-electrolyte and protein on weight gain and linear growth," *Journal of Pediatrics* **74** (1969): 890–900.

27. Gordon HH, Levine SZ and McNamara H, "Feeding of premature infants. A comparison of human and cow's milk," *American Journal of Diseases of Children* **73** (1947): 442–452.

28. Lucas A, Gore SM, Cole TJ *et al.*, "Multicentric trial on feeding low birth weight infants: Effects of diet on early growth," *Archives of Disease in Childhood* **59** (1984): 722–730.

29. Lucas A, Morley R, Cole TJ, Gore SM, Lucas PJ, Crowle P *et al.*, "Early diet in preterm infants and developmental status at 18 months," *Lancet* **335** (1990): 1477–1481.

30. Hess JH, "Oxygen unit for premature and very young infants," *American Journal of Diseases of Children* **47** (1934): 916–917.

31. Goldman NI, Maralit A, Sun S and Lanzkowsky P, "Neonatal cyanosis and arterial oxygen saturation," *Journal of Pediatrics* **82** (1973): 319–324.

32. Klaus M and Meyer BP, "Oxygen therapy for the newborn," *Pediatric Clinics of North America* **13** (1966): 731–752.

33. Kumar RM, Kabra SK and Singh M, "Efficacy and acceptability of different modes of oxygen administration in children: Implications for a community hospital," *Journal of Tropical Paediatrics* **43** (1997): 47–49.

34. Shohat M, Reisner SH, Krikler R, Nissenkorn I, Yassur Y and Ben-Sira I, "Retinopathy of prematurity: Incidence and risk factors," *Pediatrics* **72** (1983): 159–163.

35. Maheshwari R, Kumar H, Paul VK, Singh M, Deorari AK and Tewari HK, "Incidence and risk factors of retinopathy of prematurity in a tertiary care newborn unit in New Delhi," *National Medical Journal of India* **9** (1996): 211–214.

Chapter 22

AUDIT — A TOOL TO IMPROVE THE QUALITY OF PERINATAL CARE

Sophie Mancey-Jones
Research Fellow, London School of Hygiene and Tropical Medicine

Introduction

This chapter reviews the process of perinatal audit and evidence of its value in improving the quality of perinatal health care in developing countries.

The World Health Organization (WHO) estimates that globally there were 7.6 million perinatal deaths in 1995, of which 98% occurred in developing countries.[1] Ecological studies have shown an inverse relationship between the perinatal mortality rates (PNMRs) of different countries and the percentage of deliveries attended by a trained attendant. While confounding may contribute to this association, the report stated that it is likely that up to half of the perinatal deaths per year occur as a direct consequence of poorly managed deliveries.[1] Attention should be focussed on making competent attendants accessible to all, with effective referral when needed. However, unfortunately, there is evidence that even women who deliver in institutions may not receive the best care given the resources available. In developing countries, sub-optimal care has been identified in up to 77% of perinatal deaths in hospital based studies.[2] By improving the quality of care overall, perinatal audit aims to reduce these avoidable adverse outcomes.

Audit aims to improve care through ongoing, critical examination of activities against an agreed standard, leading to identification of opportunities for improvement so as to facilitate appropriate change and bring practice closer to the standard. Audit is now common in industrialised countries and there is increasing interest in its potential in developing countries.[3] Reports of apparently successful audit activities have been published from India,[4,5] China,[6] the Caribbean[7] and Africa.[2,8-10]

Before instituting an audit, policy makers and practitioners need to reach an agreement in understanding its purpose, process and limitations. There are many perceptions of what is meant by audit and this chapter clarifies some of the issues surrounding audit — concentrating on the process of local, hospital based audit of perinatal health care.

Definition of audit

Audit has been defined as "a systematic, critical analysis of the quality of medical care, including the procedures used for diagnosis and treatment, the use of resources and the resulting outcome for the patient".[11] A broader understanding of audit also includes the specific identification of deficiencies compared to a defined standard and the implementation and ongoing evaluation of recommended changes.

Once an area is chosen for audit there are five components common to all models of audit, known as the "audit cycle" (Figure 1).

The overall aim of audit in the health services is to achieve optimal health outcomes in the most efficient way.

The mechanisms by which audit may achieve higher quality of care are by:

1. Identifying errors in current activities and changing practice towards an agreed standard.
2. Ongoing education of health workers, leading to improved attitudes, skills and knowledge.
3. Motivating health workers and increasing accountability.
4. Improving communication between different specialities involved in health care.

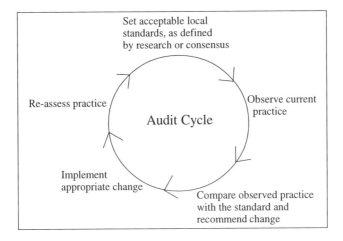

Figure 1 The audit cycle.

5. Improving the reliability and validity of data, to be used for needs assessment and planning for resource allocation.
6. A stimulus for further research.

The Perinatal Audit Process

Perinatal audit may involve looking at the process and outcomes of perinatal care. Monitoring perinatal outcomes is useful for the evaluation of interventions and may identify broad problem areas but, alone, outcome monitoring cannot identify the specific underlying constraints to high quality care and therefore has limited potential in informing appropriate, targeted recommendations.

Audit of and setting standards for outcome of perinatal care

Maternal and perinatal mortality rates have been used as indicators of the impact of perinatal health care. The analyses of maternal and neonatal morbidity rates have also been explored as an alternative,[12,13] but there are difficulties, particularly in developing countries, in valid comparisons of morbidity levels; a lack of standard definitions leads to misclassification and there may be reporting bias and inadequate methods for validation of data.

Unfortunately, in developing countries, perinatal deaths remain common enough events for the PNMR to be a sensitive and responsive indicator for measuring health status. Within any one setting it may not be possible to set definitive "acceptable" standards for levels of crude or cause-specific PNMRs and therefore comparison should be against recent PNMR trends and rates in other similar facilities.

Observation of the outcome of perinatal care

The reliability of perinatal mortality data may be low. It has been estimated that one-third of the world's population is not included in vital registration collection systems[1] and even in developed countries there may be inconsistencies in reporting.[14–17]

Livebirths may be more likely to be reported than stillbirths and early neonatal deaths, e.g. in Cameroon only 6% of perinatal deaths and 62% of births were picked up by the routine registration system[18] and in a study in Thailand there was 100% under-reporting of perinatal deaths in one district.[19]

If a delivery register is maintained it should be possible to more accurately monitor institution based perinatal outcome although there is some ambiguity in the classification of early stillbirths and abortions. At the local level, all deliveries with birthweights over 500 gm should be recorded as a stillbirth, but for international comparison only birth weights over 1,000 g are included.[1] First-week neonatal deaths may be missed if they occur after early discharge.

Comparing observed perinatal outcomes

Even when accurate, variations in the institutional crude PNMR may not be a valid reflection of the quality of perinatal health services. Observed differences may be due to substantial variations in the characteristics of the case-mix presenting for maternity care, especially in developing country settings, where only a minority of deliveries occur in institutions. Review of institutional PNMR trends is useful only if considered in the context of the differences in other contributory factors. Detailed data on case-mix characteristics are rarely available but the burden of "high risk" presentations is reflected in the proportion of deliveries which are "unbooked" patients,[20] emergency referrals-in or low birth weight (LBW) deliveries. In the search for a more valid indicator of the quality of perinatal care there was a move to standardise perinatal death measures according to birth weight, calculating a single birth weight-standardised PNMR[21] based on the rationale that birth weight is determined, in large part, by social factors rather than quality of care.[22] However, it is now recognised that the risk of low birth weight can be reduced by effective antenatal care and, therefore, a single, birth weight-standardised PNMR may not be responsive to differences in the quality of antenatal care. It is more useful to present birth weight specific mortality rates.[23]

Formulation of recommendations

If all other potential factors influencing perinatal outcome are equal the observed differences in the crude PNMR may reflect true differences in the quality of care but cannot identify the possible areas of difficulty in care provision.

Categorising further into sub-groups by cause of death provides more specific information. The most detailed diagnosis is classified by the International Classification of Diseases which lists over 300 conditions related to perinatal morbidity and mortality.[24] Apart from the common problem of lack of skills and resources to make very specific diagnoses, such detailed information may not be necessary for effective monitoring of quality of care or for informing planning of future interventions. The aim is to allocate the perinatal deaths into appropriate aetiological categories that have direct clinical implications. A number of broad groupings have been suggested over the years and Wigglesworth's classification[25] is probably the most feasible and useful for developing countries because the five wide groups are easy to recognise and are relevant for planning.

Table 1 Wigglesworth's classification of perinatal deaths and the clinical implications.

Wigglesworth's Classification	Major determinants/clinical implications
1. Congenital malformations	Influenced by genetic and environmental factors, early screening and intervention
2. Normally formed macerated stillbirth	Influenced by events before labour: environmental factors and antenatal care
3. Intrapartum asphyxia (includes birth trauma, fresh stillbirths and neonatal deaths)	Influenced by intrapartum care
4. Conditions associated with immaturity	Influenced by environmental factors and antenatal and neonatal care
5. Specific conditions other than above	

Presentation of perinatal mortality statistics by cause of death in birth weight groups provides information on the probable problem areas. For example, a high proportion of perinatal deaths of normal birth weight from intrapartum asphyxia and birth trauma indicates specific problems with intrapartum care. Further audit of the process of care for these deaths by sentinel event audit with topic audit of problems identified is needed.

Audit of the process of perinatal care

To be effective in improving and maintaining quality care, perinatal audit should concentrate on the process of care and include all components of the audit cycle (Figure 2).

Setting standards for the process of perinatal care, and practice guidelines

Ideally, what is accepted as "standard practice" should be based on evidence from research — considered in the context of available resources and skills.

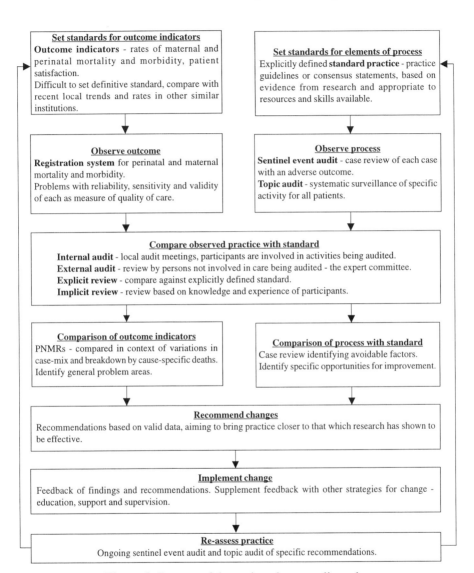

Set standards for outcome indicators
Outcome indicators - rates of maternal and perinatal mortality and morbidity, patient satisfaction.
Difficult to set definitive standard, compare with recent local trends and rates in other similar institutions.

Set standards for elements of process
Explicitly defined **standard practice** - practice guidelines or consensus statements, based on evidence from research and appropriate to resources and skills available.

Observe outcome
Registration system for perinatal and maternal mortality and morbidity.
Problems with reliability, sensitivity and validity of each as measure of quality of care.

Observe process
Sentinel event audit - case review of each case with an adverse outcome.
Topic audit - systematic surveillance of specific activity for all patients.

Compare observed practice with standard
Internal audit - local audit meetings, participants are involved in activities being audited.
External audit - review by persons not involved in care being audited - the expert committee.
Explicit review - compare against explicitly defined standard.
Implicit review - review based on knowledge and experience of participants.

Comparison of outcome indicators
PNMRs - compared in context of variations in case-mix and breakdown by cause-specific deaths.
Identify general problem areas.

Comparison of process with standard
Case review identifying avoidable factors.
Identify specific opportunities for improvement.

Recommend changes
Recommendations based on valid data, aiming to bring practice closer to that which research has shown to be effective.

Implement change
Feedback of findings and recommendations. Supplement feedback with other strategies for change - education, support and supervision.

Re-assess practice
Ongoing sentinel event audit and topic audit of specific recommendations.

Figure 2 Process of the perinatal care audit cycle.

A consensus based on the best clinical judgement needs to be reached where no conclusive research evidence is available.

To facilitate effective audit written statements of acceptable "standard practice" should be available in the form of practice guidelines or protocols. Where no written guidelines exist the "standard" against which current practice is compared is defined, retrospectively, as how competent colleagues would have acted in the same circumstances — this is known as "implicit" review. Such a "standard" can be ambiguous and subjective — it may be biased by differences in the professional opinions and experience of the assessors. Such review of care depends on the knowledge and expertise of those involved in the review and may be less productive if there is no specialist, as in many health centres and hospitals in developing countries.

Formulating effective, appropriate and feasible guidelines is not easy.[26,27] The clinicians need to have access to valid research findings and to the skill needed to apply these in their given context. Where such expertise is not widely available it is most appropriate that a central panel of experts produce national level guidelines that can be adapted to local needs.

There may be resistance to the introduction of explicit treatment guidelines if they are seen as being insensitive to the needs of individual patients, as compromising the professional autonomy of the clinician, discouraging innovation or "providing ammunition" for lawyers in alleged negligence cases.[28] However, in developing countries, where health workers' knowledge and skills may be limited, there is a particularly strong argument for using treatment guidelines[29] where they can lead directly to improved quality of care as well as facilitating audit.

Observing the process of perinatal care

The process of care can be assessed by the analysis of sentinel events or by a topic audit.

Sentinel event audit

Sentinel event audit involves reviewing cases that have resulted in a pre-specified, usually adverse, outcome. The sentinel events taken for analysis are usually perinatal and maternal deaths, but near-miss episodes and cases resulting in maternal or neonatal morbidity also may provide useful information. The case review is mainly informed by case note review and, therefore, is dependent on the quality and honesty of note keeping. Further information is obtained by interviewing the relevant health workers, the patients, and their relatives.

Sentinel event audit is the more common type of audit reported from developing countries where resources are often limited for the monitoring of quality of care. By concentrating on cases with adverse outcomes it is the most efficient way to identify potentially correctable problems.

Topic audit

Topic audit is the systematic surveillance of an activity for all patients and can provide more data to inform targeted recommendations for this specific activity. The activity chosen for a topic audit may be identified during the sentinel event audit. For example, if one perinatal death was deemed avoidable because antepartum syphilis was not treated, the underlying reason for this error may be unclear. A topic audit looking at the ascertainment of syphilis serology status and treatment in all patients will provide more information on difficulties with current practice. Topic audit is also valuable for the follow-up of recommendations and for maintaining motivation. Often, sentinel event audit focusses on adverse outcomes and can be demoralising; topic audit can also highlight the positive impact of care.

The close monitoring involved in topic audit requires extra organisation and resources. While it may not be feasible to continue the topic audit in the long term at least one cycle must be completed, i.e. to the stage where recommendations from the first review have been implemented and performance has been re-assessed. Where unsatisfactory improvements are noted after this second review a further cycle may be needed. As more problems are identified during ongoing sentinel event audit, new topic audits exploring these areas can be instituted.

Simply as a response to the surveillance involved in a topic audit, performance may improve: the Hawthorne effect. This is not a problem since this is the ultimate aim of the audit process but where long-term, systematic surveillance of a number of different activities is not feasible and monitoring stops, practice may deteriorate again. Therefore, future intermittent surveillance of specific activities in random cases is recommended.

The forum for the analysis of audit information

The most appropriate forum for the analysis of information collected during perinatal audit depends on its context. "External audit" — the national or regional "expert committee" — has the advantages of the superior knowledge, experience and objectivity of the experts and, in having more cases for review, can reach more generalisable conclusions. However, "internal audit" — the local, multi-disciplinary, perinatal audit meeting — has more advantages. The participants have more local knowledge on which to base appropriate recommendations. The inclusion of persons directly involved in the patient care has a direct impact on furthering their education and may facilitate change since staff feel "ownership" of the recommendations.[30]

Although internal audit should be an integral part of the work of the department there should also be a nominated co-ordinator who is allowed "protected time" for audit work. The timing of the meetings depends on balancing the "cost" of preparing for and attending regular meetings against the "cost" of information that may be lost if there is too long an interval between meetings. The shorter the time lag from an event to feedback, the greater the impact on implementing change.[31] Everyone involved in perinatal care, including referring clinic staff, should attend the meetings. This improves communication between health workers and allows further exploration of the different inputs into the care process. Junior medical and nursing staff should be encouraged to contribute with case presentations, feedback and suggestions and a senior should act as chairman to ensure that the discussion remains focussed, objective, and professional. Confidentiality is essential for protecting the patients' privacy and for facilitating more open and less threatening discussion, and reduces concern that the material could be used in medical negligence claims.

Process of comparison of observations and standard

Provided explicit treatment protocols exist, even relatively unskilled staff can identify observed departures from these guidelines and discuss reasons for these errors. Such divergences from the guidelines may be defined as "sub-optimal care". Where it may have contributed to the death such an episode may be known as an "avoidable factor". There are problems with the concept of "avoidablity". In identifying an adverse factor in care, one cannot be certain if, in the absence of that factor, death would have been prevented. The identification of "avoidable factors" may be perceived by health workers as being too judgmental and, therefore, review must be maintained on an objective level, ensuring that the process is seen to be corrective, not punitive, with emphasis on evolving a policy to prevent recurrence of the mistake, not on apportioning blame.

Formulation of recommendations

Recommendations that evolve as a result of the findings of audit must be based on valid information. The limitations of audit need to be borne in mind. The aim is to ensure that interventions found to be effective by research are included in practice; audit cannot provide valid data on which to base a new treatment, although it may generate a hypothesis on which to base further research. The recommendations must aim at remedying the underlying problems that have been identified as preventing implementation of effective interventions.

The recommendations must be feasible and appropriate to the resources available. For example, in one audit in Singapore[32] the presence of a lethal congenital malformation that could have been diagnosed by effective antenatal screening is categorised as avoidable and a resulting recommendation is for an improved system of antenatal screening. In a rural African hospital such a perinatal death would not be deemed avoidable and advocating universal ultrasonic antenatal screening would not be a practical recommendation.

Implementing change

The activity of audit up to this stage of the cycle may in itself have some benefit by the Hawthorne effect and by providing a forum for education and improved communication between colleagues. However, there is no point in audit unless action results.[33] The "action" should be determined by the rational and appropriate recommendations formulated at the multi-disciplinary audit meeting.

The potential for successful change depends on the people involved and on the context, content and process of the proposed change.[34] The health workers must recognise the need for improvement and be willing to participate in the audit process. They must have an understanding of the concept of audit as a problem-solving exercise — imposing an audit on unwilling health workers is unlikely to have a positive impact. Successful change has occurred where the implementers are involved in the decision making and have a sense of ownership of the process.[30,35,36] A good internal audit process which involves everyone should, therefore, facilitate implementation.

The local cultural context influences the approach to change — where it is non-threatening, open and accepting of the concept of "constructive criticism" there is a better chance of successfully implementing the proposed change. Success is also more likely where the recommendations are simple, recognised as effective and represent only a small incremental change from current practice, are appropriate to the level of resources, and compatible with current beliefs and practices.[37]

Even when there is systematic feedback to all the relevant practitioners and they acknowledge the need for the change, they may fail to change practice.[38] In recommending change a number of parallel strategies should be used which may include recognition of positive behaviour, education activities with presentation of supportive evidence from research, supervision, and follow-up audit. Rarely, administrative regulations may be needed.

Re-assessing practice

To complete the audit cycle, practice must be observed again after the recommendations have been implemented. Ideally, any recommendations resulting from sentinel event audit should be followed up with a specific topic audit, however, as discussed earlier, this is often not feasible with available resources. Continuing sentinel event case review is more practical — identifying new problems and incidences when the same difficulties recur.

Does Perinatal Audit Work?

In the UK, the first Royal College of Physicians report on clinical audit stated that measuring the benefits of audit is difficult and "it is a matter of faith that it benefits clinical practice"[33] but, as for any activity that has opportunity costs, assessment of the utility of audit is needed to inform policy makers whether audit is worth the investment of resources and, if it is effective, which features contribute to its success.

Evaluations of impact of perinatal audit in developing countries

Rates of maternal and perinatal mortality and morbidity can be taken as impact indicators for the effectiveness of audit in improving quality of care. Most published reports are from Africa and have been observational time series studies. These have used variations in the perinatal mortality rates as the main outcome measure (Table 2).

A significant reduction in crude PNMRs is reported after the introduction of some audits.[8,10,39,40] Variations in the case-mix of patients presenting were thought to have affected the crude PNMR in some hospitals, therefore, further analysis by cause of death is presented. Intrapartum deaths are commonly associated with sub-optimal care[2,10,44,45] and therefore the proportion of intrapartum deaths may be taken as a proxy indicator for sub-optimal care[10] and Bugalho and Bergstrom[9] report significant reductions in the proportion of intrapartum deaths during the course of their perinatal audits. In South Africa, Wilkinson reports a significant reduction in the

Table 2 Reported impact of published perinatal audits in developing countries.

Country (reference)	Audit process and outcomes	Authors conclusions
Zimbabwe 1984–1986 (2)	Analysis of 319 perinatal deaths in a district hospital and clinics. PNMR = 30.6/1,000 and 76% had avoidable factors	"By identifying avoidable factors in perinatal deaths, interventions could be targeted to reduce perinatal mortality."
Lebowa, South Africa 1988–1989 (8)	Over two years of internal audit the the PNMR decreased (60/1,000 to 41/1,000: $p < 0.005$). The proportion with avoidable factors decreased (28% to 13%: $p < 0.05$)	"Perinatal audit … is an effective method of detecting preventable deaths' and can increase efficiency."
Mozambique 1982–1991 (9)	Over 10 years of routine internal audit the PNMR did not change significantly (75.1/1,000 to 78.5/1,000) despite an increase in the proportion of high risk presentations. Decrease in proportion with avoidable factors (11% to 5%: $p < 0.001$)	Audit constitutes the "very basis of the sustainable improvement of existing perinatal services."
Hlabisa, South Africa 1991–1993 (39, 40)	Over a two-year audit of 288 perinatal deaths in hospital and village clinics the PNMR increased (29/1,000 to 39/1,000) as the proportion of high risk presentations increased, but the proportion with avoidable factors decreased (19% to 3%; $p < 0.01$)	"Regular feedback of results demonstrating improvement maintains motivation and interest amongst staff."
Port Elizabeth, South Africa 1991–1992 (10)	Over a two-year audit of 444 perinatal deaths in a central and 2 district hospitals the PNMR decreased (52.8/1,000 to 40.6/1,000: $p < 0.05$) and the proportion with avoidable factors decreased (20% to 9%: $p < 0.001$)	"Careful audit and increased vigilance are, in themselves, an intervention of value."

Table 2 (*Continued*)

Country (reference)	Audit process and outcomes	Authors conclusions
Pretoria, South Africa 1991–1994 (44, 45)	Over a two-year audits of 202 perinatal deaths in all facilities in an urban area the PNMR decreased (26.6/1,000 to 16.6/1,000)	"The use of this system of classification of avoidable factors has enabled the detection of problem areas that can be improved immediately and at very little cost."

proportion of perinatal deaths associated with avoidable factors after the introduction of perinatal audit in a couple of hospitals.[8,39,40]

These reports all conclude that perinatal audit process lead to improved perinatal care, but care needs to be exercised in generalising the results. Their success may be dependant on the commitment and enthusiasm of the co-ordinating clinicians; imposing perinatal audit on poorly motivated health workers may not meet with similar positive results. The reports contain limited information on the previous local trends in PNMRs, the national or neighbouring trends during the same period, or on concurrent interventions or changes in case-mix. Also, a review of published audits is open to publication bias — audit that has been unsuccessful is less likely to be reported or published.

Evaluations of the process of perinatal audit

The processes by which audit aims to achieve optimal care — changing practice towards a standard, improving practitioner education, motivation and accountability, and improving communication — could be assessed by measures of change in knowledge, attitudes, and practice.

None of the identified reports of perinatal audit in developing countries included a systematic evaluation of the effect of the audit on specific elements of practice. Reports from industrialised countries suggest that the effect of the feedback on practice is highly dependant on the context and content of the audit and so generalisation of the results is difficult.[31,41–43] However, they do conclude that while feedback is necessary in maintaining high quality clinical care, alone it may not be sufficient. "Passive feedback", the circulation of data with no stated recommendations, was found to have no impact on clinical practice. "Active feedback", data with specific recommendations, would appear to be successful in changing practice, although this may be only short term if there is no follow-up.

The audit reports from developing countries often identified avoidable factors relating to poor health worker skills and, as a result, targeted education programmes and explicit practice guidelines were instituted, but the impact of these on actual practice is not reported. There are a number of statements on the role of audit in improving motivation and communication, but these are not substantiated with qualitative data. On discussion with key informants with experience of perinatal audit in developing countries, most felt that involvement in audit activities was of overall benefit to them, stimulating interest and motivating good practice. However, there were reservations. The repetitive nature of meetings with the identification of recurrent, apparently intractable, problems had a demoralising effect, especially when these problems were related to resource constraints. Also, discussion on health workers' performance was sometimes seen as threatening, leading to worsening relations rather than improved communication.

Conclusion

If perinatal audit is generated internally and conducted by well-informed, committed people with an understanding of the process and its limitations, it has the potential to improve quality of care. However, effective audit is not simple and a poorly structured audit may detract from care, if energy and time are wasted on collecting unused data or if poorly managed meetings create a punitive atmosphere resulting in the breakdown of staff relations.

Despite methodological problems with their evaluations, reports of perinatal audit in developing countries are encouraging, showing a positive impact on crude and cause-specific PNMRs. However, any positive impact of audit is dependent on the participants' understanding and acceptance of the audit process, their commitment to change and improvement, and to the time and resources available to implement it.

In a developing country context:

1. Audit must be acceptable to the health workers. Before instituting audit, the participating health workers must be fully informed about the purpose and limitations of audit. Attitudes about self-evaluation need to be positive and it must not appear threatening or punitive.
2. Health workers should be involved at all stages and have a sense of ownership of the process.
3. The process, structure, and content of the audit must be well planned and appropriate to the resources available and the level of services being audited.
4. There should be a nominated audit co-ordinator who is allowed time away from other duties for audit work.
5. Comparison of PNMRs can be a valid indicator of quality of care only if considered in the context of variations in the case-mix presenting.
6. In most facilities in developing countries, the formulation of practice guidelines is required; implicit review by relatively unskilled and poorly informed health workers is of limited value.
7. Sentinel event audit identifies episodes of sub-optimal care but must be supplemented by topic audit to follow-up recommendations and to present evidence of positive practice.
8. Recommendations from audit must be appropriate and aim to bring practice closer to that which research or consensus on best clinical judgement indicates to be effective.
9. Other supplementary strategies are required to implement the changes recommended by audit. The feedback of recommendations from audit alone may not be sufficient to successfully change practice.

References

1. WHO, "Perinatal mortality. A listing of available information," World Heath Organization FRH/MSM/96.7, Geneva (1996).

2. De Muylder X, "Perinatal audit in a Zimbabwean district," *Paediatric and Perinatal Epidemiology* **3** (1989): 284–293.
3. Maher D, "Clinical audit in a developing country," *Tropical Medicine and International Health* **1** (1996): 409–413.
4. Bhatt RV, "Professional responsibility in maternal care: The role of medical audit," *International Journal of Obstetrics & Gynecology* **30** (1989): 47–50.
5. Srinivasan V, "Peer review among district health officers in Maharashtra, India," *International Journal of Obstetrics & Gynecology* **30** (1989): 33–36.
6. Yan RY, "How Chinese clinicians contribute to the improvement of maternity care," *International Journal of Obstetrics & Gynecology* **30** (1989): 23–26.
7. de Caunes F, Greg RA, Berchael C *et al.*, "The Guadeloupean perinatal mortality audit: Process, results, and implications," *American Journal of Preventive Medicine* **6**(6) (1990): 339–345.
8. Wilkinson D, "Perinatal mortality — An intervention study," *South African Medical Journal* **79** (1991): 552–553.
9. Bugalho A and Bergstrom S, "The value of perinatal audit in obstetric care in the developing world: A ten-year experience of the Maputo model," *Gynecological Obstetric Investigation* **36** (1993): 239–243.
10. Ward HRG, Howarth GR, Jennings OJN and Pattinson RC, "Audit incorporating avoidability and appropriate intervention can significantly decrease perinatal mortality," *South African Medical Journal* **85**(3) (1995): 147–150.
11. Secretary of State for Health, "Working for patients," Cmnd 555, HMSO, London (1989).
12. Field DJ, Smith H, Mason E and Milner AD, "Is perinatal mortality still a good indicator of perinatal care?" *Paediatric and Perinatal Epidemiology* **2** (1988): 213–219.
13. Stones W, Lim W, Al-Azzawi F and Kelly M, "An investigation of maternal morbidity with identification of life-threatening 'near-miss' episodes," *Health Trends* **23**(1) (1991): 13–14.
14. Scott MJ, Ritchie JWK, Mc Clune BG *et al.*, "Perinatal death recording: Time for a change?" *British Medical Journal* **282** (1981): 707–710.
15. Mugford M, "A comparison of reported differences in definitions of vital events and statistics," *World Health Statistic Quarterly* **36** (1983): 201–205.
16. Kleineman JC, "Underreporting of infant deaths: Then and now," *American Journal of Public Health* **76** (1986): 365–366.
17. Keirse MJNC, "Perinatal mortality rates do not contain what they purport to contain," *Lancet* **26** (1984): 1166–1167.

18. Ndong I, Gloyd S and Gale J, "An evaluation of vital registers as sources of data for infant mortality rates in Cameroon," *International Journal of Epidemiology* **23** (1994): 536–539.

19. Lumbiganon P, Panamonta M, Laopaiboon M *et al.*, "Why are Thai official perinatal and infant mortality rates so low?" *International Journal of Epidemiology* **19** (1990): 997–1000.

20. Fawcus SR, Crowther CA, van Balen P, Marumahoko J, "Booked and unbooked mothers delivering at Harare Maternity Hospital, Zimbabwe: A comparison of characteristics and fetal outcome," *Central African Journal of Medicine* **38** (1992): 402–408.

21. Mallet R and Knox EG, "Standardised perinatal mortality ratios: Technique, utility and interpretation." *Community Medicine* **1** (1979): 6–13.

22. Ashford JR, Read KLQ and Riley VC, "An analysis of variations in perinatal mortality amongst local authorities in England and Wales," *International Journal of Epidemiology* **2** (1973): 31–46.

23. Chalmers I, Newcombe R, West R *et al.*, "Adjusted perinatal mortality rates in administrative areas of England and Wales," *Health Trends* **10** (1978): 24–29.

24. *WHO International Statistical Classification of Diseases and Related Health*, 10th ed., WHO, Geneva (1992).

25. Wigglesworth JS, "Monitoring perinatal mortality. A pathophysiological approach," *Lancet* (1980): 684–686.

26. Grimshaw JM and Russell IT, "Achieving health gain through clinical guidelines I: Developing scientifically valid guidelines," *Quality in Health Care* **2** (1993): 243–248.

27. Grimshaw JM and Russell IT, "Achieving health gain through clinical guidelines II: Ensuring guidelines change medical practice," *Quality in Health Care* **3** (1994): 45–53.

28. Barron SL, "Audit in obstetrics," *British Journal of Obstetrics and Gynecology* **98** (1991): 1065–1072.

29. Larsen JV, "Reducing the perinatal mortality rates in developing countries," *Tropical Doctor* **22** (1992): 49–51.

30. Stocking B, "Promoting change in clinical care," *Quality in Health Care* **1** (1992): 56–60.

31. Mugford M, Banfield P and O'Hanlon M, "Effects of feedback of information on clinical practice: A review," *British Medical Journal* **303** (1991): 398–402.

32. Biswas A, Chew S, Joseph R *et al.*, "Towards improved perinatal care — Perinatal audit," *Annals of the Academy of Medicine (Singapore)* **24**(2) (1995): 213–216.

33. The Royal College of Physicians, "Medical audit: A first report," What, why and how?" The Royal College of Physicians, London (1989).
34. Walt G, *Health policy: An Introduction to Process and Power*, Zed Books, London (1994).
35. Atkinson C and Hayden J, "Managing change in primary care. Strategies for success," *British Medical Journal* **304** (1992): 1488–1490.
36. Greco PJ and Eisenberg JM, "Changing physicians practices," *New England Journal of Medicine* **329** (1993): 1271–1273.
37. Cleaves P, "Implementation amidst scarcity and apathy: Political power and policy design," In: *Politics and Policy Implementation in the Third World*, Grindle M, ed., Princeton University Press, New Jersey (1980).
38. Lomas J, Enkin M, Anderson GM *et al.*, "Opinion leaders vs audit and feedback to implement practice guidelines," *Journal of the American Medical Association* **265**(17) (1991): 2202–2207.
39. Wilkinson D, "Statistics of perinatal mortality due to error or omission: A suggestion of how to improve care," *Tropical Doctor* **23 July** (1993): 119–121.
40. Wilkinson D, "Avoidable perinatal deaths in a rural hospital: Strategies to improve quality of care," *Tropical Doctor* **25** (1995): 16–20.
41. Mitchell MW and Fowkes FGR, "Audit reviewed: Does feedback on performance change clinical behaviour?" *Journal of the Royal College of Physicians of London* **19** (1985): 251–253.
42. Mooney G and Ryan M, "Rethinking medical audit: The goal is efficiency," *Journal of Epidemiology and Community Medicine* **46** (1992): 180–183.
43. Robinson MB, "Evaluation of medical audit," *Journal of Epidemiology and Community Health* **48** (1994): 435–440.
44. Pattinson RC, Makin JD, Shaw A and Delport SD, "The value of incorporating avoidable factors into perinatal audits," *South African Medical Journal* **85** (1995): 145–146.
45. Pattinson RC, de Jonge E, Pistorius LR *et al.*, "Practical application of data obtained from a Perinatal Problem Identification Programme," *South African Medical Journal* **85** (1995): 131–132.

Chapter 23

TRAINED TRADITIONAL BIRTH ATTENDANTS AND ESSENTIAL NEWBORN CARE IN SOUTH ASIA

Marta J. Levitt-Dayal
*Country Director, Centre for Development
and Populations Activities (CEDPA), India*

Introduction

Neonatal morbidity and mortality is probably the least understood and most neglected health issue in the developing world today. Each year five million newborns die in the first month,[1] 1.7 million in South Asia alone.[2] South Asian newborns have a ten times greater risk of dying before the first month of life than those in developed countries. In the past 15 years, infant mortality has fallen by one-third in South Asia as a result of sharp reductions in deaths due to infectious diseases.[3] Since 1980 deaths due to neonatal tetanus have been halved throughout the world, but generally, post-neonatal infant mortality is declining at a faster pace than neonatal deaths. In Nepal, for example, neonatal mortality now accounts for two-thirds of all infant deaths.[4]

South Asia is a region of cultural, geographic and socio-economic diversity. There is wide variation in literacy rates, gross national incomes, maternal and infant mortality rates, contraceptive prevalence, and fertility levels[5] (and see Chapters 1 and 2). The proportion of births attended by a trained health worker varies from 9% in Nepal to 94% in Sri Lanka. Access to health services also varies within countries depending on transportation availability, infrastructural development, remoteness, urbanisation, and socio-economic development of the area. In Sri Lanka, where educational levels are high, access to health care is relatively high except in areas of civil unrest; in India, there is a strong infrastructure which provides access to health care even though people may not be as highly educated. In Nepal, with low literacy rates, extreme geographic remoteness and a low level of infrastructure, you find poor access to health care.

Traditional Birth Attendants and Training in South Asia

Definition

Traditional birth attendants, known as TBAs or local/village/lay midwives, are persons (usually women) who attend deliveries and provide other maternity-related services, without formal training. They usually learn from experience or under the tutelage of an older, more experienced TBA. Once a TBA receives formal training from an organisation or health professional, they are known as a trained TBA, or TTBA. Often the abbreviation TBA has been confused with the term 'trained birth attendant'. For clarity, trained traditional birth attendants will be referred to as as TTBAs and untrained traditional birth attendants as TBAs. Levitt and Minden describe the history and current situation of TBA training:

"The value of village midwives as a local maternal health resource was recognized as early as the 1920s. By the 1970s and 1980s training of TBAs had become an integral component of 'mother and child' health programmes, ...their role... [focussed] on child survival... In less developed countries, TBAs remain the major provider of care for childbearing women at the community level. The vast majority of women (73%) in the least developed world and 45% in developing countries deliver without the assistance of any trained birth attendant, compared to only 2%...in developed countries... The training of TBAs in community health has expanded over the past 10 years to include immunisation, identification and treatment of diarrhoea and ARI, and community-based distribution of oral rehydration therapy (ORT) packets and safe birth kits."[9]

Coverage

It is difficult to generalise about the use of and potential or actual impact of training TBAs. In South Asia, the types of TBA vary considerably in different communities: in some TBAs are used almost universally, in others relatives attend to most deliveries, and in more urban or developed areas, such as Sri Lanka, most deliveries are in institutions. In some communities, TBAs are only cord cutters, while in others the TBA plays a larger role in the delivery process. For example, in the southern belt of Nepal and adjoining areas of Northern India, TBAs are from untouchable castes and are called to cut the umbilical cord and clean soiled items from the delivery; in other areas of Nepal and India, TBAs attend the delivery but may not cut the cord. In Tibetan or Buddhist societies, such as Bhutan, there is usually no tradition of a TBA.

TBA training has been one strategy used in to reduce perinatal mortality rates for over a century, especially in India, Pakistan, Bangladesh and Nepal where the use of TBAs is widespread. In India, TBA training is well established and TTBAs receive a monetary incentive for each delivery they conduct and register. In Bangladesh, TBA training is conducted by both government and non-governmental organisations in a concerted manner, with the government providing training materials and supplies for NGOs training TBAs. In Pakistan from 1981 to 1990, health professionals trained 50,000 TBAs. In Nepal, the national TBA programme covers 55 of the 75 districts and, since 1973, approximately 15,000 TBAs have received training.

Content of TBA training

The content of TBA training varies but, generally, includes referral of mothers for tetanus toxoid immunisation, referral for high risk or complicated cases, clean delivery, discouragement of harmful practices, immediate care of the mother and newborn infant, and promotion of immediate and exclusive breastfeeding. Some programmes teach TBAs how to do antenatal and postnatal exams, provide family planning counselling and contraceptive distribution, and distribute or market disposable clean delivery kits. In India, special projects have even taught TBAs to manage birth asphyxia using mask-to-mouth resuscitation and the use of mucus suction traps, and to weigh newborns to identify low birth weight (LBW) babies.

TTBAs and Essential Neonatal Care in South Asia

While the Safe Motherhood Initiative (SMI) includes care of the newborn infant, as illustrated in the WHO publication "The Mother-Baby Package", many interventions proven to benefit the newborn, but which do not save the life of the mother during an obstetric emergency, are given relatively low priority. Prenatal care, for example, has been shown in many studies to increase neonatal survival yet is a low priority intervention for Safe Motherhood (SM) programmes as it has been found to have little value in predicting obstetric emergencies. TBA training has been proven to reduce neonatal deaths but many SM proponents devalue its usefulness since TBAs are unable to manage obstetric emergencies that require surgery, blood transfusions, or chemotherapy.

In order to identify appropriate neonatal interventions, it is necessary to be aware of the factors which are directly and indirectly related to neonatal death and survival:

- The nutritional health status of mother and health care received during pregnancy,
- The birth process,
- Care after birth.

The mother's physical condition, as well as complications of pregnancy and delivery, directly and indirectly affect the survival of the newborn as shown in Table 1.

According to the WHO the major causes of neonatal deaths in developing countries in 1993 included birth asphyxia, birth injuries, neonatal tetanus, pneumonia, congenital abnormalities, and prematurity (see Table 2).[11] Of these almost half (42%) were due to infections such as neonatal tetanus, sepsis, meningitis, pneumonia and diarrhoea. Two-thirds of infections in newborns were contracted during the birth process. Most of the neonatal deaths are early neonatal deaths as indicated in a recent Demographic and

Table 1 Effects of maternal complications on the newborn infant.[13]

Maternal complications in pregnancy and delivery	*Adverse effects on the newborn*
Severe anaemia	LBW, asphyxia, stillbirth
Haemorrhage	Asphyxia, stillbirth
Hypertensive disorders	LBW, asphyxia, stillbirth
Unclean delivery	Neonatal tetanus, sepsis
Obstructed labour	Asphyxia, sepsis, stillbirth, disabilities
Unwanted Pregnancy	Increased risk of morbidity, child abuse, neglect, abandonment
Infection during pregnancy, such as STDs or malaria	Prematurity, neonatal eye infections, blindness, pneumonia, stillbirth and congenital syphillis, LBW

Health Survey conducted in Nepal which found that 63% of neonatal deaths occur in the first six days of life.[12]

As part of the Safe Motherhood Program, essential elements of newborn care are recommended. These include:[14]

- clean and safe delivery,
- clean cord cutting and care,
- drying and wrapping the baby,
- establishing breathing, resuscitation if necessary,
- keeping the baby warm,
- putting the baby to the breast,
- preventing blindness,
- keeping mother and baby together, and
- immunisation against tuberculosis and polio.

Most of these neonatal-specific interventions have been included in TBA training to increase the chance of neonatal survival and reduce neonatal deaths in the South Asian region. In fact, the region has been a leader in developing and testing these interventions. Table 2 lists the major causes of neonatal deaths in developing countries, indirect causes of neonatal deaths and what skills TBAs in South Asia have been taught in order to reduce the chances of these deaths.

Table 2 Causes of neonatal deaths in developing countries (WHO, 1993) and interventions taught in TBA training,

Causes of neonatal death	% of all neonatal deaths	Indirect factors causing death	Skills taught to TBAs
Birth asphyxia	21	Obstructed or prolonged labour, severe maternal anaemia, haemorrhage, birth attendant does not know how to clear air passages or manage when cord is around neck	Referral for labour > 12 hours or bleeding in pregnancy; identification of signs of anaemia, provision of iron/folate tablets and nutrition advice; clearing of air passages, physical stimulation, resuscitation, and mucus suction
Pneumonia	19	Newborn hypothermia, aspiration of birth fluids, withholding colostrum	Drying and wrapping after birth, discouraging early baths; Kangaroo method; mucus suction, counselling about early breastfeeding; ARI case detection and referral; provision of antibiotics for ARI treatment
Tetanus	14	Unhygienic cord cutting and care, no tetanus immunisation, unclean surfaces or dirty clothes for infant	Counselling family on hygienic preparation of the delivery room; hand washing; use of sterilised cord cutting implements; discouraging application of substances; counselling hygiene for the newborn

Table 2 (*Continued*)

Causes of neonatal death	% of all neonatal deaths	Indirect factors causing death	Skills taught to TBAs
Congenital anomalies	11	Use of drugs, alcohol or tobacco; iodine deficiency; older mothers	Discouraging the use of unprescribed medication, alcohol and tobacco during pregnancy; promoting iodised salt; counselling on family planning
Birth injury	11	Harmful traditional practices like pulling on limbs, or the head, pushing on fundus, external inversion	Allowing the baby to be born without interference; detection and referral of malpresentations and multiple births; discontinuation of harmful practices
Prematurity, LBW	10	Anaemia, poor diet, age < 18 or > 35 years, presence of an STD; inappropriate care of a premature/LBW newborn resulting in poor feeding, hypothermia, infections	Pre-pregnancy family planning advice; prenatal nutrition advice and iron/folate; identification of STDs and referral; teaching Kangaroo method; expressing breast milk and spoon feeding of premature newborns
Sepsis	7	See neonatal tetanus	Use of the three or six cleans during delivery and cord care; advice on personal hygiene; detection of signs of infection and referral

Table 2 (*Continued*)

Causes of neonatal death	% of all neonatal deaths	Indirect factors causing death	Skills taught to TBAs
Diarrhoea	2	Poor hygiene of mother or newborn, giving non-breast milk products, dirty bottles, withholding colostrum, or restricting fluids during diarrhoea	Promotion of early, exclusive breastfeeding 0 to 4 months; strong discouragement of bottle feeding; advice about hand washing; advice to increase breastfeeding during diarrhoea; preparation and use of ORS
Other causes	5	Lack of prenatal care	Provision of routine prenatal care and referral if concern; identification of high risk pregnancies.
Total:	100%		

Cord Care

To prevent infections due to tetanus and cord sepsis, disposable clean home delivery kits (DDKs) are produced and distributed or marketed in India, Bangladesh and Nepal and imported and used in Bhutan. DDKs contain the essential items needed to follow the "three, or more recently the six, cleans" recommended by the WHO, i.e. clean hands, clean surface and clean cord. These kits contain items such as soap, clean cord ties, a plastic sheet for the delivery surface, a new razor blade, a gauze piece or instructions not to put anything on the cord, a nail stick and pictoral insert.[15] In Nepal, a clean plastic disc is put to replace the use of a betel nut or coin used for the cord cutting surface.

In India, a WHO study investigated the incidence of cord and puerperal sepsis among three types of DDKs and a control group. It was found that those using both the gamma-irradiated DDK and a clean DDK had significantly lower rates of both cord and puerperal infections. For example, they found that the occurrence of cord infection occurrence when a trained TBA used the clean or gamma-irradiated kits was 1.3 and 2.4% respectively, while the rate for the control group (untrained persons using traditional equipment) was 21.5%.[16]

Hypothermia and Maintenance of Body Temperature

Neonatal hypothermia is a serious problem in South Asia, especially in northern parts of India, Bangladesh, and Pakistan, and in Bhutan and Nepal. A village-based study of hypothermia in Nepal, for instance, taught TBAs to take rectal temperatures of newborns using thermometers marked at 35°C. This study found that 58% of the newborns born between the months of January–March had a rectal temperature of < 35°C within 12 hours of birth.[17] In addition to climatic reasons for hypothermia, and probably more important, are the birthing and newborn care practices which put the newborn at risk of hypothermia; practices such as leaving the baby, still wet from the birth, on the floor immediately after birth while awaiting the delivery of the placenta; or immediately bathing the newborn regardless of the time or weather conditions. During training TBAs are taught to immediately dry and wrap the newborn, and to keep the head covered (40% of heat is lost via the head) and the newborn away from cold surfaces like walls and floors.

Birth Asphyxia and Establishment of Breathing

It is estimated that 840,000 newborns (3%) suffer from mild to moderate birth asphyxia in developing countries and that they account for 25% of birth-related neonatal deaths.[18] Of those who survive birth asphyxia, many suffer from brain damage and lifelong disabilities. In northern India, TBAs have been trained in neonatal resuscitation, using a resuscitation mask and a mucus suction trap. During 1989–1991, 100 TBAs in 54 villages of Chandigarh, India, were trained in modern methods of resuscitation for birth asphyxia.[19] Resuscitation methods taught included gravity drainage of secretions, physical stimulation by flicking the soles of the feet, cleaning of secretions from the mouth with a gauze piece wrapped around the finger, cardiac massage, mouth-to-mouth breathing, and prevention of heat loss by wrapping the baby. In addition, 31 TBAs were trained in more advanced methods including the use of a mucus extractor and mask-and-bag ventilation. To determine the impact of training on resuscitation by TBAs, the project conducted a resuscitation survey of 31 asphyxiated newborns and 30 recently stillborn babies delivered by trained TBAs. The study found that TBAs can be trained to adopt modern resuscitation methods: in 73% of the cases, the trained TBAs had used a modern resuscitation method, and the TBAs who had received more advanced training had used the mucus trap and mask-and-bag techniques in 33% and 43% of the cases respectively.

Prevention of Neonatal Sepsis and Tetanus

On the subject of neonatal infection, a Technical Working Group on Essential Newborn Care organised by the WHO in 1994 concluded: "Increasing coverage of pregnant women with tetanus toxoid can and does reduce neonatal tetanus deaths but babies may still die of other bacterial infections caused by lack of hygiene at birth and during the newborn period. Women and infants delivered at home without a trained birth attendant and without precautions of hygiene are particularly at risk".[20]

Therefore, to reduce neonatal deaths resulting from infection, the group recommended that a two-pronged approach be used:

• tetanus toxoid immunisation to the pregnant woman, and
• promotion and adoption of clean delivery practices.

In a study in Bangladesh, it was found that clean delivery is critical to preventing neonatal tetanus since tetanus toxoid vaccine may not be potent. Samples of vaccines were tested and it was found that three consecutive lots of the vaccine were not potent. Clean delivery techniques reduced the risk of tetanus despite the ineffectiveness of the vaccine.[21]

A controlled trial of 2,482 women conducted in 1982 in Bangladesh found that in one study area where TBAs had been trained and in another where tetanus toxoid was given, the tetanus-specific neonatal mortality rates were 5.6 and 1.3 per 1,000 live births, respectively, in comparison to 24 in the control area where neither intervention was available. This indicated that both interventions in themselves contribute to reductions in neonatal tetanus. TBAs were also found to be the key to greatly reducing neonatal tetanus in Faisalabad, Pakistan.[22]

Improvements in the Use and Quality of Maternity Services

In Lalitpur, Nepal, 15 years after the first TBA training, records kept for 1990–1991 found a much reduced infant and maternal mortality rate, and 27% of women attending antenatal clinics had been referred by TTBAs with 6.5% of deliveries in hospital being referred by TTBAs.[23]

In a Pathfinder project area of Pakistan TTBAs appeared to be effective in providing family planning services with the Contraceptive Prevelance Rate (CPR) increasing from 12.1 to 41.7% in 1989–90.[24]

In India, a study conducted in three primary health centres of Bassi, Bhanpurkalan and Rajasthan to determine the impact of TBA training[25] found that TTBAs were significantly superior in their work in comparison with untrained TBAs in advising on immunisation, anaemia, and family planning. Furthermore, the TTBAs used cleaner and safer cord cutting instruments with 50% using a razor blade and 30% using bamboo splinters whereas 48% of the untrained TBAs used bamboo splinters and only 15% used blades.

An in-depth qualitative study of the work of trained and untrained TBAs in Nepal clearly showed that TTBAs used cleaner and safer techniques and were far more knowledgeable than their untrained counterparts.[10]

Identification and Treatment of Pneumonia by TBAs

In Gadchiroli, India, a community based intervention trial to reduce infant mortality due to pneumonia included mass education about pneumonia and case management through the recognition of signs and treatment with co-trimoxazole by paramedics, village health workers, and TBAs. Case-fatality rates were greatly reduced in the intervention villages with equal success by TBAs as well other health workers. In addition, a significant reduction of neonatal mortality due to birth injury and prematurity was unexpectedly found in the intervention area "owing to the combination of better maternal and neonatal care by the TBAs trained in the project and the availability of treatment for pneumonia".[26]

Conclusions

Recently, there has been much controversy over the cost-effectiveness of TBA training in relation to Safe Motherhood. This debate has been documented in detail by Minden and Levitt.[27] Opponents of TBA training argue that there is little a TBA can do to prevent maternal deaths, except perhaps reduce maternal sepsis. The evident contribution TTBAs play in the reduction of neonatal deaths due to infection, birth trauma, and birth asphyxia is downplayed. It seems ironic that while improved survival of the neonate is part of the Safe Motherhood Mother-Baby Package developed by the WHO and the training of TBAs is considered an appropriate approach to reducing neonatal mortality, many leaders of Safe Motherhood programmes argue against TBA training. This paper has shown how TTBAs in South Asia have been very effective in improving neonatal outcomes through a variety of interventions, innovations, and simple technologies.

South Asian countries have led the way in training TBAs and developing simple technologies to reduce neonatal deaths. The WHO TBA Training Package, produced in 1992, and the WHO Disposable Clean Delivery Kit Guidelines were developed in South Asia. The social marketing of disposable delivery kits was first tested in Bangladesh, and shortly after in Nepal. India was the first to test color-coded weighing scales to detect low birth weight, TBA training for detection and management of birth asphyxia by neonatal resuscitation, and the use of a mucus suction trap.

Currently, the Ministry of Health in Nepal is developing a Neonatal Essential Care Training package for TBAs with assistance from neonatologists. This package includes information on the simple management of and referral for neonatal infection, hypothermia, jaundice, care of premature and LBW newborns, and birth asphyxia. Perhaps this can be a model for neonatal care packages appropriate to the village level, which can be used for TBAs and other village health workers.

So is TBA training cost-effective? TBAs are still actively practising and millions of mothers are relying on their services. Intuitively, as well as based on the evidence collected, it seems sensible and cost-effective to train them to adopt safe and potentially life-saving practices and to give up harmful traditions. What price can we put on a newborn's life? If a TTBA saves one newborn's life, is it worth the $60 it cost to train her? We believe so.

References

1. WHO, The World Health Report, Geneva (1996).
2. Extrapolated from data on number of births and IMR in UNICEF's State of World's children, 1997, and by estimating that neonatal deaths comprise 60% of infant deaths in the region.
3. WHO, The World Health Report, Geneva (1996): p. 43.
4. New Era. The National Health and Fertility Survey, 1996 Preliminary Report. Ministry of Health, Nepal. Kathmandu (1997).
5. UNICEF, *State of the World's Children, 1997*, Oxford University Press, Oxford.
6. UNICEF, *State of the World's Children, 1997*.
7. "Children and women of Nepal: A situation analysis," UNICEF/Nepal Kathmandu, Nepal (1992).
8. Levitt M and Doma U, "Motherhood in Bhutan: Maternal health practices among postpartum Bhutanese women," Thimpu UNICEF/Bhutan, December (1993).
9. Minden M and Levitt M, "The right to know: Women and their traditional birth attendants," In: *Midwives and Safer Motherhood*, Murray S, ed., London: Times Mirror International Publications (1996).
10. Levitt M, "From sickles to scissors: Birth, traditional birth attendants and perinatal health development in Nepal," Ann Arbor, Michigan University dissertation, Microfilms (1998).
11. WHO, "Maternal and newborn health: Essential newborn care report of a technical working group," Trieste, 25–29 April 1994, Geneva (1996).
12. Pradhan A, Nepal Family Health Survey, 1996 Kathmandu, Nepal and Calverton, Maryland: Ministry of Health [Nepal], New Era, and Macro International Inc.

13. From WHO, "The newborn baby needs special care," *Safe Motherhood: A Newsletter of Worldwide Activities*, Issue 12, July–October 1993: p. 5.

14. Anonymous, "The newborn baby needs special care," *Safe Motherhood: A Newsletter of Worldwide Activities*, Issue 12, July–October 1993: p. 4.

15. PATH. Regional Delivery Kit Workshop Proceedings. Seattle, Washington: Program for Appropriate Technology in Health and SWACH (1994).

16. SWACH, "Development, use and health impact of simple delivery kits in selected districts of India," Unpublished Report, Chandigarh, India: Survival for Women and Children Foundation (1992).

17. Johanson R, Rolfe P, Spencer SA and Rai R, "Should thermometers be issued to birth attendants in Nepal (Letter)?" *Journal of Tropical Pediatrics* **38**(4) (1992): p. 202.

18. WHO, "Maternal and newborn health: Essential newborn care," Report of a Technical Working Group, Trieste, 25–29 April 1994, Geneva (1996): p. 1.

19. Kumar R, "Effect of training on the resuscitation practices of Traditional Birth Attendants," *Transactions of the Royal Society of Tropical Medicine and Hygiene* **88**(2) (1994): 159–160.

20. WHO, "Maternal and newborn health: Essential newborn care," Report of a Technical Working Group, Trieste, 25–29 April 1994, Geneva (1996): p. 1.

21. Anonymous, "But clean delivery is important too," *Safe Motherhood: A Newsletter of Worldwide Activities*, Issue 13, November 1993–February 1994: p. 9.

22. Kamal I, "Traditional Birth Attendant training: Sharing experiences," *International Journal of Obstetrics and Gynecology* **38**(Suppl) (1992): S55–58.

23. Hale C, "The incorporation of Traditional Birth Attendants in a primary health care programme in Lalitpur District, Nepal," Health Services Office, United Missions to Nepal (1987) (with addendum 1991).

24. Ibid.

25. Benara SK and Chaturvedi SK, "Impact of training on the performance of Traditional Birth Attendants," *Journal of Family Welfare* **36**(4) (1990): 32–35.

26. Bang AT, Bang RA, Tale O, Sontakke P, Solanki J, Wargantiwar R and Kelzarkar P, "Reduction in pneumonia mortality and total childhood mortality by means of community based intervention trial in Gadchiroli, India," *Lancet* **28** [336 (B709)] (1990): 201–206.

27. Minden M and Levitt M, "The right to know: Women and their TBAs," In: *Midwives and Safer Motherhood. International Perspectives on Midwifery*, Murray S, ed., London Mosby (1996).

Chapter 24

TBA TRAINING: COST-EFFECTIVE?

Carole Presern

Health Adviser, Department for International Development, UK

The heated debate about when, or whether, it is cost effective to train TBAs is fuelled by the polarised positions of the pro- and anti-debaters (community development versus crisis management).[1] This polarisation is unhelpful. Pragmatically, a mix of strategies is needed to achieve the desired outcomes: healthy mothers and children.

The cost effectiveness debate was really crystallised by the publication of the World Development Report (WDR) in 1993.[2] Cost effectiveness can be defined as "the selection of interventions which improve health at least cost or which maximise health gain for a given budget".[3] Therefore, interventions are chosen if they can lead to the same outcome at lower cost, or a better outcome at the same cost. Although sometimes criticised for its rather mechanistic and formula type approach, the 1993 WDR did open the debate about what public money should be spent on which interventions, and also stated "just because a particular intervention is cost-effective does not mean that public funds should be spent on it".

The most cost-effective investments for resource-poor countries are identified as being in public health (immunisation, information, family planning, and prevention of killer diseases), at a cost of between US$25–75 per Disability Adjusted Life Year (DALY) gained and on essential clinical services (for pregnancy, family planning, TB control, control of STDs, and control of illnesses amongst young children). This would cost less than

US$50 per DALY gained. The total cost of implementing these interventions in a low-income country is estimated at US$12 per capita.

Choices must be made about the financing of training. The training of primary care providers is a priority so subsidies may have to be removed from specialised training. It is less clear whether the state (or donors) should subsidise TBA training. Should they be included as primary care providers, or seen as essentially private practitioners who will receive personal benefits from publically subsidised training?

The WDR suggested possible choices between investments. Longer term investment in girls schooling would have bigger effects on health than investments in health *per se*. For example, seven years of maternal education reduces child deaths by up to 65%. Maternity services probably require high subsidies until there is greater gender equality, and women have greater control over household resources. In the WDR section on making pregnancy and delivery care safe the focus is on information, community based obstetrics with trained nurse midwives, and district hospital care for emergencies.

Cost Effectiveness and TBA Training

One major constraint to economic analyses (of TBA training and other interventions) is a lack of information on the relative effectiveness, impact, and cost of different interventions.[4] There have been few attempts in low-income countries to apply cost effectiveness analysis to health because it is difficult, and also because provision of basic health care is seen as a fundamental human right, so cost becomes a secondary consideration. However, cost effectiveness is not incompatible with equity. The objective is to offer services to those who most need them, at least cost, and without compromising quality. The aim is not to subsidise services which can be essentially considered as private goods.

Empirical evidence

The cost of training might outweigh a net benefit in terms of health gains. A study in Bangladesh concluded that although the use of trained TBAs was high, their presence at delivery did not affect maternal outcomes, and perinatal mortality, which was also high, was strongly related to adverse events at TBA-assisted delivery.[5]

There is little empirical evidence on the actual costs of training related to outcomes — both maternal and neonatal. However, the cost effectiveness of certain interventions in terms of deaths averted is very low. For example, the cost per (maternal) death averted of antenatal care has been estimated at US$17,692, TBA trained care at US$11,500, while health centres linked to rural hospitals are very cost effective (US$3,735 per death averted). The analysis indicates that providing family planning and obstetric care at rural health centres, in conjunction with transportation to nearby hospitals, are the most cost effective interventions. This study points out the real scarcity of hard data on costs but does not estimate the cost effectiveness of preventing neonatal deaths.[6]

Others suggest that "improving nutrition, expanding family planning, increasing girl's access to education... may well be more likely to reduce maternal morbidity and mortality than will ineffective TBA training programmes".[7]

Are TBAs naturally dying out?

One Indian study noted that although 27% of TBAs inherited their profession only 4% were passing it on.[8] This would perhaps make any TBA training intervention somewhat artificial. Indonesia is gradually replacing TBAs with midwives posted at village level. A study in Kenya noted that TBAs were doing less than three deliveries per year, which made any investment in training expensive.[9]

Do TBAs reduce neonatal tetanus?

One review of the evidence concluded that "the evidence that the training of TBAs does lead to a reduction in neonatal tetanus is by no means conclusive".[10] In Indonesia, "33% of TBAs were unaware that neonatal tetanus can be prevented by hygienic delivery; in this respect there was no difference between trained and untrained TBAs".[11] A study from Krabi in Thailand showed that neonatal tetanus fell not only in areas where TBAs were trained but also in those where they were not. The key interventions were mass immunisation and overall strengthening of the health service network.[12]

Does training improve other aspects of perinatal care?

There are effective TBA programmes, and Dr. Marta J. Levitt has given examples of where they can have an impact on neonatal health. In most cases, the effective TBA programmes have been those in which both transport systems and essential obstetric services have been implemented in addition to the TBA component. In addition, they are well targeted and implemented only in geographical areas where there is a definite need. Levitt and Minden[13] have listed the ways in which TBAs can practically help beyond a narrow definition of their ability to deal with obstetric emergencies, and have come some way to developing indicators that could allow a cost effectiveness analysis, which would include their potential contribution to perinatal and neonatal health.

Some studies evaluating the effectiveness of TBA training programmes have found that there is no difference in the knowledge of trained and untrained TBAs and that significant changes, which may not be justified by the cost, would have to be made to ensure effectiveness.[14,15] Lynch and Derveeuw show no difference in knowledge and practices of trained and untrained TBAs. This was mainly due to inappropriate training and poor supervision. They conclude that in remote areas TBA training could still be valid, but great care has to be taken over training content and supervision. Other studies show that while reductions in maternal mortality are difficult to assess, reductions in neonatal mortality can be made.[16] A key failure has been inadequate evaluation of TBA training programmes. 580,000 TBAs have been trained in India but it is not known what effect this has had on maternal or neonatal health.[17]

Do TBAs have a role in child health?

In India, TBAs were assessed to be the most cost-effective option in managing Acute Respiratory Infections (ARI). Mortality from ARI in the control areas fell by 20%. The cost of saving one child's life was US$2.64 — highly cost effective.[18] Giving TBAs additional skills in child health interventions may ultimately be more cost effective than trying to equip them to deal only with obstetric emergencies.

Where there is regular supervision and a link to referral, TBA training can be valuable. The sad fact is that many birth attendants remain untrained and many do few deliveries, making the numbers that need to be trained far in excess of any useful outcome.

What is Left Out of Cost Effectiveness Analysis?

There is very limited data on whether the same outcomes (e.g. improved neonatal health) could be achieved with different strategies. However, it would be useful to look more at the role of information to the wider community, particularly on environmental risks to the newborn. If women and family members knew what to do for the neonate, and the skills are not necessarily sophisticated, and if they knew when to refer there could also be significant impact on maternal and child health.

The problem with providing information is an often inappropriate desire then for "modern" care which results in overloading of facilities. For example, it is known that the number of women who actually seek institutional care in the Kathmandu valley is 2.5 times more than those who actually need care (if it is assumed that 20% of women need referral care). This can lead to poor quality care at overloaded institutions and reallocation of resources to cope for the demand for care at referral facilities.

There has been limited attention by recipient governments to the recurrent cost implications of donor funded programmes, and most TBA training programmes are donor financed. Long after the donors have left the government is expected to fund a programme which has not even been assessed against basic cost effectiveness criteria. TBA programmes often fail soon after donor support is withdrawn, indicating poor design of the programme, and the subsequent inability by government to pick up recurrent costs and the ongoing commitments of supervision, resupply of kits and the labour-intensive effort needed to link TBAs with the referral systems (personal observation in Pakistan).

What is not discussed is the explicit policy choice that has to be made in resource-poor situations. If TBA training is needed, how can it be done most cost effectively and in which areas? If properly linked with a workable decentralised planning system choices could be made at the local level about whether TBA training is a cost effective and viable option in any given district. Some TBA programmes are centrally planned and without due recognition of geographical and social variables.

Debate

Dr. Levitt explains convincingly that TBA training has a place, but it is one item in a menu of policy options. Also, explicit choices should be made about whether the TBA intervention will ultimately be more cost effective than other interventions, for example, increasing the number of trained midwives. A disadvantage of the way some TBA training programmes have been implemented has been their vertical, centrally-led planning. Pragmatically parallel strategies have to be followed, especially in counties such as Nepal and Bhutan where remoteness can mean that the only person available at the time of birth is a TBA.

A further key disadvantage, not much discussed by researchers, is the actual cost of training and supervision. TBA training is a cost-intensive initial investment which has to be continuously followed up, both in recruiting "new" TBAs and in refreshing and supervising "old" TBAs. It can be surmised that the aggregate expenses of training older women (with shorter working lives) is in excess of the costs of training younger women as professional midwives. Lynch and Derveeuw assess that it costs US$44 to train a TBA against US$150 for midwives (US$60 for TBA training in Nepal).[14] In areas where the gross availability of funding is an issue (as in most developing countries) a choice might need to be made between training someone with a potentially short working life and few deliveries, against a younger person who, when trained will do more deliveries over a longer time-scale. However, more flexible options have to be found to allow midwives either to work independently, to take career breaks without penalty, to job share, or to legitimately work in both the public and private sectors. Ways have to be found to retain these women in remote and poor areas.

Results have been mixed and overall the evidence is contradictory. While there have been successes, there have also been disappointments and certain lessons have been learned: supervision is critical; follow-up immediately after training needs improving; stipends and kits continue to cause problems; the length and content of training is not always assessed; and respect from health professionals towards TBAs is often lacking. Most importantly, TBA training should not be undertaken at the expense of supplying more adequate midwifery and obstetric care services to people in need.[19] The training of TBAs is a necessary but temporary step in improving maternal and child health.[20]

Conclusion

Evidence is still needed to state conclusively whether the training of TBAs is cost effective. TBAs will continue to exist in poor rural areas of many parts of South Asia. They should be trained to do the best possible job. However, if funds are limited (and in most parts of the region they are) then explicit choices will have to be made about the relative impact of this intervention over any other. Training will probably have to be much better targeted to women who are younger, who will continue to practice, and who will do sufficient numbers of deliveries every year to make the investment worthwhile. The training of nurse midwives must have higher priority, as do changes in the environment which will allow them to take on more flexible employment.

NB: The views expressed in this article are the author's and do not necessarily reflect the policy of the United Kingdom Government Department for International Development.

References

1. Minden M and Levitt MJ, "The right to know: Women and their traditional birth attendants," In: *Midwives and Safer Motherhood*, Murray S, ed., Mosby, London (1996).
2. WHO. *World Development Report 1993: Investing in Health*, Oxford University Press.
3. Mills A, *"Improving the Efficiency of Public Sector Health Services in Developing Countries: Bureaucratic Versus Market Approaches*, Public Health and Policy publications no. 17, London School of Hygiene and Tropical Medicine (1995).
4. Tinker A and Koblinsky MA, "Making motherhood safe," WB report no. 202, WHO (1993).
5. Goodburn EA, Chowdhury M, Gazi R, Marshall T, Graham W and Karim R, "An investigation into the nature and determinants of maternal morbidity related to delivery and the puerperium in rural Bangladesh," Research and Evaluation Division, BRAC, Dhaka (1994).
6. Maine D, *Safe Motherhood Programs: Options and Issues*, School of Public Health, Colombia University (1991).
7. Starrs A and Measham D, *Safe Motherhood in South Asia: Challenge for the Nineties*, the World Bank and Family Care International (1990).
8. Singh SL, "Profile of traditional birth attendants in a rural area of north India," *Journal of Nursing and Midwifery* **39**(2) (1994): 119–123.
9. Boerma JT and Baya MS, "Maternal and child health in an ethnomedical perspective: Traditional and modern medicine in coastal Kenya," *Health Policy and Planning* **5**(4) (1990): 347–357.
10. Ross D, "The trained traditional birth attendant and neonatal tetanus," In: *The Potential of the Traditional Birth Attendant*, Mangay Maglacas A and Simons J, eds., WHO, Geneva (1986).
11. de Haas I, Moes N and Wolffers I, "Prevention of neonatal tetanus in developing countries hampered by local organisation and limited knowledge of health personnel and traditional midwives, North Sulawesi, Indonesia," From Medline citation, translated. *Ned Tijdschr Geneeskd* **138**(20) (1994):1032–1035.
12. Chongsuvivatwong V, Bujakorn L, Kanpoy V and Treetrong R, "Control of neonatal tetanus in southern Thailand," *International Journal of Epidemiology* **22**(5) (1993): 931–935.
13. See ref. 1, *op. cit.*
14. Lynch O and Derveeuw M, "The impact of training and supervision on traditional birth attendants," *Tropical Doctor* **24** (1994): 103–107.

15. Fleming JR, "What in the world is being done about TBAs? An overview of international and national attitudes to traditional birth attendants," *Midwifery* **10**(3) (1994): 142–147.

16. Kwast BE, "Building a community based maternity program," *International Journal of Obstetrics & Gynecology* **48** (1995): 67–82.

17. Leedham E, cited in Maine (1991) (*op. cit.*).

18. Bang AT, Bang RA and Sontakke PG, "Management of childhood pneumonia by traditional birth attendants," *Bulletin of the World Health Organization* **72**(6) (1994): 897–905.

19. Royston E and Armstong S, eds., *Preventing Maternal Deaths*, WHO, Geneva (1989).

20. Levitt MJ, "From sickles to scissors: Birth, traditional birth attendants and perinatal health development in rural Nepal," unpublished PhD dissertation, University of Hawaii (1988).

Chapter 25

WHAT TO DO ABOUT REFERRAL AND TRANSFERS OF HIGH RISK MOTHERS AND NEWBORNS?

Daljit Singh

Professor of Pediatrics, Dayanand Medical College, Ludhiana, India

Introduction

A well organised system of referral and transfer of high risk mothers and newborns to a centre equipped with adequate facilities for specialised care is a key factor in reducing neonatal mortality and morbidity.[1-3] Several vital elements are involved: organisational aspects, trained manpower, equipment, and modes of transport.[4,5]

Socio-economic conditions and financial constraints preclude the establishment of an ideal system in countries with limited resources, and compromises are inevitable. It should, however, be possible to build up infrastructure and facilities of a higher order in an optimum number of specialised centres to cater for larger populations connected effectively through a network.[3] An integrated system is particularly needed in India and other South Asian countries where the arrangements for the care of high risk mothers and neonates are far from ideal.

Current Status of Neonatal Referral in India

In India, about 70% of deliveries take place in rural areas. Home deliveries are predominant (90–95%) in rural areas, but also common in urban areas.

503

Only 33% of all births in India are conducted by trained birth attendants (TTBAs) or medical personnel, and the situation is similar in many other developing countries.[6]

The present status of referral and transport is far from satisfactory. No organised system exists for co-ordinated referral from primary to secondary or tertiary levels. The concept of maternal transport to a referral centre in high risk pregnancy is not propagated. Many loopholes exist in the timely detection of high risk situations in the mother. It is a common observation that preterm infants are referred soon after birth rather than transported *in utero*.[7] Level-3 care is available at only a few selected centres. Non-availability of high level neonatal care in nearby places involves travel over long distances by road; organised neonatal air transport, as occurs in Australia, is a distant dream. Journey conditions are unsatisfactory and roads are rough and bumpy in most areas. Skilled transport teams are simply not available. Commonly, newborn infants are received at referral centres in an unstable and often critical condition.

A clinical audit of neonatal referral in the Punjab

In a study of 110 referred neonates in the Punjab (one of the wealthier and better-resourced states in India), we observed that medical personnel, emergency kits and monitoring of the infant's condition during transportation were invariably absent.[7] The incidence of hypothermia at the time of admission has been reported in two studies to be about 15%, occurring even in the summer months.[7,8] Hot weather accounted for hyperthermia in nearly 20% of infants.

Grossly inadequate information was generally made available to the referral centre. Communication of relevant clinical details was usually conspicuous by its absence. Complete pre-transport information was obtainable in only 2% of the referred neonates in our study.[7] The distance travelled was more than 100 km in 54% of cases. As no exclusive vehicles/ambulances were available for optimum neonatal transport, parents had to fend for themselves and were compelled to use unsuitable vehicles. In our experience cars and trucks were commonly used, and often, open vehicles like jeeps, tractors, bullock carts, and rickshaws.

Numerous steps are required to eliminate the existing weaknesses, and there is an urgent need for developing an integrated system of referral in the region. The recommendations pertain to

- prerequisites at the referring centre,
- requirements in transit, and
- responsibilities of the referral centres.

Prerequisites at Referring Centres

Identification of high risk cases

Early recognition of high risk pregnancy would enable *in utero* referral, which is more desirable than transfer of a sick newborn, and is associated with better neonatal outcome.[9-11] Moreover, postnatal transport of a infant requires a highly evolved system of skilled care which is not easy to achieve.[12]

Identification of risk would mostly be carried out by traditional birth attendants (TBAs) who should screen the pregnant women with regard to maternal age, height, weight, parity, medical illnesses, previous obstetric history including neonatal deaths, and present obstetric problems. Important indications for maternal referral include obstetric complications like antepartum haemorrhage and severe preclampsia, maternal complications like renal disease, infection, class 3/4 heart disease and diabetes, and surgical complicaticons like trauma or an acute abdomen.

Recognition of high risk in a neonate requires consideration of the infant's weight, gestational age, evidence of asphyxia, poor feeding, evident illness, and the maternal background. Infants may be categorised as low, moderate, high, and very high risk and requiring different levels of care, as shown in Table 1.[13] Neonatal mortality can be lowered by timely referral to the appropriate level[14] (see Tables 1 and 2).

Communication

A reliable communication system between the referring person and the receiving hospital is necessary. Apart from confirmation of bed availability, the estimated arrival time should be intimated.

Table 1 Classification of newborn infants at risk.

	Neonatal risk			
	Low	*Moderate*	*High*	*Very high*
Gestation	FTND	Term	33–36 weeks	< 33 weeks
Weight	> 2.5 kg	2–2.5 kg	1.5–2 kg	< 1.5 kg
Birth asphyxia	No	No	Moderate	Severe
Feeding	Good Sucking Breastfed	–	Not sucking well, but tolerating tube feeds	Not feeding
Maternal background	Experienced, educated mother	Teenaged, uneducated, primigravida, or ill during pregnancy	–	–
Illness	No major congenital malformation or illness	–	–	Sick neonate*

*Lethargy, hypothermia, fever, early or deep jaundice, respiratory distress, cyanosis, irritability, seizures, apnoea, vomiting, diarrhoea, abdominal distension, bleeding, gross congenital malformations.

Table 2 The levels of risk and care for newborns.

Group	Mortality rate compared to average	Population incidence (%)	Care needed
Low risk	Less	50	Level-1
Moderate risk	Up to 5 times	30	Level-1
High risk	5–10 times	15	Level-2
Very high risk	10–50 times	5	Level-3

Clinical details

Specific clinical information regarding the newborn and the mother should also be communicated precisely.[3,13] Details regarding the condition of the infant should include:

- Gestational age and birth weight,
- APGAR score and type of resuscitation,
- Reason for transfer,
- Vital signs: heart rate, blood pressure (BP), respiratory rate and their changes since birth,
- Any indication of sepsis,
- Results of investigations, especially chest X-ray,
- Treatment given, e.g. intravenous (IV) fluids, drugs, or oxygen.

Other referral items

The following items should be sent along with the infant:

- A copy of case records including investigation reports,
- X-rays,
- Blood sample from the mother, if relevant.

The parents should be informed regarding the exact condition of the infant and the reason for referral. The details of the referral centre, including location, route and names of concerned personnel, must also be conveyed. Information regarding the expected duration of stay at the referral centre and the estimated cost of treatment should also be given.

Pre-transport stabilisation

Stabilisation before transport is a critical aspect of inter-hospital care, since identification and management of complications during transit is difficult. Establishment of a satisfactory respiratory and circulatory status before transport facilitates an optimum haemodynamic status during the journey, especially in preterm infants.[15]

Thermal stabilisation

Regular recording and maintenance of temperature is vital.[16] Heat loss can be prevented by measures like warm blankets, heat shields, bubble plastic, or foil.[17] Skin-to-skin contact with the mother is a satisfactory method of keeping the infant warm.[18] If the infant is hypothermic, gradual rewarming is necessary because rapid rewarming may result in shock and apnoea.[19] A radiant heater is the most effective and safe method for rewarming a hypothermic infant at the referring centre.[20] During hot summer months hyperthermia should be avoided.

Respiratory and circulatory status

The airway must be kept patent, keeping the neck slightly extended and frequently suctioning out secretions. If intubation is anticipated during transport it is advisable to carry it out in advance. If there is inadequate respiratory effort or respiratory distress with a respiratory rate > 70 per minute or retraction, intubation and ventilation with bag should be commenced. Ventilation should also be considered for infants below 30–32 weeks of gestation and with a birth weight < 1,500 g.[3] Oxygenation is required in all these situations. If a pneumothorax is identified chest tube drainage should be considered. Blood pressure, peripheral pulses and capillary refill time should be monitored. A reliable IV line should be instituted.

Specific measures

Blood glucose should be checked and maintained, and vitamin K injection (1 mg) administered. Special interventions are required for infection, seizures, anaemia, or hydrops. Surgical conditions like tracheo-esophageal fistula, neural tube defects, omphalocele, or diaphragmatic hernia require specific care before transfer.[21,22] Tests should be carried out only if the results would be obtained in time and will influence the care during transport.

Referral for tertiary care

Regional centres capable of providing tertiary care for newborns must be identified. Ideally, these would cater for an area not more than 90–100 km radius, since air transport is hardly a feasible alternative in these regions. Round-the-clock facilities with regard to transport vehicles, equipment, and trained personnel should be under the charge of the centre which would be required to transport the patients from the referring hospital.

Referral for secondary care

Since these would be the more common form of transfer, facilities should be available at district level. Provisions should be on the same line as for referral for tertiary care, but expensive equipment like transport incubators and vital signs monitors may not be feasible. A closed van may serve as an ambulance. One trained person in the transport team would be acceptable.

Requirements in Transit

Organisation of transport

A one-tier referral and transfer system would not be appropriate. Tertiary centres cannot take responsibility for transport for all cases. Infrastructure for transport has to be developed at district as well as regional levels.

Transport vehicle

The transport vehicle should have adequate space to accommodate the team as well as the equipment, with adequate lighting and sound insulation. As turbulence of the road and distance of transport are important considerations, a "tempo traveller" would be an appropriate vehicle, which should be driven smoothly with minimum jolting. Arrangements for heating should be available. A transport incubator would be ideal, but a thermocol box with hot water bottles will serve the purpose.

Equipment and drugs which should be available in the vehicle are:

- Vital sign monitors for heart rate, respiratory rate, blood pressure and a pulse oximeter to estimate the pO2 saturation.
- Oxygen cylinder with head box and tubing.
- Emergency procedures kits, e.g. for intubation and chest tube insertion.
- Basic items: stethoscope, thermometer, hot water battles, mucus extractor, ambu bag and mask, infant laryngoscope, endotracheal tubes, catheters, syringes, needles, feeding tubes, adhesive tape, flash light, clip board, paper.
- Drugs: spirit, betadine, injectable (inj) adrenaline, inj phenobarbitone, inj diazepam, inj calcium gluconate, inj sodium bicarbonate, inj Frusemide, inj normal saline, 10% dextrose.

Personnel

The transport team should include at least two competent persons who have expertise in IV cannulation, intubation, chest tube insertion, and appropriate use of drugs. They should be thoroughly familiar with the equipment, as any malfunction en-route must be handled by them.[23] A minimum of eight months to one year training is deemed necessary for the physician or nurse accompanying the transport.

Care during transport

The problems that need special consideration during transport include hypothermia, hypoglycaemia, respiratory arrest, and seizures. These problems can be minimised by anticipating them and stabilising the patient prior to transport and discussing the required appropriate measures with the transport team.

Complications related to turbulence during road transport include vomiting, apnoea and intraventricular haemorrhage.[15] Endotracheal tube dislodgement, hypoventilation, and pneumothorax also need to be watched out for. If problems do arise, the vehicle should be stopped while interventions are carried out. Important aspects of care during transit include:

Maintenance of temperature

In the absence of a transport incubator, thermocol boxes with hot water bottles are practicable, provided hot water in a thermos flask is available for refilling.[24]

Monitoring

Colour, heart rate, respiratory rate, and temperature should be checked every 10–15 minutes and documented. Urine output should be maintained at around 1 ml/kg/h. Heart rate should be kept between 100–180/min.

Respiratory support

Oxygen, suction, and intermittent positive pressure ventilation (IPPV) must be provided as indicated. Oxygen saturation should be 88–92% but electronic equipment like pulse oximeter do not always function well on the road when there is turbulence or electrical disturbances. The flow rate of oxygen should take into account the duration of the journey and the size of the oxygen cylinder.

Glucose homeostasis and feeding

A glucometer should be used to check blood glucose every four hours. The infant should be fed en-route if not contraindicated and if the duration of journey is long. However, in most practical situations feeding is not feasible and the stomach should be kept empty, especially since vomiting may occur. A nasogastric tube should decompress the stomach and be left open. Ideally, a mechanical drip regulator with microdrip set should be used. IV plastic cannulae are preferable to butterfly cannulae which are more likely to extravasate during transport.

Completion of transfer

The personnel receiving the infant must be prepared to manage promptly any unresolved or new problems. Monitoring and care must not be compromised during transfer from the vehicle to the nursery. Complete information, including events during transfer, should be handed over by the transport team, who should also recheck equipment and prepare for the next call.

The referral centre should keep the referring physician informed regarding the progress of the infant. At discharge or even following the death of the infant, a detailed note about the events should be communicated.

Strategies for Improving Referral and Transfer Programmes in Developing Countries

A thoroughly integrated approach needs to be adopted to improve the referral system which necessarily demands cost-effective preventive and therapeutic strategies. A supportive political and economic environment would greatly improve the transport system. National neonatology bodies need to take up the matter with the government for appropriate fund allocation for perinatal care and development of organised referral.

Educational programmes

Maternal education is a prerequisite for improving neonatal care. Extensive use of the media is required to promote antenatal care and safe delivery, and to inform mothers about risk factors in pregnancy and the availability of perinatal services.

Out-reach educational programmes for health personnel need to be systematically implemented. The importance of early risk identification, *in utero* transport, pre-transport stabilisation, and the role of skilled manpower during transport needs to be stressed during these programmes.[8]

The training of birth attendants must include identification of high risk pregnancy, and a pictorial scoring system as devised by the National

Neonatology Forum (NNF) of India may be useful. Feedback from the referral centre incorporating suggestions for future referrals of mothers as well as newborn infants would go a long way to eliminating the more easily preventable adverse factors.

Regionalisation of care

Optimal utilisation of limited resources is possible by appropriate channelling of patients to various levels of care. Although the need for skilled transport for sick neonates must be recognised, it cannot be regarded as a satisfactory alternative to regionalisation of perinatal care.[3,25] Services need to be improved. The availability of neonatal resuscitation by trained doctors, nurses or TBA skilled in the procedures including ambu bag ventilation should be ensured not only at primary health centres but also at home. Death in the first hours of life closely reflects skills in intrapartum management and neonatal resuscitation.[26]

Using the state of Kerala in India as a model, primary health centres should function as Level-1 care and be upgraded to provide a "foetal kick chart" to the mother for surveillance of high risk pregnancies, and equipped with a good resuscitation corner.

District hospitals should be able to provide Level-2 care while a medical college or an apex institute in the area should provide tertiary care with ventilatory services.[27]

Categorisation of risk

Categorisation of risk and the consequent decision regarding place of transfer should be clear to the referring personnel. With improvement of assessment, the actual need for referral may decrease. The utility of transport to another centre would have to be weighed against the problems for transport, and a decision not to refer might be more appropriate in many cases.[28]

Inter-hospital care requires a high degree of co-ordination and co-operation of many skilled persons, and should be required only in situations where antenatal identification of risk is not possible. If referral is necessary it should be carried out as early as possible.[29]

Early transportation is critical, especially in infants with respiratory distress, carried out by a skilled team trained in a level-3 centre, and transported with the recommended guidelines. Organisation of a transport system by the tertiary care centre, including a transport vehicle, equipment and personnel, is a high priority and might initially have to be funded from charitable sources.

Formulation of a model system

A model system can act as a stimulus for others to replicate. A specific area can be selected for intensive input to create a model referral and transfer system with the best possible methodology and facilities. This would provide an example to others and give insight into financial and logistic requirements and feasibility.

Data collection and analysis, perhaps using audit methodology (see Chapter 22), is essential to provide feedback to staff and to monitor the progress of the referral programme.

Conclusion

Advances in technology and communication, improved transport facilities, and better understanding of the immediate needs of the sick newborn have resulted in great refinement of neonatal transport in the developed world. Concerted efforts in bringing about similar changes could help to reduce neonatal morbidity and mortality in developing countries. A high priority is to audit existing systems and procedures, because our own audit of neonatal referrals in Punjab (by no means the worst area in India) has revealed serious problems.

References

1. Brann AW and Cefalo RC, "Guidelines for perinatal care," AAP committee on foetus and newborn. American Academy of Pediatrics, Evanston (1983): 185–198.

2. Chance GW, G'Brien MJ and Swyer PR, "Transportation of sick neonates 1972: An unsatisfactory aspect of medical care," *Canadian Medical Association Journal* **109** (1973): B47–851.

3. Chiswick ML, "Regional organisation care," In: *Textbook of Neonatology*, Roberton NRC, ed., Churchill Livingstone, London (1992): 1136–1146.

4. Chance GW, Mathew JD, Gash G *et al.*, "Neonatal transport: A controlled study of skilled assistance," *Journal of Pediatrics* **93** (1978): 662–666.

5. British Association of Perinatal Medicine, "Referrals for neonatal medical care in the United Kingdom over one year," *British Medical Journal* **298** (1989): 169–172.

6. *The State of the World's Children, 1989.* Table 7, UNICEF, Oxford University Press (1989): p. 79.

7. Singh H, Singh D and Jain BK, "Transport of referred sick neonates: How far from ideal?" *Indian Pediatrics* **33** (1996): 851–853.

8. Mir NA and Javied S, "Transport of sick neonates: Practical considerations," *Indian Pediatrics* **26** (1989): 755–764.

9. Modantou HD, Dorchester W, Freeman RK and Rommal C, "Perinatal transport to a regional perinatal center in a metropolitan area: Maternal versus neonatal transport," *American Journal of Obstetrics and Gynecology* **138** (1980): 1157–1164.

10. Modantou HD and Dorchester W, "Evaluating the impact of perinatal transfer an patient care," In: *Emergency Transport of the Perinatal Patient*, MacDonald MG and Miller MK, eds., Little Brown, Boston (1989): 125–142.

11. Miller TC, Densberger M and Krogman J, "Maternal transport and the perinatal denominator," *American Journal of Obstetrics and Gynecology* **147** (1993): 19–24.

12. Lamont RF, Dunlop PDM, Crowley P *et al.*, "Comparative mortality and morbidity of infants transferred *in utero* or postnatally," *Perinatal Medicine* **11** (1993): 200–203.

13. Bhakoo ON, "Identification, referral and transport of high risk neonates," *Bull NNF* (1987): 1–4.

14. Vogt J, Chan L, Wu P *et al.*, "Impact of a regional infant dispatch center on neonatal mortality," *American Journal of Public Health* **71** (1981): 577–582.

15. Lazzara A, Kanto WP, Dykes FD *et al.*, "Continuing education in the community hospital and reduction in the incidence of intracerebral hemorrhage in the transported pre-term infant," *Journal of Pediatrics* **101** (1982): 757–761.

16. Bhargava SK, Kumari S, Saxena HMK *et al.*, "Primary cold injury in the newborn," *Indian Pediatrics* **8** (1971): 827–831.

17. Besch NJ, Perlstein PH, Edwards NK *et al.*, "The transport infant bag: A shield against heat loss," *New England Journal of Medicine* **284** (1971): p. 121.

18. Cattaneo A, Davanzo R, Uxa F and Tamburlini G, "Recommendations for the implementation of Kangaroo Mother Care for low birth weight infants," International Network on Kangaroo Mother Care, *Acta Paediatrica* **87**(4) (1998): 440–445.

19. Tafari N and Gentry J, "Aspects on rewarming newborn infants with severe accidental hypothermia," *Acta Pediatr Scand* **63** (1974): 595–597.

20. Yeh TF, Lilien LD and Pyatis J, "Thermoregulation in neonates," In: *Textbook of Neonatology*, Vidyasagar D, ed., New Delhi, Interprint (1987): 356–367.

21. Warner LD, "Before transfering a newborn infant for surgery: A check list of dont's and do's," *Am Med Wom Assoc* **19** (1964): 1051–1061.

22. Reys HM and Burrington JD, "Neonatal surgical problems," In: *Atlas of Perinatology*, Aladiem S and Vidyasagagar D, eds., Philadelphia, WB Saunders (1987): 345–378.

23. Frank HD, Ballowitz L and Schachinger M, "Ambulance with intensive care facilities for the transport of infants at risk," *Journal of Pediatric Medicine* **1** (1973): p. 125.

24. Daga SR, Chandrashekhar L, Pol PP and Patole S, "Appropriate technology for keeping infants warm in India," *Annals of Tropical Paediatrics* **6** (1996): 23–25.

25. Mir NA, "Regionalization of reproductive medical and perinatal mortality," *Indian Journal of Pediatrics* **53** (1986): 335–338.

26. Paneth N, Kiely JL and Susser M, "Age at death used to assess the effect of interhospital transfer of newborns," *Pediatrics* **73** (1984): 854–861.

27. Kanto WP, Johnson G, Sturgill C *et al.*, "Performance of a level-2 nursery in a neonatal regional program," *South Med J* **75** (1982): 1043–1050.

28. Branger B, Chaperon J, Mouzard *et al.*, "Hospital transfer of newborn infants in Loive-Atlantic area," *Rev Epidemiol Sante Publique* **42**(4) (1994): 307–314.

29. Cordero LP, "Transport of the very sick infant: Time factor analysis," *Pediatric Research* **8** (1974): 444–446.

Chapter 26

MAKING PERINATAL SERVICES MORE USER-FRIENDLY

Susan F. Murray
Lecturer in International Maternal Health,
Institute of Child Health, University College, London

The Baby Friendly Hospital Initiative (BFHI) to protect, promote, and support breastfeeding has been extraordinarily successful in changing entrenched routines in many hospitals, and has introduced the notion of "friendly" services into international health care terminology.

The broader issue of the "user friendliness" of perinatal services has also come to prominence in its own right recently. There are three principal reasons for this. The first is the increased awareness of maternal mortality rates in developing countries and of the need to minimise any delay to women with complications reaching appropriate obstetric or midwifery care. The second reason is the current emphasis on evidence based medicine and the realisation that the human environment in which services are provided may have a real effect on outcomes. Finally, the move towards fees for service as part of cost recovery mechanisms has inspired new interest in quality of care, and with this the notion of "willingness to pay" for a particular service or carer.

This last reason requires little explanation, arising as it does from the current economic climate and the self interest of institutions and facilities in generating income. The relationship that "user friendliness" may have with safer motherhood or with the effective care revolution, however, may need exploration in more detail, not least because they concern the needs of the most vulnerable sectors of the society.

Safer Motherhood

It has been estimated that 89% of maternal deaths are avoidable with appropriate medical management.[1] We know that many women in developing countries, if they had received appropriate obstetric health care *in time* would not have died from complications of pregnancy and childbirth. We can only begin to guess at how many perinatal deaths might also have been averted.

Phases of delay

Thaddeus and Maine's conceptual framework of the Three Phases of Delay[2] has enabled major steps forward in the understanding of that road to maternal (and perinatal) death and of the possible intervention points for reducing unnecessary delays.[3]

- Phase 1:   Delay in deciding to seek care, on the part of the individual, the family or both.
- Phase 2:   Delay in reaching an adequate health care facility.
- Phase 3:   Delay in receiving adequate care at that facility.

Phase 3 delays may be due to inadequate internal referral systems, shortages of supplies and equipment and shortages of competent personnel. They may be addressed by additional in-service training of staff in life-saving essential obstetric skills, by drugs and equipment audits and supply systems, by routine use of the partograph to monitor labour, by appropriate staffing rotas etc.

Phase 2 delays may be due to lack of transportation, difficult terrain, the high cost of travel and so on, and may be partly remedied by the construction of maternity waiting homes near urban facilities, by the relocation of skilled practitioners and resources to provide 24 hour essential obstetric care at district hospital level, by local emergency transport systems and by community emergency transport funds.

Phase 1 delays may be due to a lack of understanding of danger signs in pregnancy and labour, the characteristics of the illness, the absence of the decision maker from the household, the low status of the woman, low self-esteem leading to the belief that suffering is womens' lot,[4] hesitation on setting out on a journey that may be difficult and costly, previous experience with the health care system and perceived quality of care.

In rural settings, the consequences of Phase 1 and Phase 2 delay are often obvious. The majority of deliveries happen at home, and those women who do come in with complications often come in the advanced stages when little can be done to help them. Urban maternity units may think they have no problem with attracting customers: they are busy, overstretched and under resourced, and have a large "turnover" of deliveries per year. However, any complacency may be misplaced, the problem of the Inverse Care Law still exists even in the urban context — those who need the care are often the least likely to seek it. Sheer turnover numbers may tell us little about the service's ability to provide essential obstetric care in a timely manner to those who require it most.

Interventions to reduce delay at each stage are essential if maternal and perinatal mortality are to be reduced, but it is the issues around *delay in care-seeking due to reluctance to use health services* that are of particular concern in this paper.

Dissatisfaction with care

Far less work has been done on dissatisfaction and poor uptake of maternity services than has been done on quality of care issues within family planning services in developing countries. In the "post-Cairo" era the latter have a strong incentive to persuade the public that their primary concern is individual reproductive rights rather than population control.

The studies that do exist in the maternity care sector make salutary reading. These are the reasons that women in studies from different countries gave for being dissatisfied with, or not using available maternity services:

- "undignified" care[5]
- no labour companion permitted[5]

- would prefer a female care provider[5,6]
- long waiting times and rushed antenatal care consultations[6]
- the use of routine episiotomy, pubic shaving, and repeated vaginal examinations[7]
- the use of horizontal positions for labour and delivery[5]
- mistreatment by hospital staff[7]

Unpopular hospital routines may have developed out of convenience to the providers, or out of notions of "clinically appropriate" practice which may or may not have any evidence base. Many have simply converted into habit "the way it has always been done". Health professionals often comment on traditional healers' use of ritual to promote status or convey a sense of mystique about their remedies, but we need to acknowledge that Western medicine has developed its own rituals — and obscure language — with aims that are not that dissimilar.

We, however, claim our medicine to be a science based discipline, and thus have a responsibility to our users to constantly take stock, to review the evidence base for our activities, to way up costs and benefits (social and physiological as well as financial) of our care provision, and to update practice accordingly.

Evidence Based Practice

Midwifery and obstetric care have come under the most extraordinary and exciting review process internationally in the last decade, with the publication of "Effective Care in Pregnancy and Childbirth" in 1989, which systematically reviewed the effects of care during pregnancy and childbirth.[8] With this came the establishment of regularly updated meta-analyses of specific care practices on an electronic database now known as the Cochrane Library Database of Systematic Reviews.[9]

Birth position

We can access good scientific reviews that support the 90% of women interviewed in the Ecuador study who would prefer to use upright positions rather than be recumbent for birthing. There are no data to justify restricting women to a supine position during the second stage of labour, indeed there is tendency for recumbency to lengthen the second stage of labour, reduce the incidence of spontaneous births, increase the incidence of abnormal foetal heart rate patterns, and reduce umbilical cord pH.[10]

Episiotomy

The women from Bolivia who objected to routine episiotomy also have evidence on their side. A British randomised controlled trial (RCT) comparing restricted or liberal use of mediolateral episiotomy found no difference between the two groups in the amount of sutured perineal trauma, episiotomy extensions or post partum pain, nor in the occurrence of urinary incontinence or dyspareunia three years after the initial study.[11,12]A Canadian RCT comparing routine versus restricted median episiotomy policies also that there was no evidence that routine (liberal) use of episiotomy prevented perineal trauma or pelvic floor relaxation.[13]

Perineal shaving

Routine pre-delivery pubic shaving is practised on the assumption that it lessens the risk of infection and makes suturing easier. The two randomised trials and several non-randomised cohort studies that have been done, however, have been unable to detect any effect of perineal shaving on lowering puerperal morbidity. Indeed, there was a tendancy towards an increased morbidity in the shave groups. For this reason pubic shaving is now classified as a "form of care likely to be ineffective or harmful" in *A Guide to Effective Care in Pregnancy and Childbirth*.[14]

Companionship in labour

The women who would like someone to accompany them through labour have very strong evidence to support their case. Thornton and Lilford[15] reviewed the results of 23 randomised controlled trials and concluded that of active management of labour's four elements: strict diagnostic criteria, early amniotomy, early use of oxytocin, and continuous professional support, it is only the last element (the one most often neglected when the model has been copied for use in developing countries) which improves outcomes and should therefore be encouraged.

The reviewers found there was no evidence that oxytocin and amniotomy gave any significant benefit in early labour. There have, on the other hand, been ten randomised controlled trials in different settings (industrialised and developing countries) demonstrating that having the continous presence of a trained female support person can reduce the need for pain relief, the length of labour, the rate of operative vaginal delivery, the likelihood of caesarean delivery, and the likelihood of a five minute Apgar score of below seven. As Hofmeyr and Nikodem,[16] who ran the South African trial put it, companionship in labour seems to be an important and fundamental human need. "When it is lacking labour is adversely affected... the nature of these effects may vary according to the extent to which the birth environment is experienced as threatening, frightening, intimidating or unsupported." Hofmeyr and Nikodem argue that enormous attention has been paid to ensure the physical safety of mothers and their babies during childbirth, but similar attention now needs to be paid to the human environment, "which may impact both at a physiological and a psychological level on the outcome of childbirth."

The explanatory mechanism for why the presence of a supportive female during labour (with no previous social bond with the woman) should reduce the length of labour is fascinating. Fear and anxiety have long been thought to increase the pain experienced and there have been studies in human and animal mothers that suggest that they can cause disturbances in the progress of labour. One theory is that an increased level of catecholamines decreases uterine contractility. Some studies on monkeys suggest that uterine and placental blood flow reduction resulting in foetal distress has also been related to increased catecholamine levels.[17] If this is the case then the techniques and the environments which reduce maternal anxiety and fear should be of great interest to all those providing perinatal care.

Hofmeyr and Nikodem's randomised controlled trial found that the presence of a female companion in labour significantly increased breastfeeding success at six weeks post partum, and the authors hypothesised the following explanation for their results: "Labour in a clinical environment may undermine women's feelings of competence, perceptions of labour, confidence in adapting to parenthood and initiation of successful breastfeeding. These effects may be reduced by the provision of additional companionship during labour aimed to promote self esteem".[16]

Staff attitudes

But how often do health personnel see the promotion of self esteem in their patients as part of their task? It is a sad fact that complaints about staff attitudes to patients abound in the existing literature. Minden in her qualitative study of care in a Nepal maternity unit described women crying in pain being ignored by staff, or being shouted at and told "It's normal to have pain".[18] In Smith and Estrada-Claudio's account from the Philippines "women said that hospital staff had shouted at them. Worst of all, some women were on the receiving end of sarcastic comments about their sex lives. A typical comment of this type was: It isn't as much fun now as when you were making the baby, is it?"[19]

In a Jamaican study carried out for MotherCare it was reported that "staff attitudes to patients is the greatest problem. This they describe as not even coldly professional but openly hostile, demeaning, disrespectful, lacking in empathy, condemnatory, condescending, harsh".[20]

It seems that those inhuman environments, which undermine the women being "cared" for, not only discourage timely use of services, but may also unnecessarily complicate the labour process. This makes it more important that women perinatal service users (and non-users) are listened to. It is not only a basic human right to be given a service that is genuinely caring, respectful and dignified, but it is a physiological imperative for the health of both mother and baby.

What do women want in labour?

Research so far on "what women want" from their perinatal services indicates two important aspects. Firstly, women want to be accorded dignity and kindness, and secondly most women do not want to be interfered with unnecessarily. While vigilance in the detection of complications during pregnancy and labour is vital especially in vulnerable and poorly nourished populations, we need to remember that labour and birth are effective physiological processes in the great majority of women and that those processes should be facilitated, not hampered. "First do no harm" is a still a basic tenet of good medical practice and care providers might do well to take Nicky Leap's advice "to respect the extraordinary nature and intricacy of the many interacting hormonal cascades and surging polypeptide chains that trigger feedback mechanisms in a swirling dance of purpose".[21] Any intervention in or interruption of that intricate process by providers needs to be rationally justified. It was recognition of this and concerns about "the temptation to treat all births routinely with the same high level of intervention required by those who experience complications" that recently prompted the World Health Organization to convene a technical working group with representation from childbirth experts from each of the WHO regions to clarify, in the light of current knowledge, what they consider to be good practice in the management of non-complicated labour and delivery.[22]

Taking Action for Change

Data collection

Information gathering from users and their families is a necessary first step to change. Methods of data collection may include structured surveys, depth interviews, observation methods and group activities such as focus group discussions, group interviews and "autodiagnosis" semi-structured discussion within organised community groups.[23] It is often better to use more than one method in order to get a full picture. If women and/or their relatives are to be interviewed in the health facilities it is important that they are clearly told that their responses will not affect in any way the treatment they are about to receive. This explanation has to be part of the informed consent process. Exit interviews get around that problem to a degree but are still often difficult to interpret because of most patients' natural desire to appear polite and to express appreciation. In some settings the users may also have started out with very low expectations of the service and therefore are easily "satisfied" on a rating score. Observational work by researchers using checklists can be useful in gauging the extent to which good communication and interpersonal relations between staff and users may be occurring. Because of a likely "Hawthorne effect" of the provider knowing that she/he is being watched, these tend to give a picture of "best practice" as it stands at the facility, but there is usually still considerable visible room for improvement and these types of methods have been used with effect in both family planning and gynaecology clinic assessments.[24]

What it is that women (and their families) do not like or that discourages them from using a service will not always be ascertained by interviewing the attenders, of course. As I suggested at the beginning of this paper, it is often the case that "dissatisfaction with services is often expressed through tacit rejection of those services rather than vocal expression at the service site".[25] It is therefore useful to interview both service users and non-users in the community. This has the added advantage of taking place on home territory where honest opinions may perhaps be more readily expressed. It is also preferable to use non-health workers as the interviewers.

The idea of developing observational checklists and scoring systems for assessing the *technical* quality of antenatal services is not particularly new, Srinivasa *et al.* developed one such tool for use in primary health centres in India over 15 years ago.[26] What has been added more recently is the idea of an observation checklist for the interpersonal elements of the service. The Population Council, for example, uses these within a range of assessment tools to produce a comprehensive appraisal of family planning service delivery points including the sub-systems (logistics, facilities, staffing, supervision, and training and record keeping) as well as elements of quality.[27]

Placing "user friendliness" within a conceptual framework

Building on Judith Bruce's work on quality of care in family planning, Semeraro and Mensch suggest five general dimensions for assessment of quality of care in relation to women's health services: choice, provider–woman information exchange, provider competence, interpersonal relations, and mechanisms to encourage continuity of medical care.[27] It is important to view the five dimensions named above as complementary. The development of better interpersonal relations, information exchange and continuity of care, cannot in any real way be separated from the improvement in the technical quality of care. Services could not in any legitimate sense be termed "user-friendly" if the technical aspects of care were not informed and competent, and as Donabedian, one of the most influential writers on quality of care has pointed out, "interpersonal process is the vehicle by which technical care is implemented and upon which its technical success depends".[28]

Strategies for change: National and local initiatives

In Namibia, when the BFHI was launched in 1992, it was named the Baby and Mother Friendly Initiative with the understanding that in order to promote breastfeeding there must be a suitable environment for mother and baby at birth. Attention was therefore paid in their BMFI Guidelines to the attitudes of personnel towards their patients, to whether fathers or other family members were allowed to attend and support mothers in labour, and whether mothers were permitted to give birth in the position of their choice. The obligation of staff to provide and maintain a supportive atmosphere in the labour ward was emphasised.[29]

In December 1996, Indonesia launched a national Mother Friendly Movement. One of its proposed elements was "Ten Steps for a Mother Friendly Hospital".[30] Mirroring the Baby Friendly Hospital initiative's ten steps, these were:

1. Develop policy and guidelines on management that support mother friendly health services.
2. Provide comprehensive essential obstetrics services.
3. Antenatal care provision.
4. Safe delivery provision.
5. Adequate postpartum care.
6. Family planning services.
7. IEC on maternal health.
8. Referral service and referral network.

9. Maternal and perinatal audit.
10. Quality of care assessment and improvement mechanisms.

These steps not only specify a high level of technical quality in service provision, but specifically mention the human environment in which this care should be given:

- Under step 3: "Consider actions taken by mothers based on beliefs or religion, and tradition or local custom".
- Under step 4: "Health providers are kind, patient and polite in guiding the patient and her family." "Allow patient to be accompanied by husband or a member of the closest family during delivery".
- Under step 5: "Give the family a chance to visit and greet the newborn infant".
- Under step 10: "Conduct regular evaluation on patients' wishes and satisfaction with hospital service".[30]

It is not necessary, however, to wait for national policies of this nature. Smaller scale, more focussed initiatives are also valuable. What does seem to work is dual innovation in the technical *and* human environment areas. A MotherCare funded project in two Nigerian states that combined Life Saving Skills *with* Interpersonal Communication and Counselling Skills training was found to provide the combined skills that a midwife needed to do her job well.[31]

Some changes may be small but significant. They may mean working to redevelop a language that can be understood by the lay person, or respecting local traditions such as burial of placenta by the family. However, "user friendliness" may not be as relatively simple as holding a hand or putting up curtains between beds. Large units with enormous volumes of users may actually need to consider new ways of organising their work if they are to provide space for satisfactory information exchange between provider and user, and for the possibilities for continuity of care. In some situations this may involve abandoning the practice of involving doctors or obstetricians in the care of every pregnant woman, and (as is beginning to happen in the UK) allowing the care of the normal childbearing woman to be the role of the professional midwife. It may mean changing clinic hours to meet the needs of working families, or devolving some antenatal and delivery care responsibilities to satellite clinics, as has occured in Lusaka, Zambia.

Finally, as with the BFHI, genuine local, facility based initiative is essential if things are to change in a real and sustained manner. "Ownership" of the review and change process by staff is essential, as is leadership by example. In their preface to the book *Perinatal Health Care with Limited Resources* Bergstrom and colleagues say that our principal task is to "treat every pregnant woman as if she was your own wife, and the newborn as if it was your own child".[32] While at first glance this may not seem particularly helpful advice to the female care providers amongst us, their message is still an essential one. The everyday nature of our work and its intimacy with the beginnings of life and with death and pain should not make us immune to the anxiety, suffering, or to the happiness of others.

References

1. "WHO Maternal Mortality: Helping women off the road to death," *WHO Chronicle* **40** (1986): 175–183.
2. Thaddeus S and Maine D, *Too Far to Walk: Maternal Mortality in Context*, Columbia University (1990).
3. Fawcus S, Mbizvo M, Lindmark G and Nystrom A, "A community-based investigation of avoidable factors for maternal mortality in Zimbabwe," *Studies in Family Planning* **27**(6) (1996): 319–327.
4. Timyan J, Griffey Brechin SJ, Measham DM and Ogunleye B, "Access to care: More than a problem of distance," In: *The Health of Women: A Global Perspective*, Koblinsky, Timyan and May, eds., Oxford: Westview Press (1993).
5. Pino A, Reascos N, Villota I, Landázuri X and Yépez R, "Mortalidad materna en el ecuador y aspectos culturales en la atención de la mujer embarazada" *Revista del Instituto Juan César García* **1**(1) (1991): 33–56.
6. Kazmi S, Marketing and Research Consultants (MARC), Association of Business Professional and Agricultural Women. 1991 Safe Motherhood: Consumer View Points, sample survey: Pakistan (Unpub.).
7. CIAES Qualitative research on knowledge, attitudes, and practices related to women's reproductive health, Cochabamba: MotherCare (1991).
8. Chalmers I, Enkin M and Keirse M, *"Effective Care in Pregnancy and Childbirth*, Vols. 1 and 2, Oxford University Press, Oxford (1989).

9. Cochrane Database of Systematic Reviews. London: BMJ Publishing Group/ Update Software.

10. Sleep J, Roberts J and Chalmers I, "Care during the second stage of labour," In: *Effective Care in Pregnancy and Childbirth*, Chalmers, Enkin and Keirse, eds., Oxford University Press, Oxford (1989): 1129–1144.

11. Sleep J, Grant A, Garcia J, Elbourne S, Spencer J and Chalmers I, "West Berkshire perineal management trial," *British Medical Journal* **289** (1984): 587–590.

12. Sleep J and Grant A, "West Berkshire perineal management trial. Three year follow-up," *British Medical Journal* **295** (1987): 749–751.

13. Klein MC, Gauthier RJ, Jorgensen SH *et al.*, "Does episiotomy prevent perineal trauma and pelvic floor relaxation?" *Online Journal Current Clinical Trials* (1992): p. 1.

14. Enkin M, Keirse M, Renfrew M and Neilson J, *A Guide to Effective Care in Pregnancy and Childbirth*, 2nd ed., Oxford University Press, Oxford (1995). Table 6, p. 410.

15. Thornton J and Lilford R, "Active management of labour: Current knowledge and research issues," *British Medical Journal* **309**(6951) (1994): 366–369.

16. Hofmeyer GJ, Nikodem VC, Wolman WL, Chalmers BE and Kramer TR, "Companionship to modify the clinical birth environment: Effect on progress and perceptions of labour, and breastfeeeding," *British Journal Obstetrics and Gynaecology* **98** (1991): 756–764.

17. Kennell J, Klaus M, McGrath S, Robertson S and Hinkley C, "Continuous emotional support during labour in a US hospital. A randomised controlled trial," *Journal of the American Medical Association* **265** (1991): 2197–2201.

18. Minden M, "In whose interest? Women's experiences of hospital birth in Nepal," In: *Baby Friendly/Mother Friendly*, Murray SF, ed., London, Mosby (1996): 101–113.

19. Smith DG and Estrada-Claudio S, "Women organize their own health care: A case study from the Philippines," In: *Baby Friendly/Mother Friendly*, Murray SF, ed., London, Mosby (1996): 122–134.

20. Wedderburn M and Moore M, "Qualitative assessment of attitudes affecting childbirth choices of Jamaican women," Arlington: MotherCare project Working Paper 5 (1990) Report prepared for Agency for International Development Project 5936–5966.

21. Leap N, "Woman-led midwifery: The development of a new midwifery philosophy in Britain," In: *Baby Friendly/Mother Friendly*, Murray SF, ed., London, Mosby (1996).

22. WHO, *Care in Normal Birth: A practical Guide*, Geneva: WHO/FRH/MSM96.24 (1996).

23. Brems S and Griffiths M, "Health women's way: Learning to listen," In: *The Health of Women: A Global Perspective*, Koblinsky, Timyan and May, eds., Oxford, Westview Press (1993).

24. Adamu A, "Women's experiences of gynaecological care in a government hospital in northern Nigeria," Dissertation submitted in partial fulfilment of Masters in Mother and Child Health, Institute of Child Health (University of London) (1996).

25. Atkinson SJ and Correia L, "Quality of Primary Health Care in urban Brazil: A case study of prenatal care," Department of Public Health and Policy, London School of Hygiene and Tropical Medicine (1993).

26. Srinivasa DK, Danabalan M and Rangachari R, "Methods to assess quality of services in antenatal clinics of primary health centres," *Indian Journal of Medical Research* (1982): 458–466.

27. Semeraro P and Mensch BS, "The quality of care in maternal and reproductive health services: Definition, assessment and improvement," In: *Baby Friendly/Mother Friendly*, Murray SF, ed., London, Mosby (1996): 48–158.

28. Donabedian A, "The quality of care: How can it be assessed?" *Journal of the American Medical Association* **260**(12) (1988): 1743–1748.

29. Viljoen EH and Amadhila JN, "A case study from Namibia: The National Mother Baby Friendly Initiative," In: *Baby Friendly/MotherFriendly*, Murray SF, ed., London, Mosby (1996): 53–60.

30. Affandi B, "The role and implementation of a mother friendly hospital," A paper prepared for the Xth Donor Agency Coordination Meeting on the Safe Motherhood Initiative in Indonesia, Ministry of Health, Republic of Indonesia Jakarta, 12 December (1996).

31. Payne AO, "The MotherCare Project, Nigeria: A step in a revolution in midwifery education and practice," In: *Midwives and Safer Motherhood*, Murray SF, ed., London, Mosby (1996): 122–131.

32. Bergstrom S, Hojer B, Liljestrand J and Tunell R, *Perinatal Health Care with Limited Resources*, Macmillan Press: London and Basingstoke (1994).

Commentary

IMPROVING THE USER-FRIENDLINESS OF DISTRICT PERINATAL SERVICES

Shameem Ahmed

Health Scientist, Operations Research Project,
International Centre for Diarrhoeal Disease Research,
Bangladesh (ICDDR,B)
Dhaka, Bangladesh

Each year at least half a million women die from causes related to pregnancy and childbirth — more than 99% in developing countries.[1] India has more maternal deaths in one day than there are in the entire affluent world in one month.[2] In Bangladesh, the maternal mortality ratio is among the highest in the world at 4.7 per 1,000 live births.[3] Research shows that most deaths are avoidable with access to simple basic maternity care.[4]

Most home deliveries in developing countries like Bangladesh are assisted by untrained traditional birth attendants or relatives who have no midwifery training.[3] These deliveries take place in very unsafe and unhygienic conditions. Although TBAs may be trained to perform normal deliveries, their utilisation is often poor, with only 6–8% of the deliveries being conducted by TTBAs in Bangladesh.[5] TBAs can, however, play an important role in preventing unhygienic deliveries, thereby reducing the risk of neonatal infections.

Improving Antenatal Care

Although antenatal care is an acknowledged requirement for the prevention of perinatal deaths, most women in developing countries do not perceive its necessity. In Bangladesh, only about a quarter of the women who gave birth in 1993–1994 received antenatal care.[3] Information on the importance of antenatal and delivery care needs to be underscored. Antenatal care is an important meeting place for pregnant women and exchange of information can take place here. Pictorial cards showing the symptoms of complications of pregnancy and childbirth for which the woman should go to hospital can be used both at the static clinics and on the doorstep. The ICDDR,B in Bangladesh is using a pictorial card to raise awareness in its study areas[6] where about 97% of the pregnant women are now aware of at least one obstetric complication. It must, however, be remembered that risk classification of pregnancy tends to have a low predictive value.[7] This fact indicates clearly that antenatal care must be supplemented with access to emergency care in case of unforeseen complications.

Institutional Delivery in Bangladesh

Despite a reasonably good infrastructure for providing free-of-charge maternal and child health services in rural areas of Bangladesh, utilisation is poor. The district hospital is supposed to provide comprehensive obstetric services, but usually services are poor: government-employed doctors may not be available for duty, through poor accountability, and equipment is neglected or in need of repair. The sub-district hospitals, serving a population of 200,000 to 400,000, are supposed to provide basic emergency obstetric services. However, the proportion of deliveries carried out at these facilities are far below the expected 15–20% of complicated births which need medical assistance.[8] The biggest problem is that women do not go to the hospital until it is too late. In a recent community based study[6] in Bangladesh showed that most of the women who had perinatal complications did not go to the hospital because they did not think they needed the extra attention. Other reasons included fear, taboos about delivering in a hospital, lack of awareness, distance, cost, family objection, and lack of family support to look after the home during the woman's absence. The need, therefore, is to remove the barriers to hospital utilisation.

Although there is a system of referral and linkage in the government health structure, it is almost non-functional, so patients are rarely sent to the district or upgraded sub-district hospital in due time. Pregnant women should be introduced to the health care system during antenatal care. She can be told about what to expect at the district hospital in case a need arises. This introduction should foster confidence to encourage the woman to utilise the hospital when needed.

Also, the cost of hospital delivery is too high, the service providers not adequately trained, and essential drugs and equipment are not available. Neonatal issues are rarely addressed in the district hospital until the baby is critically ill. Breastfeeding support in the postpartum period is also lacking.

The crucial role of rural hospitals in preventing maternal deaths is beyond doubt. To ensure that appropriate technologies, including caesarean sections, reach the masses might mean revolutionary improvement. An example is the ICDDR,B-designed comprehensive EOC service programme at a sub-district hospital in Bangladesh, which serves a population of about 400,000.[6] This has addressed the needs of the community and appears to be extremely useful and popular.

Improving the Quality of Care

Improving the quality of care by addressing issues like waiting time of patients, technical competence of the service providers, client–provider interaction, availability of adequate equipment and drugs, and effective follow up mechanisms would increase the utilisation of perinatal services. Qualified medical staff are needed to inspire and maintain efforts for the better care of patients in the district hospitals. One problem is that specialised doctors, such as obstetricians, anaesthetists and paediatricians only rarely work outside the big cities.[9] Efforts need to be made and incentives devised to increase the commitment of these specialists to provide services not only among the urban but also among the rural community, who equally need their expertise.

The district hospital managers should supervise the quality assurance mechanism by setting performance standards and establishing a system of surveillance with appropriate measurements to detect deficiencies.[10] Standards and periodic assessment by independent outside groups can also help to prevent the internal laxity to which hospitals tend to fall victim. Quality assurance should be seen as the responsibility of all health workers and not of a person or unit. It is important to find out why one district hospital is performing better than the other, and to implement the necessary changes in service provider behaviour. Another important aspect of quality assurance of district hospital to improve perinatal care[9] is to have *perinatal audits*. This action-oriented review monitors what has happened in a health unit over a certain period to identify the causes of bad outcomes like perinatal deaths or maternal disease or death (sentinel audit, see Chapter 22). Regular audit sessions at which all staff are present are essential for good perinatal care.[11]

Improved quality of care seldom involves significant cost increases. It may relate to aspects such as friendliness of staff, cleanliness of facilities, and good equipment.[10] It is important that everyone at a district hospital is motivated to make the best of their resources and concentrate on client satisfaction.

References

1. Royston E and Armstrong S, eds., "Preventing maternal deaths," Geneva, WHO (1989).
2. World Health Statistics Annual, 1986, Geneva, WHO (1986).
3. Bangladesh Demographic and Health Survey 1993–1994. National Institute of Population Research and Training (NIPORT). Mitra and Associates, Demographic and Health Surveys Macro International Inc.
4. Mahler H, "The safe motherhood initiative; A call to action," *Lancet* i(8534) (1987): 668–670.
5. Mirza T, Khanam PA, Juncker T *et al.*, "Utilization of Trained Birth Attendants," Working Paper No. 84, MCH-FP Extension Project, ICDDR,B (1993).
6. Ahmed S, Khanum PA, Islam A *et al.*, "Strengthening maternal and neonatal health: Results from two rural areas of Bangladesh," Working Paper No. 86, ICDDR,B (1997).

7. Maine D, "Too far to walk," New York: Columbia University Center for Population and Family Health (1991).
8. UNICEF, "Emergency obstetric care. Intervention for the reduction of maternal mortality," Obstetrical and Gynaecological Society of Bangladesh. September (1993).
9. Bergstrom S, "Maternal health: A priority in reproductive health," In: *Health and Disease in Developing Countries*, Lankinen KS, Bergstrom S, Makela PH and Peltomaa M, eds., The Macmillan Press Ltd. (1994).
10. Vienonen MA, "Health systems and their management," In: *International Maternal Health Care 1992 — The Challenge Beyond the Year 2000*, Bergstrom S, Molin A and Povey GW, eds., Uppsala: University of Uppsala (1993).
11. Ali L, Kifle H, Mbaruku G *et al.*, "Audit of maternal health care," In: *International Maternal Health Care 1992 — The Challenge Beyond the Year 2000*, Bergstrom S, Molin A and Povey GW, eds., Uppsala: University of Uppsala (1993).

Chapter 27

HOW TO IMPROVE INFORMATION, EDUCATION AND COMMUNICATION FOR BETTER NEWBORN CARE

27.1 PLANNING A CME PROGRAMME ON NEONATAL CARE AT THE DISTRICT LEVEL

O. N. Bhakoo

Former Professor of Paediatrics, PGIMER Chandigarh, India

The aim of continuing medical education (CME) training programmes is to improve neonatal care at district medical centres. Although most of the elements required to improve level-1 and level-2 neonatal care are relatively simple, they do require additional resources and changes in administrative procedures.

It is important to actively involve the administration at the decision-making level when planning such programmes. The level of training and awareness in neonatal care amongst medical staff in different district medical centres is quite variable. Before planning a CME programme, it is important to evaluate the current level of training of the medical professionals and to assess the existing neonatal care facilities. The problem of neonatal care can then be discussed with the administrator of the medical centre, and the changes which can be implemented assessed. The CME programme should then be designed with these objectives in mind.

The programme can be planned as a one week educational programme, followed by one or more weeks of training in special skills. The programme director (PD) should make a follow-up visit to the centre a few months after the CME to assess the improvement in neonatal care and provide help and advice on further improvements.

Steps Involved in Planning a Typical CME Programme

The steps involved in planning a typical CME programme are:

1. Select the CME programme director (PD) and the training centre(s).
2. Prepare a plan for assessing the facilities available and the level of training of medical and nursing staff in neonatal care (see Table 1).
3. Identify the district medical centres from where the staff will attend the CME programme.
4. Visit (PD) the selected district medical centres for discussions with paediatric, obstetric and nursing staff, and the hospital administrator. Assess the facilities and the level of staff training according to the plan prepared in Step 2.
5. Prepare a plan for the CME programme and post-CME training for both doctors and nurses.

Table 1 Components of neonatal care in a hospital setting.

Physical facilities	Infection control
Staff available	Monitoring and therapeutic facilities
Neonatal resuscitation	Investigative facilities
Neonatal transport	Neonatal follow-up
Thermoregulation	Teaching
Nutrition	Administration

(For details see "Norms for accreditation of Level 2 special care units", National Neonatology Forum, India, New Delhi, 1991.)

6. Prepare a workbook for the CME and send it to participants at least two to four weeks in advance to prepare them for the programme.
7. Plan a post-CME visit (PD) to the target centres three to six months after the CME programme. The observations should be recorded on a form prepared specifically for this purpose and the results discussed with the hospital administrator.

The CME Programme

The CME programmes for nurses and doctors should be held at the same time. If possible all the neonatal doctors and nurses from the selected district centres should attend the programme. It is also helpful to invite the hospital administrators to a one-day discussion about their role in augmenting neonatal care.

Table 2 List of proposed sessions for the CME programme.

Introduction — Review of the neonatal care facilities available at the selected medical centres and the objectives of this CME

Care of the normal newborn

Breastfeeding

Care of LBW — temperature and infection control

Care of LBW — feeding and hypoglycaemia

Fluid therapy

Birth asphyxia and resuscitation

Post-resuscitation care and HIE

Respiratory problems — diagnosis and monitoring

Respiratory problems — prevention and treatment

Infections

Diarrhoea

Jaundice

Surgical problems

Care during transport of a sick neonate

Equipment — requirements, specifications, and cost

Equipment — maintenance

Maternal education and home care

Immunisations and follow-up care

Open session for miscellaneous questions

Concluding session including the post-CME training plan and its objectives

---

The one-week CME programme should comprise 20–22 sessions of up to 90 minutes each, and must include discussions on equipment maintenance, maternal education and neonatal care at home (see Table 2). The educational objectives of each session should be clear. Each session should start with about 30 minutes introduction to the subject by an expert highlighting the essential requirements. This should be followed by an extended discussion of 40–50 minutes in which the participants identify their problems and attempt to evolve a practical solution. The last ten minutes can be used to summarise the lessons from the session.

The theoretical programme should be followed by at least one week of training (preferably more) in a well-developed neonatal unit. Discussions should be held with the participants and a list of the skills which each needs to learn prepared (see Table 3). This information should be shared with the director of the host neonatal unit and his/her staff to ensure good co-ordination.

Table 3 List of necessary skills for district medical staff.

Assessment of normality in the neonate, assessment of gestation, cord care, bathing.
Breastfeeding techniques, manual expression of breast milk, gavage feeding.
Diagnosis of thermal stress, methods of keeping a baby warm including incubator care.
Methods for asepsis (including hand washing) and for decontamination of rooms, furniture and equipment.
Doing a suprapubic tap, setting up an IV line.
Testing for PCV and hypoglycaemia, micro ESR, CRP, and gastric aspirate cytology.
Resuscitation techniques including the use of a face mask, resuscitation bag, endotracheal intubation, manual IPPR and draining a pneumothorax.
Use of a heat shield, head box, pulse oximeter, and BP, heart rate respiration and apnoea monitors.
Assessment of peripheral circulation and shock.
Clinical assessment of jaundice, use of phototherapy, and performing and monitoring exchange transfusion.
Monitoring and care during transport.
Teaching mothers about keeping baby warm, spoon feeding, breast milk expression, asepsis, assessment of adequate nutrition, and identifying early signs of illness.
Assessment of growth and development during follow-up visits.

27.2 EFFECTIVE DISSEMINATION OF HEALTH LEARNING MATERIALS

Hemang Dixit

Professor in Child Health, Director,
Health Learning Materials Centre, Kathmandu, Nepal

According to the 1991 Nepal Fertility Health Survey, only 5.5% of deliveries in the country were attended by medical doctors and 1.9% by trained nurses or midwives.[1] Infant mortality is high, the IMR and the U5MR for 1994 were 84 and 118 respectively. A substantial proportion of infants die in the neonatal period.[2] A significant reduction in neonatal deaths must be achieved to reduce both the IMR and the U5MR. The Health Learning Materials Centre in Kathmandu has an important role to play in the promotion of teaching/learning (T/L) materials related to neonatal care for health workers.

Health workers at all levels, including those providing primary health care, often work in remote areas where teaching and learning materials are hard to obtain. Although many manuals are produced for health workers, distribution is difficult. Furthermore, even when books and manuals have reached a health institution, staff who are leaving often remove them so that new staff may find no information resources unless they come prepared with their own set of materials.

Developing countries should aim to produce their own T/L materials, adapted to their own needs, in sufficient amounts, and at a cost health workers can afford.[3]

Current Situation

Health learning materials in Nepal

The Health Learning Materials Centre (HLMC) in Kathmandu was set up in 1985. It was designated as a WHO Collaborating Centre in 1989, and in 1990 was selected as the regional centre for a South-East Asia network responsible for promoting the exchange of materials and expertise between HLM Centres.

Communication

Communication is used to transfer knowledge about an idea, elicit a response to the idea, and bring about a change in behaviour. The message may be passed on orally, through pictures, or through the written word. Printed or electronic media may be used.

HLMC currently produces a variety of printed materials (posters and books), audio tapes, and visual materials such as slides with commentaries, films and videotapes.

Literacy and comprehension

A major difficulty in disseminating health learning materials is knowing whether the message has been received and comprehended, and whether it will affect knowledge and behaviour. Literacy is a common problem in most developing countries. The written word can be ineffective as a means of communication because it cannot be read by the intended audience. Similar problems apply to visual materials. Tests of visual materials with pre-literates have shown that there is such a thing as "visual literacy".[4] What educated people take for granted may not be understood by those less privileged. Equally, messages which are spoken may not actually be comprehended. And if messages sent by radio are to be heard, the intended audience must be listening when the message is transmitted. In all cases the first requirement is that the materials to be used are properly field-tested and adjusted accordingly. Materials should only be mass produced and disseminated when it is sure that they will be accepted by the target audience.

Radio

In South Asia the radio remains the best medium for reaching a large number of people. The aim with audio materials is to send messages as often as possible, ideally during prime time, in such a way that the recipient does not switch off. In Nepal, there are regular weekly programmes on family planning and health care. Some series have had to be repeated by popular demand. The series "From the Teaching Hospital to the Health Post", prepared as a form of continuing education for basic, and middle-level health workers, was on the air for a number of years. The audience can be increased by "piggy-backing" onto a programme which is already popular. This was done with the UNICEF series on "Facts for Healthy Living" which was linked to a popular BBC programme broadcast from London.

TV

More recently, the HLMC has collaborated in the production of a TV soap opera produced by UNICEF and the Ministry of Health. The programme, entitled "Devi", uses the story of a village girl to raise issues of gender bias, female literacy, and health. It is shown as part of a regular programme on health care. It is hoped to reissue the whole series as a combined set of video cassettes to be used for disseminating knowledge on health care at the community level. The United Mission to Nepal has shown that this is possible with their video "Sanu Maiya's Baby" which is being used as a T/L aid.

Books

A World Bank study has shown that books are the best choice in terms of cost effectiveness. Nevertheless, in developing countries books are often too expensive for most centres, even for the libraries of teaching institutes. It has been difficult in Nepal to produce books on general medicine, and even more problematic for specialities. Paediatrics is only just coming into its own as a separate subject.[5] Good-quality T/L materials for paediatrics are gradually being produced, but there is very little on care of the newborn. Some major textbooks have been brought out, but these tend to focus on less common conditions.

A series of posters on Safe Motherhood was brought out in Nepal as a calendar. This was initially planned as T/L material for mothers-in-law, but is now being used by NGO workers, nurses, and midwives at the grassroots level. Different versions in different languages were made for different areas and ethnic groups.[6]

Conclusion

Up to 90% of people in Nepal live in rural areas and a substantial percentage receive primary health care services from grassroots level workers. T/L materials including guidelines on the care of the newborn should be available to doctors at district hospitals and to those involved in the delivery of primary health care services if the health of newborn infants in Nepal is to improve.

References

1. "Common framework — Third monitoring of progress," MOH/WHO, Kathmandu (1994).
2. *The State of the World's Children*, UNICEF (1996).
3. Dixit H, "Towards self-sufficiency in health learning materials," *World Health Forum* **15** (1994): 93–95.
4. McBean G, "Rethinking visual literacy, helping pre-literates learn," UNICEF Nepal (1989).
5. Dixit H, "Health learning materials in paediatric education," In: *Current Concepts in Paediatrics*, Puri RK *et al.* eds., New Delhi, Jaypee Brothers (1994): 122–125.
6. Thapa M and Shrestha S, "Pictorial aid on Safe Motherhood components," *Journal of the Institute of Medicine* **14** (1992): 306–317.

27.3 DISSEMINATION OF HEALTH INFORMATION

Matthew Ellis
Research Fellow in International Child Health, Kathmandu

Who Needs What Information?

A conference held by the British Medical Journal (BMJ) Publishing Group in London in 1994 was entitled "Getting Information from the Developed to the Developing World".[1] The starting point was the problem faced by developing country clinicians in accessing relevant up-to-date information. One participant estimated that only 15% of doctors in India regularly read a journal. The problems of cost and poor communications faced by potential subscribers in developing countries are obvious. However, the conference soon reached the conclusion that the title was inappropriate as some of the information needed by developing countries, for example epidemiological data, needs to be generated by the countries themselves. There is also a growing recognition that developing countries have information of relevance to the global medical community. It has been estimated that only 2% of international scientific discourse as represented by indexed journals is contributed by developing country scientists.[2] This hugely underestimates the increasingly high quality of scientific output which originates in developing countries. North-South information flow should be supplemented by South-North flow. As development proceeds at widely differing pace both within and between neighbouring countries there is also a growing need for both intra-regional and intra-country exchange of information, so called South-South flow.

Health Informatics and the Communication Revolution

The collection, management and transmission of information in the medical field is all subsumed within the term *health informatics*.[3] There have been important advances in information and communication technology in the last decade that are revolutionising health informatics in industrialised countries. Paper-based information systems which are liable to high transportation and storage costs are giving way to electrical information systems which are far cheaper to convey, store, and retrieve information. The key cost — telephonic transmission — is coming down in real terms all the time. What is the relevance of these changes to developing country health professionals?

The communication revolution offers great opportunities to progressive developing country health professionals. It would be naive to ignore the obvious problems relating to telephone line availability, unreliable electricity, outlay costs for the hardware, and lack of technical support. But despite these constraints the information technology industry has established a huge foothold in South India which is spawning imitators in Kathmandu and elsewhere in South Asia. Communication is a key component in the broader trend towards globalisation and appears set to reach all but the most remote areas in the coming years. As many commentators have noted, electronic media are biased towards urban centres and the more technically sophisticated members of society. Health professionals are a potential bridge between technocrats and ordinary people and should become familiar with the new technology. It has huge potential for both the professional and the patient.

Electronic Information

What do you need?

So what are the requirements to participate in the new technology? A personal computer (PC) is the first prerequisite. Either of the two main operating systems, IBM clones or Apple Macintosh, are now available for under $1,000. A modem is required to connect the computer to a telephone line. This can be piggy-backed on an existing telephone line if necessary. You now need a telephonic connection to a server, esssentially another computer with access to the internet, an enormous worldwide network of computers. There are increasing numbers of commercial companies offering varying charging structures for internet access. These internet servers usually provide the client with the appropriate software to enable the desired operations. There are various types of service available via the internet. Which type of service you wish to use determines the amount of access you require and hence the charges you will pay.

E-mail

Firstly, you can use this computer network to send and receive "e" (for "electronic") mail. For this you will require some sort of e-mail software package. This will enable you to cut and paste documents into an appropriate format for mail transfer. The more sophisticated e-mail packages permit transfer of attached files, but especially for image or data files these can run into compatibility problems. When you want to send or receive e-mail you visit the server via your computer and modem. Your e-mail is stored for you at the server, which acts exactly like a post office. The exchange of information "online" typically lasts a minute or so, and you are charged accordingly.

Your e-mail may include one-to-one information from/to colleagues at home or abroad. It may also include discussion forums/usergroups/conferences where people with similar interests post comments which can be read and responded to by anyone in the group. These exchanges do not occur in real time, but rather at the contributors' convenience. The overall effect is of receiving (and contributing to if you so choose) an ongoing international newsletter written by enthusiasts in your field which comes out everyday or so. The possibilities for human networking leading to collaborative working relationships are limitless.

The internet

Other internet services all require real time access to the internet. The most well known of these is the World Wide Web, an enormous computer-networked resource base for just about any topic you can think of. To find your way around the web (so called "surfing") you will need some sort of search engine software which your server company will provide. To make the most of the information opportunities you may want to download files from sites you visit, for which a file transfer protocol (FTP) software package is essential. Other services include newsgroups for catching up with the latest news, chat servers for real time, online discussion with other users as well as one-to-one conversations equivalent to telephone conversation. Searching for information on the internet is more akin to visiting a virtual library and browsing the shelves, the online discussion groups being the coffeeroom where you exchange news with colleagues. It takes time until you know your way around, and time on line is the biggest expense. Recurrent costs for full internet access are of the order of three times those for e-mail connection alone.

Academic and health links, including healthnet forums

In addition to the commercial sector the academic world are big users of communication technology. Indeed the internet was largely the creation of the academic community in the USA. This technology lends itself to the economies of scale and the addition of a single hospital or health centre access line to a university based server will make no overall difference to the economics of the system. Therefore it is always worth asking your academic colleagues in attached or neighbouring institutions if they have an internet link.

Even more appropriate is the healthnet service provided by SatelLife. Very active in Africa this North American based NGO has developed a low-cost e-mail system for use locally, regionally and internationally. In effect thay act as a server company through local management committees and provide startup software and continuing technical support at low cost. They also act as a distributor for a number of moderated forums to which access is open for all via e-mail. To illustrate the range of these forums to date I quote their respective aims below:

AFRO-NETS

The main purpose of the conference is exchange of information between the different networks active in Health Research for Development in the Eastern and Southern African Region. By this better collaboration between the networks is expected in the fields of capacity building, planning and conducting research, transformation of research recommendations into action, etc. We also hope to avoid duplications and save the scarce resources.

ProCAARE

The goal of this electronic conference is to provide a forum for discussion among researchers and clinicians both in the industrialized and the developing world who are engaged in the fight against the HIV epidemic. Discussions will be segmented into specific areas of research and treatment with particular relevance to the developing world. For example, there will be sub-conferences on epidemiology, vaccine development, therapies, HIV and women, paediatric AIDS, and opportunistic infections such as tuberculosis and Kaposi's sarcoma.

ProMED

The Program for Monitoring Emerging Diseases (ProMED) was proposed by the Federation of American Scientists specifically to create a global system of early detection and timely response to disease outbreaks.

E-Drug

E-Drug is an electronic conference to allow health professionals to share information in the field of essential drugs. Colleagues in developing countries often cannot afford to communicate by telephone or facsimile. And normal postal services are often too slow and unreliable. Many have already discovered the usefulness of electronic mail as an affordable tool for communication.

ProCOR

ProCOR, an international electronic conference on emerging cardiovascular diseases in developing countries, is a collaborative effort between The Lown Cardiovascular Center and SatelLife. The goal of the conference is to create a platform for exchanging information and engaging in dialogue related to cardiovascular health in the developing world.

Nepal has been the first entry point into Asia for healthnet thanks to a returning Nepali software engineer in 1996 and has proven to be a resounding success. The author has practical experience in helping to identify and set up an internet link for our research programme in Nepal and found the healthnet to be a highly cost-effective and appropriate entry point for medical informatics in developing countries. I have been unable, however, to identify a moderated discussion group dedicated to perinatal health in developing countries.

Useful sources of information

Useful sources of relevant information are:
SatelLife, the providers of Healthnet can be contacted at:
126 Rogers Street, Cambridge, MA 02142, USA.
Fax: (617)868 6647; E-mail: hnet@usa.healthnet.org

Free medline access at Johns Hopkins (one of many sites)
http://www.sts.org/repos/medl/

Useful reference site for other medical databases
http://www.gen.emory.edu/medweb/medweb.db.html

Possibly the first major "southern" database site dedicated to the National Bibliographic Database on Tuberculosis and Chest Diseases comprising Indian biomedical literature
http://tbindia.info.nih.gov/

Health related resources including discussion groups by speciality
http://www.clearinghouse.net/tree/hlthmed.html

International Neonatal Network, formed in 1992 to improve neonatal intensive care and encourage large multicentre randomised controlled trials. From more than a hundred collaborating centres only four are situated in developing countries!
http://www.inn.org/inn/inn.htm

Pedinfo, a web site dedicated to paediatric resources
http://www.vab.edu/pedinfo/international.html

Appropriate Health Resources and Technologies Action Group
Information resource centre good for access to paper based materials
http://www.poptel.org.uk/ahrtag/
E-mail: ahrtag@gn.apc.org

References

1. Kale R, "Health information for the developing world," *British Medical Journal* **309** (1995): 939–942.
2. Zielinski C, "New equities of information in an electronic age," *British Medical Journal* **310** (1995): 1480–1481.
3. Coiera E, "Medical informatics," *British Medical Journal* **310** (1995): 1381–1387.

Section 5:

Challenges for Future Policy Implementation and Research

Chapter 28

CHALLENGES FOR FUTURE POLICY IMPLEMENTATION AND RESEARCH

Anthony Costello and Sophie Mancey-Jones
Centre for International Child Health,
Institute of Child Health, London

This chapter was developed from a plenary discussion at the Kathmandu workshop which explored potential future needs in research, audit, and human resource development in the area of newborn care in developing countries. The views of participants were elicited using a goal-orientated programme planning method. There was agreement that audit, research, and human development are interrelated, and when practised together can contribute to the development of effective health care (Figure 1). Many of the constraints which limit effective audit, research and human resource development were identified, but participants focussed on the strategies for sustainable solutions.

Audit: Problems and Possible Solutions

Audit is not a simple process. In industrialised countries audit is widely practised but concerns have been expressed about its value and cost effectiveness in improving service delivery. Table 1 outlines some of the important problems associated with audit and potential remedial strategies. A major challenge is to spread the word about audit methods and to help

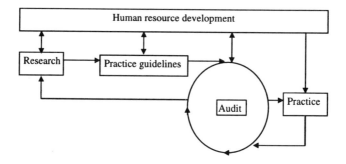

Figure 1 The interaction of research, audit, and human resource development.

Table 1 Audit: Problems and possible solutions.

Problems limiting effective audit	*Potential remedial strategies*
Misunderstanding of the term and concept of audit	Education and dissemination of information on audit
Patchy evidence to inform valid guidelines which can act as "standard" against which practice is audited	Outgoing, high quality research
Inadequate dissemination of research findings to developing countries	Effective and timely dissemination of research findings to clinicians and policy makers in developing countries
Lack of available skills to conduct systematic and critical review of published research findings to produce appropriate practive guidelines	Broad international/national level recommendations with skills training for their appropriate adaptation to produce feasible local guidelines
Lack of reliable data collection mechanisms	The development of simple data collection systems, including active feedback to those involved in data collection
Resource constraints — funds, manpower, and motivation	Promotion of issues relating to quality of health care and audit to the policy makers to encourage appropriate resource allocation
Failure to complete the audit cycle — to change practive and to re-audit	Sustained support for change from policy makers

senior clinicians and midwives develop useful guidelines for good practice. There is much useful published information about effective care in pregnancy, childbirth and the neonatal from the industrialised world. The Cochrane Collaboration based in Oxford, but with centres in Germany, Australia and the USA, is the best single source of reliable evidence about the effectiveness of health care and provides up-to-date systematic reviews of the evidence for interventions in all aspects of medicine including pregnancy and childbirth, and neonatal care. The Cochrane database may be contacted via the internet at http://cochrane.co.uk

The Cochrane Library is available on a subscription basis on CD-ROM for Windows or 3.5" disks for Windows directly from the publishers:

Update Software Ltd
Summertown Pavilion
Middle Way, Summertown
Oxford, OX2 7LG
UK
Tel: +44 (0) 1865 513902
Fax: +44 (0) 1865 516918
E-mail: info@update.co.uk

or

Update Software Inc.
936 La Rueda Drive
Vista, CA 92084
USA
Tel: +1 760 727-6792
Fax: +1 760 734-4351
E-mail: updateinc@home.com

One must remember that evidence concerning the effectiveness, or otherwise, of an intervention in well-nourished European or North American mothers may not be applicable to a population of mothers in a poor, developing country. For example, micronutrient supplementation in a developing country might have a greater marginal benefit in poor communities. However, there is a real shortage of good quality randomised controlled trial data from poor populations, and so those developing guidelines may not always be able to base their decisions on a systematic review of evidence.

Participants in the Kathmandu workshop recognised that even if agreed guidelines are drawn up, bringing about effective change in working practices to implement these guidelines presents a formidable challenge. Hospitals, health centres and primary care programmes face an array of complex and inter-related problems — resource constraints, demoralised staff, rigid bureaucracies and civil service regulations, inflexible management systems, economic turbulence, and poor data monitoring systems. Bringing about sustainable change requires a high degree of leadership and energy from the audit co-ordinators.

Research: Problems and Possible Solutions

Despite the pressing need for well designed research studies to inform policy makers about the effectiveness of interventions, major obstacles impede the design and completion of good research studies in developing countries (see Table 2). Research funding, training, and support given to national institutions from grant giving bodies and international agencies is still very limited.

Participants at the workshop agreed that international agencies and national governments should target their resources to strengthen national research institutions, and to help the best and brightest investigators to have protected time for research. Non-practice allowances for academics (to compensate them for loss of private practice earnings) need to reflect economic realities. Institutions in the industrialised world which conducted research in developing countries should ensure that national institutions were genuine partners and were strengthened by the research collaboration. Too often, the main beneficiaries of research grants were the expatriate workers and their own academic institutions.

Dissemination requires far more attention. Publishing papers in expensive and inaccessible journals will not change policy and practice. Researchers should feedback important results to communities, national institutions, and governments through informal meetings, seminars, workshops and publication in developing country national journals. Many in-country journals are now

Table 2 Research: Problems and possible solutions.

Problems limiting effective research	*Potential remedial strategies*
Resource constraints — manpower: Retaining and motivating personnel	Reward research staff with due financial support, status, and stable career structure
Inadequate training for research	Strengthen research training programme and allocate sufficient funding for training
Resource constraints — financial, conditional research funding	Award institutional research grants *rather than* programme specific research grants. Conduct a baseline survey of state of current research funding in developing countries
Inappropriate research agendas, driven by the demands of funders, not necessarily by local needs	Identify region specific research issues: e.g. neonatal asphyxia, infection, jaundice, and evaluations of low-cost interventions
Inadequate and slow dissemination of research findings	No veto by donor agencies. Allow timely dissemination of research findings to clinicians and policy makers in developing countries
Problems in getting valid research findings into practice	Central level continuing meta-analysis of all studies — once impact of intervention reaches significance — dissemination of findings to include in practice guidelines

on Medline and other journal databases, and the quality of the top journals in South Asia has improved dramatically over the past decade with the spread of rigorous peer review and the application by editors of more formal paper appraisal using the principles of evidence-based medicine.

Human Resource Development (HRD): Problems and Possible Solutions

Despite the huge unmet need for neonatal training for doctors and nurses, there has been considerable progress made, especially in India, under the auspices of the National Neonatology Forum. They have led the way in providing the national government with clear policies for the development and improvement of neonatal care and training. In other countries like Nepal guidelines for essential newborn care at different levels of the health care system have been built into national policy on maternity care.

Competency-based learning programmes, e.g. on neonatal resuscitation, with accreditation, are being developed gradually for different cadres of worker.

Nonetheless, a major problem persists with the recruitment, training, and placement of midwives and neonatal nurses, especially below district level

Table 3 Human Resource Development (HRD): Problems and possible solutions.

Problems limiting effective HRD	*Potential remedial strategies*
Newborn health given low priority at national level	Development of a national policy on perinatal and neonatal health — with specific resource allocation and defined functions and objectives
Newborn health given low priority during training	Specific newborn health training programmes to undergraduates, nurses, midwives, and TBAs
Low priority of issues concerning quality of newborn care	Raise awareness of administrators to quality issues
	Focus on competency-based learning with critical accreditation process
Poor access to continuing education and support for district based health workers	Decentralisation of training
Low motivation of health workers	Decrease isolation through effective communication and district team building
	Realistic and worthwhile career development
	Include health workers in decision making through involvement in audit

and in remote areas. In all South Asian countries it is recognised that the status of the nursing profession needs to be raised, that nurses need career opportunities especially for specialist neonatal nursing, and that decentralised planning is needed for district team building, to ensure that nurses in health centres do not feel isolated and receive active support from the district centre.

Areas for Future Research and Audit in Newborn Care in Developing Countries

A number of problems compromising optimal newborn care in developing countries were identified, and participants suggested audit activities and recommendations for research in these areas as summarised in Table 4.

These preliminary ideas have been developed further by a sub-group of participants who since the workshop have developed protocols for audit studies in their own workplace or as part of a multicentre collaborative study.

Going to Scale

There are several priorities if neonatal care programmes are to go to scale and have a significant impact on mortality and morbidity. There is always a trade-off between the impact and sustainability of a programme or intervention, and a higher priority must be given to the financial and institutional aspects of sustainability in the longer term.

Partnerships

Donors and international agencies have to co-ordinate their activities and form partnerships for large scale programmes. Governments must recognise the need for partnerships with the voluntary sector through NGOs (non-governmental organisations) and PVOs (private voluntary organisations) to achieve maximum impart. Researchers from different disciplines (neonatology, nutrition, epidemiology, social science and anthropology) must combine to ensure that interventions and packages are both efficacious and sustainable.

Table 4 Potential audit or research activities in newborn care.

Problem	Issues for audit	Research needs
Inadequate neonatal resuscitation Possible underlying causes: Untrained birth assistants Delays in getting help from trained health worker Existing guidelines not clearly understood by providers	Setting appropriate protocols for resuscitation Identifying the current incidence of asphyxiated newborn infants Assessing current outcomes to establish high risk groups Assessing the current procedures Assessing current practice in maintaining and checking equipment	Follow-up of resuscitated newborn infants Evaluate impact of hands-on training for resuscitation
Non-promotion of breast-feeding Possible underlying causes: Motivation of mothers not done by providers Importance of colostrum not impressed on mothers Expressed breast milk not used	Monitoring proportion of exclusively breastfed newborn infants on discharge Monitoring prevalence of use of expressed breast milk Case review analysis for individual newborn infants not breastfed to identify underlying reasons	Effect of lactogogues on breastfeeding patterns
Neonatal hypothermia Possible underlying causes: Lack of knowledge and awareness regarding the importance of detecting and preventing hypothermia Failure to appreciate that the baby is cold No proper guidelines	Setting standards for diagnosing cold stress and hypothermia Identifying prevalence of hypothermia at admission Identifying current practices	Comparison of temperature assessment by thermometer with provider by touch Comparison of temperature assessment using palm compared with dorsum of hand

One important area to be clarified is the position of newborn care in Safer Motherhood Programmes and the Integrated Management of Childhood Illness (IMCI) strategy developed by WHO and UNICEF. Currently neonatal care is built into the "Mother and Baby Package" linked to Safer Motherhood training packages developed by WHO, and IMCI training deals with problems affecting children older than one week of age. This situation is likely to change, and neonatal care guidelines will probably be incorporated into IMCI training in the future.

Beacon projects and champions

Health planners are more likely to learn by example than by diktat. The development of beacon projects led by newborn care champions (for example Dr Bang in Maharashtra, and many in the National Neonatology Forum in India) can be used to disseminate examples of good practice to other district level health workers.

Demand side research

Maybe too much effort has been spent on the supply side of newborn care and too little on the demand side. We need to know much more about cultural and household level constraints on care-seeking behaviour by mothers and other family members in the neonatal period.

RCTs of sustainable packages and effectiveness audits

There is a need to move from efficacy trials of single magic bullet interventions like malaria chemoprophylaxis or vitamin A supplementation towards effectiveness trials and audits of potentially sustainable packages. Even Dr Bang's successful intervention (see Introduction) using village health workers, which appears to have reduced neonatal mortality by up to 62% in a poor district of Maharashtra, will be difficult to scale up in India, and a modified approach using a less intensive intervention working with participatory methods at village level will need to be evaluated in different settings.

References

1. Foster M-C, "Management skill for project leaders: What to do when you do not know what to do," Published by the Centre for International Child Health, Institute of Child Health, 30 Guilford St, London WC1N 1EH, UK. Cost £9.99 plus overseas surface mail £2.75. Or contact cich@ich.ucl.ac.uk
2. Cassells A and Janovsky K, "Strengthening health management in districts and provinces," World Health Organization Manual. WHO/SHS/DHS/91.3

INDEX